SIRTFOOD
DIET COOKBOOK

The Most Complete Collection With 600+ Recipes To Activate Your "Skinny Gene" , Losing Weight, Burning Fat, Getting Lean, And Jumpstart Your Health! Includes A 28-Day Meal Plan

By **Brenda Loss**

Table of Contents

INTRODUCTION

The sirt diet is that the new way of burning excess body fat which will hamper the state of your health. In fact, this diet can help in losing weight with none quite experience regarding malnutrition or maybe starving. The thin genes are activated by the method of exercising and fasting. Certain food items come alongside a compound referred to as polyphenols. When such chemical compounds are consumed alongside the food items, it may result in exerting a touch of stress on the body cells. This ultimately leads to the event of the genes which will easily follow the after-effects of fasting and exercising.

Food items that are rich in polyphenols include coffee, kale, red wine, green tea, coffee. Once you consume any of the food items from this group, sirtuins are going to be released which will end in aging, mood swings, alongside enhancement of body metabolism. Any sort of diet that's rich within the consumption of sirtuins can help in triggering loss of weight with none got to expend the muscles. You'll get the prospect to realize a healthy body alongside a healthy lifestyle. This diet is predicated completely on the restriction of calorie intake that must be wiped out various phases. Calorie restriction of this type can help within the improvement of sirtuin production within the physical body. You would possibly be having thoughts about whether the diet is fit you or not, and that I am sure that this book goes to clear all of your doubts.

You ought to confine mind that each one the food items that are included within the diet plan are very healthy. The diet are going to be providing you with the specified amount of minerals, nutrients, and vitamins. The difference of the body to the present diet will improve with time as you'll keep it up following the diet. Despite the advantages of the diet, this diet is slightly restrictive naturally for specific food items additionally to calorie intake. So, the diet might end in being a touch complex for a few people to urge wont to it and follow an equivalent.

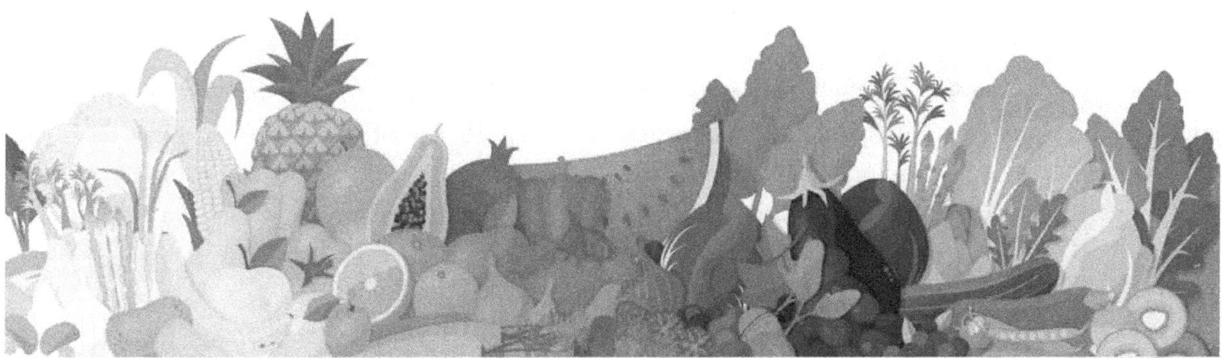

CHAPTER 1:

How the Sirtfood Diet works

The high flexibility of the Sirte diet, which according to scholars is divided into two phases, allows those who decide to follow it not to be severe in doing it, that is, the two phases of which it is characterized can be repeated even only occasionally, supporting our needs.

Phase 1 - Weight loss
Phase 1 is also known as the moment of weight loss and lasts for seven days. It is the hardest phase because they are low in calories and the diet is less varied. The first 2-3 days must not exceed 1000 kcal; therefore, the food will focus on three green or centrifuged juices accompanied by a single solid meal. From the third day onwards, the calories can increase to 1500 kcal, feeding with two green juices (or centrifuged) together with two solid meals. It is the "supersonic" phase precisely because slimming is clearly evident in this week.

Phase 2 - Maintenance
Phase 2 lasts about two weeks and is used to maintain and maintain weight loss. Nutritionists recommend three solid meals, to choose from the aforementioned Sirte foods + a green maintenance juice. The calories not to be exceeded reach 2000 kcal, but in this phase more sari is granted with glasses of wine and vegetables at will.

Exercise during phase 1

During phase 1, caloric intake is restricted ad set to 1,000. During this week and in this week only, you may decide to avoid exercise if you don't feel to. It' up to you. If you are already used to training, you may want to keep going, maybe with less intensity. If you never trained before, the suggestion is to listen to your body. Always remember that there's no need to climb a mountain during phase 1, a brisk walk will be ok and this should be sustainable for everyone.

Exercise during phase 2

During phase 2 you will gradually return to a normal calorie intake and you should feel a lot more energized so, why not put the excess energy to good use? Plenty of athletes from have tried this diet, so you can easily conclude that it works perfectly fine with training and workout. In order to maximize the fat- burning effect, workout while dieting is important, but it is up to you how intense you want to train.

The Advantages Of Sirtfoods Diet

There is growing evidence that sirtuin activators can have a good range of health benefits, additionally to putting together muscle and suppressing appetite. These include improving memory, helping the body to raised control blood glucose levels, and cleaning up damage from radical molecules which will build up in cells and cause cancer and other diseases. There is substantial observational evidence of the beneficial effects of taking food and drinks rich in sirtuin activators to scale back the danger of chronic disease. Sirtfood diet is especially suitable as an anti-aging regimen. Although sirtuin activators are present throughout the Plantae, only certain sorts of fruit and vegetables are large enough to be considered Sirtuin foods. Examples include tea, chocolate, Indian spice turmeric, cabbage, onion, and parsley. Many of the fruit and vegetables displayed in supermarkets, like tomatoes, avocados, bananas, lettuces, kiwis, carrots, and cucumbers, are quite scarce in sirtuin activators. However, that doesn't mean it's not worth eating, as they supply many other benefits. The beauty of a diet rich in sirt-based foods is that it's far more flexible than other diets. You'll simply eat healthily by adding some small amounts, otherwise you may have them concentrate by adding sirtfoods, and the diet could leave more calories on low-calorie days. A notable discovery from a sirtfood diet study is that participants lost considerable weight without losing muscle. It had been common for participants to extend muscle mass, resulting in a more defined and toned appearance. This is often the sweetness of sirtfoods; they activate fat burning but also promote muscle growth, maintenance, and repair. This is often in complete contrast to other diets where weight loss generally results from both .

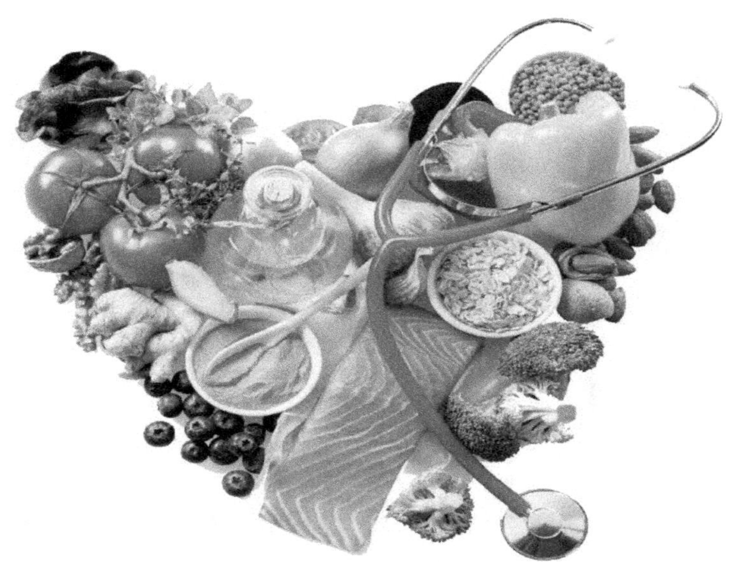

What Is The Skinny Gene ?

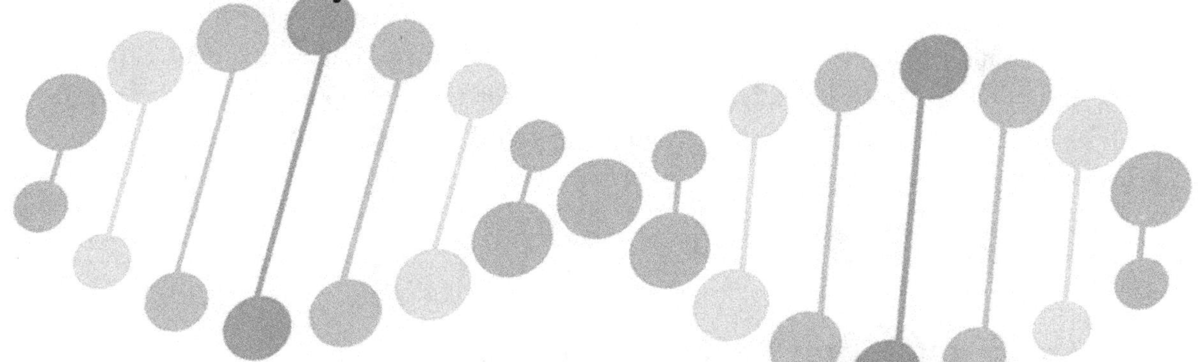

Almost 95% of individuals during this world of today aren't satisfied with the sort of body or the body shape that they possess. The dimensions of the body is taken into account to be unattractive or unappealing by the bulk of the individuals. All of this ultimately leads to the event of feeling disturbed regarding the varied ways during which the form of the body are often controlled, contoured, and altered. You want to have met someone in your life who is unable to realize some bodyweight despite the sort and amount of food that they consume.

Various studies and research are conducted to work out how some people don't have the tendency to realize any excess pounds while taking under consideration the habits of eating in contrast to all or any those people that seems to realize excessive weight with anything they consume. The right account this will actually be found in their genes. Nobody can ever find a gene that's perfect altogether possible aspects. While talking about the gain of weight and obesity, genetics is one such factor that we frequently fail to note. Genetics can actually play a really important role in weight gain, alongside obesity.

There are certain people that accompany the advantage of the thin genes. Such people can activate the thin genes whenever they desire while people cannot. Even once you belong to the not so lucky group, you'll choose certain things which will help in activating the genes that you simply desire. It's actually the way during which the genes interact with the encompassing environment. The thin genes or sirtuins add a lively way for altering the definite path by which the body cells function. Sirtuins are the foremost effective genes when it involves burning down body fat.

This group of genes is taken into account to be special as they will activate the survival mode for the cells of the body. All of those things are administered via a process named autophagy. Autophagy is additionally considered important for discarding waste materials from the body cells additionally to the varied sorts of unwanted particles that tend to urge stored up within the course of your time.

When unwanted particles tend to urge accumulated within the cells, it can cause inflammation. The general result that's associated with the method of restoration is of alarming nature. It can help in making the body cells look healthier and younger, and may also help in handling inflammation. The activation of the thin genes is that the primary key which will help within the process of weight loss. Not only that, but it also can help in preventing the body from health problems with various types.

Nutrition for activating the required Genes

It has been found that the character of food that folks consume, alongside the character of the environment during which they live, can show certain adverse effects on the makeup of the genes. The thin gene, also referred to as the sirtuins, are often found altogether folks. All that we'd like to try to be to seek out them out and just activate them. Some groups of individuals might get exposed to certain things counting on the genetic makeup in accordance with their weight, alongside another factors. It's possible to beat the genes if it's the most reason behind the increasing weight of the body. If administered within the proper way, a person can lose their bodyweight that's resulting in problems of several kinds.

But, there's no definite reason behind putting all the blame on the makeup of the genes for developing obesity. As already discussed before, the genes play a few 15 – 20% role in increasing weight. The remainder depends on various environmental factors. It's needed to form certain adjustments altogether those places wherever it's necessary without barely blaming the genetic makeup for being overweight. One among the foremost definite ways of doing so is by following the sirtfood diet can readily help in losing a substantial amount of weight. It'll not have any sort of adverse effects on your muscle mass also. All that you simply will got to do is to incorporate certain food items in your daily diet.

CHAPTER 2:

BASIC SIRTFOOD INGREDIENTS

There are various foods that can be included in your plan of Sirtfood Diet. This chapter is all about the various types of sirtfoods that you should include in the diet for getting the best results. The following twenty foods contain the highest amounts of sirtuin-activating polyphenols. The levels of polyphenol are not uniformly distributed in all these foods, and some of them contain higher amounts. Moreover, different types of polyphenols are present in each of them, and they are associated with special effects on the sirtuin gene. This is why one of the most important aspects of the Sirtfood Diet is to use a variety of foods. Each of these foods has their own impressive health qualities, but nothing compares to when they are combined.

Buckwheat

Flour that is made from buckwheat helps a lot in losing weight. The overall fat content of buckwheat is very low. In fact, the calorie count is less from normal rice or wheat. As the flour comes with a low amount of saturated form of fat, it can stop you from binge-eating or eating unnecessarily. So, it can help in facilitating and maintaining quick digestion.

Because of the low amount of fat along with a greater quantity of minerals, it can facilitate controlling diabetes of type II.

Arugula

Arugula is a great sirtfood vegetable and is low in calories. It will not only help you to lose weight but also comes with several healthy properties. Arugula is rich in chlorophyll that can help in preventing DNA and liver damage resulting from aflatoxins. For getting the best from the arugula, it is always recommended to consume this vegetable raw.

It is made of 95% water, and thus it can also act as a cooling and hydrating food for the summer days. Vitamin K plays an important role in maintaining bone health.

Capers

Caper is the unripe flower bud of Capparis spinosa. It is rich in compounds of flavonoid that also includes quercetin and rutin, great sources of antioxidants.

Antioxidants can act readily in preventing free radicals that can lead to skin diseases and also cancer. Capers can help in keeping a check on diabetes. It contains several chemicals that can keep the level of blood sugar under control.

Chilies

Consumption of chilies in your daily diet can help in burning down calories. So, adding a bit of spice to your daily diet like cayenne or bird's eye chili can help in getting rid of the extra calories and help boosting up the metabolism.
It also helps in lowering the levels of blood sugar. It has also been found that people who have the habit of consuming chili in their diet can feel full easily, and thus, it can lower your food cravings.

Celery

Celery contains very low calories and that is excellent for losing weight. It can also aid in preventing dehydration as it comes with a great amount of water and electrolytes that also helps in lowering bloating.
It comes with antiseptic properties and prevents various problems of the
kidney. Consumption of this vegetable can also help in excreting toxic elements from the body. Celery comes with great amounts of vitamin K and vitamin C, along with potassium and folate.

Cocoa

Intake of cocoa, even in its chocolate form, can help in controlling weight. Cocoa comes along with fat-burning properties and is the prime reason why most of the trainers suggest mixing cocoa in shakes before exercising.
It can help in reducing inflammation and thus can also help in proper digestion. Cocoa is rich in antioxidants like polyphenols.

Coffee

Coffee is one of the most famous beverages that can be found all over the world. Coffee comes with a very low-calorie count. Caffeine is a form of natural stimulant that is abundant in coffee.
It increases the mental functionality and alertness, making the brain alert and sharpened. Caffeine can help in improving metabolism and thus can act as a great weight loss component. But do not exceed as it can affect your sleeping patterns.

Olive Oil

Olive oil has always been popular for cooking food. Olive oil that is of the extra virgin category can help you in losing weight as it is unrefined and unprocessed. It comes with a great percentage of fatty acids of mono- saturated type that plays an important role in losing weight.
Olive oil is also rich in vitamin E that is good for the health of hair and skin. It comes with great properties of anti-inflammation as well. Olive oil helps in aiding low absorption of fat and thus makes your food healthy and tasty at the same time.

Garlic

Garlic is one of those vegetables that can be found in every kitchen. Consumption of raw garlic can help in boosting energy levels that can aid in losing weight. Garlic is well known for suppressing appetite that can help you in staying full for more amount of time. Thus, with the consumption of garlic, you will be able to prevent yourself from overeating.
A strong relationship can be found between burning fat and the consumption of garlic. Garlic helps in stimulating the process of fat burning and also helps in removing harmful toxins from the body.

Green Tea

Green tea is often regarded as the healthiest type of beverage that can be found on this planet. This is mainly because green tea is full of antioxidants, along with several other plant compounds that can provide you with several health benefits like theine. Theine effect is similar to caffeine and acts as a stimulant for burning fat.
It can also help in boosting your levels of energy at the time of exercising. Green tea comes with a high concentration of minerals and vitamins, along with low content of calories. It can help in improving the metabolic rate as well.

Kale

Kale is a very popular vegetable that comes with excellent weight loss properties. It is a vegetable that is rich in antioxidants like vitamin C that performs various important functions in the body cells, along with improving the bone structure of the body.
It is rich in vitamin K and comes with excellent capabilities of binding calcium. Kale can provide you with 2.4 g of dietary fiber and thus can help in reducing the feeling of hunger. It comes with compounds rich in sulfur and can help in detoxifying the liver.

Medjool Dates

Dates are rich in dietary fibers along with fatty acids that can help in losing the extra kilos when consumed in moderation as they are very caloric. They help staying healthy and fit thanks to their protein content.
Moderate consumption of dates daily can help in boosting the functioning of the immune system.

Parsley

Parsley is a very common herb that can be found in every kitchen. The leaves are rich in important compounds such as vitamin A, vitamin B, vitamin C, and vitamin K. Important minerals such as potassium and iron can also be found in parsley. As it acts as a natural form of diuretic, it can help in flushing out toxins along with any excess fluid.
Parsley is rich in chlorophyll, and it can effectively aid in losing weight. It also helps in keeping the levels of blood sugar under control. Parsley comes with certain enzymes that can help in improving the process of digestion and also helps in weight loss.

Red Endive

Endives are rich in fiber with a low-calorie count. They are rich in fiber that can help in slowing down the process of digestion and keeps the level of energy stable, a great combination of elements that can help in promoting weight loss.

Thanks to their water and fiber content, you will be able to consume more volume of food without the risk of consuming extra calories. It is rich in potassium and folate as well, important for the proper health of the heart. Potassium can act very well in lowering the level of blood pressure.

Red Onion

Red onion is rich in an antioxidant named quercetin. Red onions can help inadding extra flavor to your food without piling up extra calories. Quercetin helps in promoting burning down extra calories. It can also help in dealing with inflammation.

Red onion is rich in fiber and thus can make you feel full for a long period without the urge to consume extra calories. It can also help in improving the level of blood sugar and can deal with diabetes of type II.

Soy

It has been found that increasing the consumption of soy can help in reducing your body weight thanks to its essential amino-acids. It is rich in fiber that can help you to stay full for long.

Soy can also help in regulating the level of blood sugar and can have great control over the appetite. It can also promote better quality skin, hair, and nails, besides its weight loss benefits.

Red Wine

According to some recent studies, it has been found that drinking red wine in moderation can help in cutting down extra pounds. Red wine consists of a polyphenol named resveratrol that can aid in losing weight.

This polyphenol can help in converting white fat, the larger cells that store up energy, into brown fat that can deal with obesity. It can also reduce the risk of heart attack. In fact, serious problems like Alzheimer's disease and dementia can also be reduced by consuming two glasses of red wine daily. Red wine can also prevent the development of type II diabetes.

Strawberries

Strawberries are filled with fiber, vitamins, polyphenols, zero cholesterol, and zero fat. They are also a great source of magnesium. Potassium and vitamin
C. The high fiber content also assists in losing weight.

It can help you in staying full that will reduce the chances of overeating or
snacking. A hundred grams of strawberries comes with 33 calories only. Strawberries also help in improving the system of digestion and can also readily eliminate toxins from the body.

Turmeric

Turmeric is one of the primary spices in every household. It comes with an essential antioxidant called curcumin. It helps in dealing with obesity, disorders related to the stomach, and other health problems. It can help in reducing inflammation that is linked with obesity.

Remember to add some pepper when using turmeric: the absorption of curcumin will be higher.

Walnuts

Walnuts are rich in healthy fats along with fiber that can aid in losing weight. They can provide you with a great deal of energy as well.

They contain high quantities of PUFAs or polyunsaturated fats that can help in keeping the level of cholesterol under check while alpha-linolenic acid helps in burning body fat quickly and promotes proper heart health.

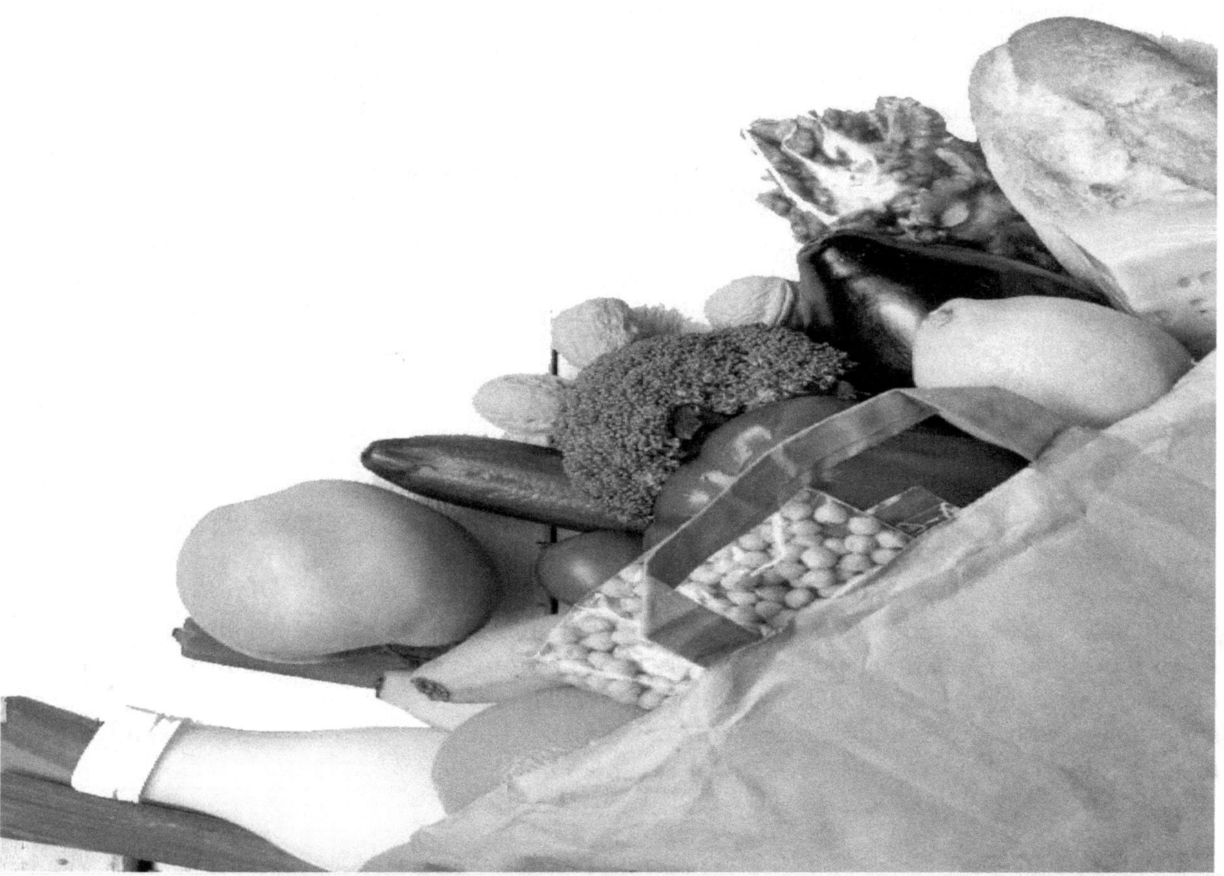

CHAPTER 3:

GETTING STARTED ON SIRTFOODS

Starting the sirtfood diet is very easy. It just takes a bit of preparation. If you do not know what kale is, or where you would find green tea, then you may have a learning curve, albeit very small. There is little in the way of starting the sirtfood diet.
Since you will be preparing and cooking healthy foods, you may want to do a few things the week you start:

1. Clear your cabinets and refrigerator of foods that are obviously unhealthy, and that might tempt you. You also will have a very low-calorie intake at the start, and you do not want to be tempted into a quick fix that may set you back. Even though you will have new recipes, you may feel that your old comfort foods are easier at the moment.

2. Go shopping for all of the ingredients that you will need for the week. If you buy what you will need, it is more cost-effective. Also, once you see the recipes, you will notice that there are many ingredients that overlap. You will get to know your portions as you proceed with the diet, but at least you will have what you need and save yourself some trips to the store.

3. Wash, dry, cut and store all of the foods that you need that way you have them conveniently prepared when you need them. This will make a new diet seem less tedious.

One necessary kitchen tool that you will need aside from the actual foods is a juicer. You will need a juicer as soon as you start the sirtfood diet. Juicers are everywhere, so they are quite easy to find, but the quality ranges greatly, however. This is where price, function, and convenience come into play. You could go to a popular department store, or you can find them online. Once you know what you are going after, you can shop around.

Here are some other tips to help you get started:

Drink your juices as the earlier meals in the day if it helps you. It is a great way to start your day for three reasons.

- It will give you energy for breakfast and for lunch, especially. By not having to digest heavy foods, your body saves time and energy usually spent on moving things around to go through all the laborious motions. You will be guaranteed to feel lighter and more energetic this way. You can always change this pattern after the maintenance phase, but you may find that you want to keep that schedule.

• Having fruits and vegetables before starchy or cooked meals, no matter how healthy the ingredients are the best way to go for your digestion. Fruits and vegetables digest more rapidly, and the breakdown into the compounds that we can use more readily. Think of it as having your salad before your dinner. It works in the same way. The heavier foods, grains, oils, meats, etc., take more time to digest. If you eat these first, they will slow things down, and that is where you have a backup of food needing to be broken down. This is also when you may find yourself with indigestion.

• Juices, especially green juices, contain phytochemicals that not only serve as anti-oxidants, but they contribute to our energy and mood. You will notice that you feel much differently after drinking a green juice than you would if you had eggs and sausage. You may want to make a food diary and note things such as this!

Be prepared to adjust to having lighter breakfasts for a little while. Most often, we fill up with high protein, carbohydrate, and high-calorie meals early in the day. We may feel that we did not get enough to eat and that we are not full at first. Oddly as it sounds, we may even miss the action of chewing. Some people need to chew their food to feel like they have had a filling meal. It is something automatic that we do not think of. Some also will miss that crunch such as with toast. Just pay attention to this, and know this is normal,
that it will pass.

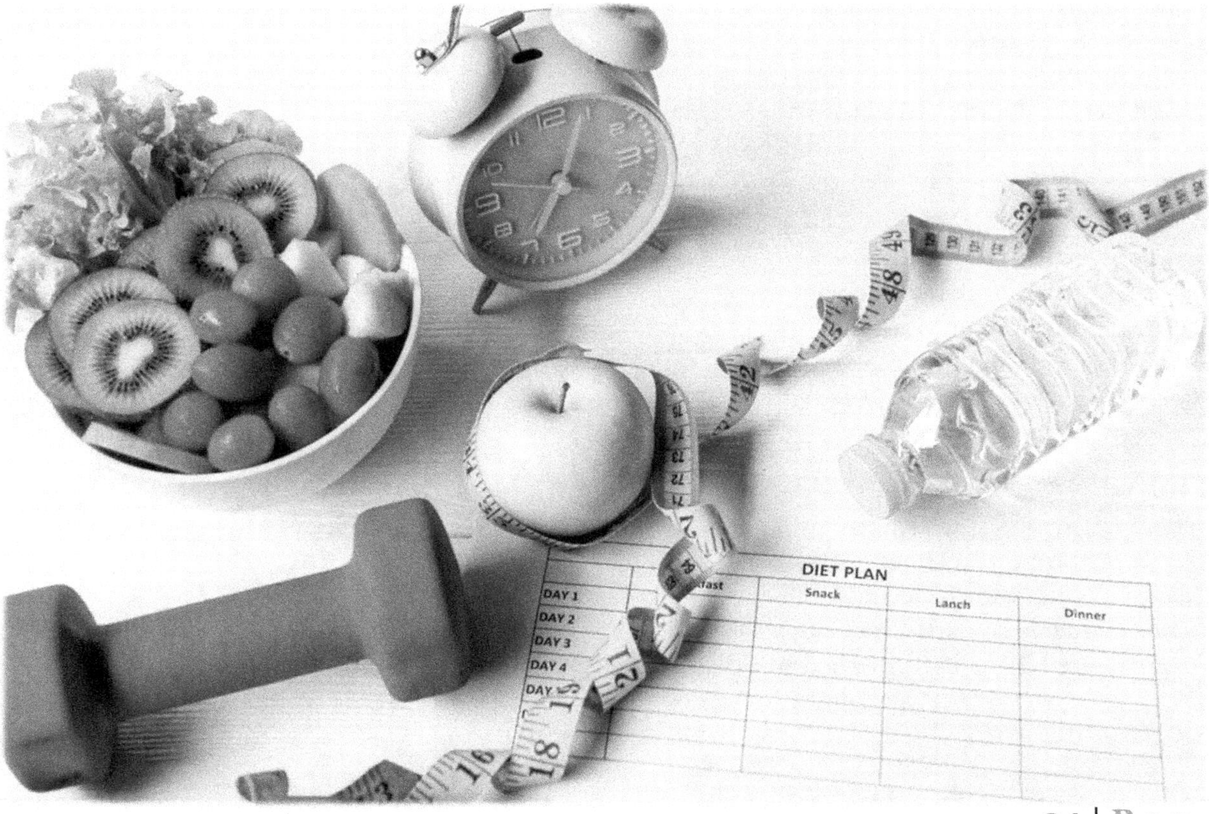

CHAPTER 4:

BASIC SIRTFOOD MEAL PLAN

Week 1

Monday
Breakfast: Sirtfood Green Juice
Snack: 2 squares of dark chocolate
Lunch: Sirtfood Green Juice
Snack: Sirtfood Green Juice
Dinner: Sweet Potato and Salmon Patties and Raw Artichoke Salad

Tuesday
Breakfast: Sirtfood Green Juice
Snack: 2 squares of dark chocolate
Lunch: Sirtfood Green Juice
Snack: Sirtfood Green Juice
Dinner: Lemon Paprika Chicken with Vegetables

Wednesday
Breakfast: Sirtfood Green Juice
Snack: 2 squares of dark chocolate
Lunch: Sirtfood Green Juice
Snack: Sirtfood Green Juice
Dinner: Tomato Soup with Meatballs

Thursday
Breakfast: Sirtfood Green Juice
Snack: Sirtfood Green Juice
Lunch: Chicken with Kale and Chili Salsa
Snack: 2 squares of dark chocolate
Dinner: Seared Tuna in Soy Sauce and Black Pepper

Friday

Breakfast: Sirtfood Green Juice *Snack:* Sirtfood Green Juice *Lunch:* Sirt Salmon Salad
Snack: 2 squares of dark chocolate
Dinner: Green Veggies Curry

Saturday

Breakfast: Sirtfood Green Juice *Snack:* Sirtfood Green Juice *Lunch:* Shrimp Tomato Stew *Snack:* 2 squares of dark chocolate
Dinner: Turkey Breast with Peppers

Sunday

Breakfast: Sirtfood Green Juice
Snack: Sirtfood Green Juice
Lunch: Goat Cheese Salad with Cranberries and Walnut
Snack: 2 squares of dark chocolate
Dinner: Spicy Chicken Stew

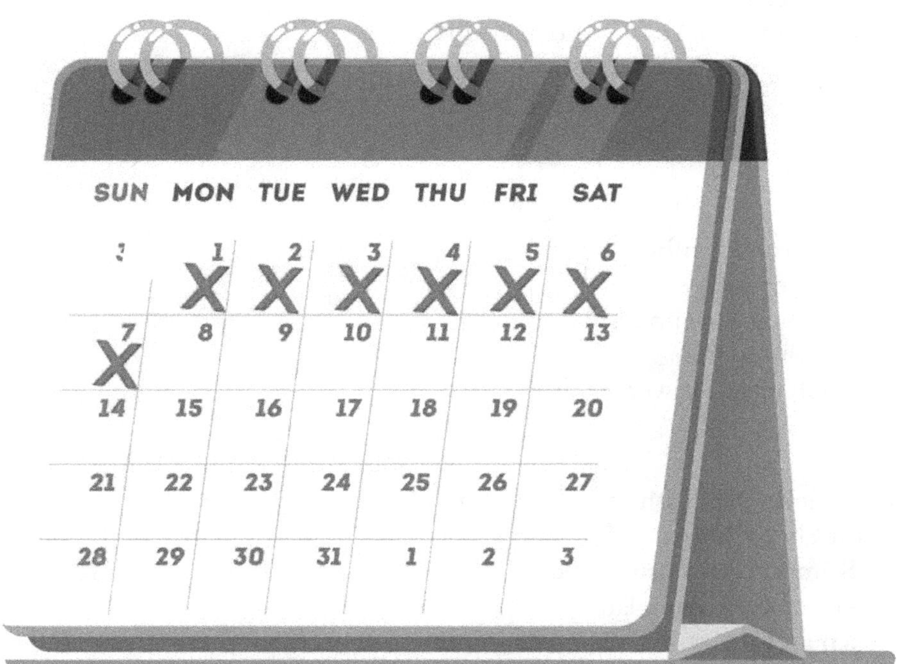

Week 2

Monday
Breakfast: Fluffy Blueberry Pancakes
Snack: Sirtfood Green Juice
Lunch: Caprese Skewers
Snack: 2 squares of dark chocolate
Dinner: Baked Salmon with Stir Fried Vegetables

Tuesday
Breakfast: Kale and Mushroom Frittata
Snack: 2 squares of dark chocolate
Lunch: Trout with Roasted Vegetables
Snack: Banana Strawberry Smoothie
Dinner: Mince Stuffed Peppers

Wednesday
Breakfast: Vanilla Parfait with Berries
Snack: Sirtfood Green Juice
Lunch: Arugula Salad with Turkey and Italian Dressing
Snack: 2 squares of dark chocolate
Dinner: Creamy Mushroom Soup with Chicken

Thursday
Breakfast: Super Easy Scrambled Eggs and Cherry Tomatoes
Snack: Sirtfood Green Juice
Lunch: Lemon Ginger Shrimp Salad
Snack: Blueberry Smoothie
Dinner: Lemon Chicken Skewers with Peppers

Friday
Breakfast: Overnight Oats with Strawberries and Chocolate
Snack: Sirtfood Green Juice
Lunch: Spicy Salmon with Turmeric and Lentils
Snack: 2 squares of dark chocolate
Dinner: Chicken and Broccoli Creamy Casserole

Saturday

Breakfast: Sautéed Mushrooms and Poached Eggs
Snack: Sirtfood Green Juice
Lunch: Asian Beef Salad
Snack: 2 squares of dark chocolate
Dinner: Creamy Turkey and Asparagus

Sunday

Breakfast: Banana Vanilla Pancake
Snack: Sirtfood Green Juice
Lunch: Shredded Chicken Bowl
Snack: 2 squares of dark chocolate
Dinner: Indian Vegetarian Meatballs

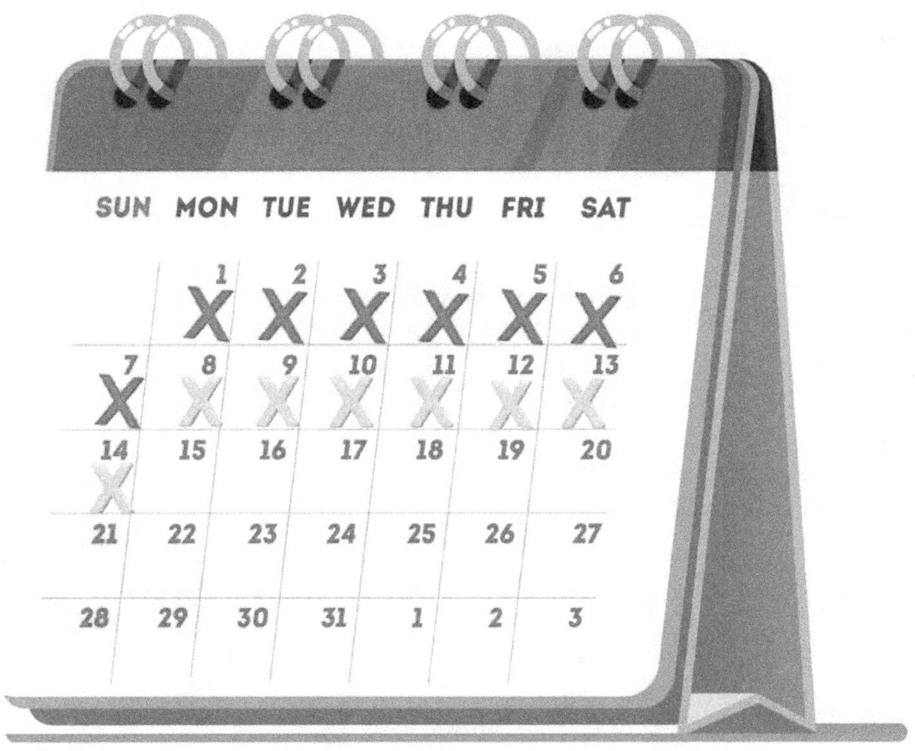

Week 3

Monday
Breakfast: Blueberry and Walnut Bake
Snack: Sirtfood Green Juice
Lunch: Shrimp Tomato Stew
Snack: Buckwheat Granola
Dinner: Turkey Bacon Fajitas

Tuesday
Breakfast: Brussels Sprouts Egg Skillet
Snack: Sirtfood Green Juice
Lunch: Orange Cumin Sirloin and Simple Arugula Salad
Snack: 2 squares of dark chocolate
Dinner: Garlic Salmon with Brussel Sprouts and Rice

Wednesday
Breakfast: Banana Vanilla Pancake
Snack: Sirtfood Green Juice
Lunch: Indian Vegetarian Meatballs
Snack: Blueberry Smoothie
Dinner: Sesame Glazed Chicken with Ginger and Chili Stir-Fried Greens

Thursday
Breakfast: Super Easy Scrambled Eggs and Cherry Tomatoes
Snack: Sirtfood Green Juice
Lunch: Brussels Sprouts and Ricotta Salad
Snack: 2 squares of dark chocolate
Dinner: Sesame Tuna with Artichoke Hearts

Friday
Breakfast: Fluffy Blueberry Pancakes
Snack: Sirtfood Green Juice
Lunch: Baked Salmon with Stir Fried Vegetables
Snack: Chocolate Mousse
Dinner: Spicy Stew with Potatoes and Spinach

Saturday
Breakfast: Sautéed Mushrooms and Poached Eggs
Snack: Sirtfood Green Juice
Lunch: Roasted Butternut and Chickpeas Salad
Snack: 2 squares of dark chocolate
Dinner: Eggplant Pizza Towers

Sunday
Breakfast: Vanilla Parfait with Berries
Snack: Sirtfood Green Juice
Lunch: Arugula Salad with Turkey and Italian Dressing
Snack: Mango Mousse with Chocolate Chips
Dinner: Greek Frittata with Garlic Grilled Eggplant

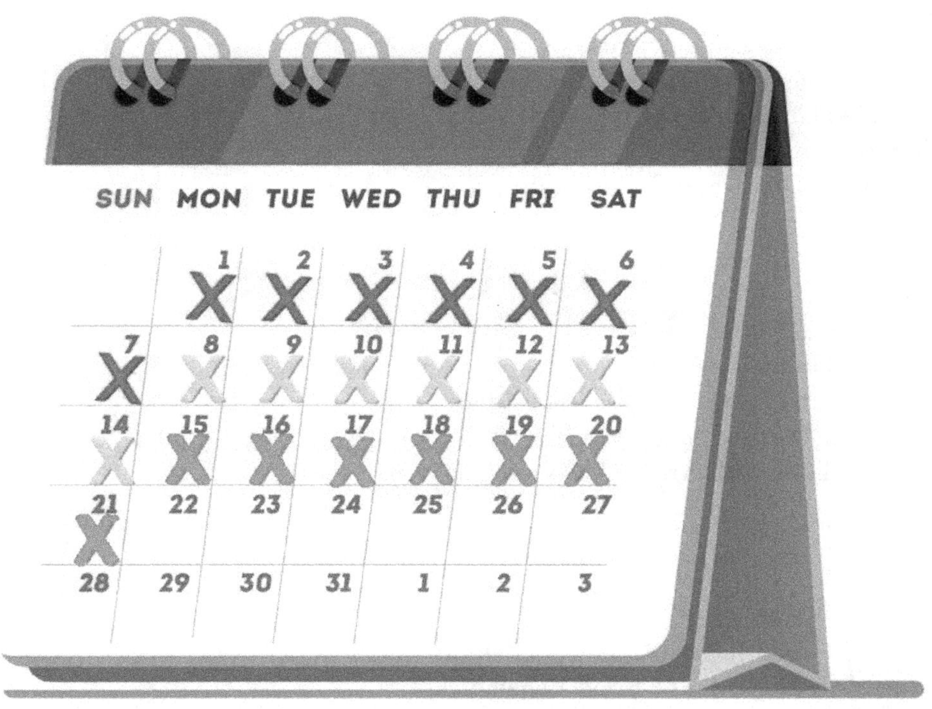

Week 4

Monday
Breakfast: Brussels Sprouts Egg Skillet
Snack: Chocolate Mousse
Lunch: Creamy Turkey and Asparagus
Snack: Sirtfood Green Juice
Dinner: Spicy Indian Dahl with Basmati Rice

Tuesday
Breakfast: Vanilla Parfait with Berries
Snack: Sirtfood Green Juice
Lunch: Lemony Chicken Burgers
Snack: Walnut Energy Bar
Dinner: Sesame Tuna with Artichoke Hearts and Baked Sweet Potato

Wednesday
Breakfast: Blueberry and Walnut Bake
Snack: Mango Mousse with Chocolate Chips
Lunch: Shredded Chicken Bowl
Snack: Sirtfood Green Juice
Dinner: Creamy Broccoli and Potato Soup

Thursday
Breakfast: Chickpea Fritters
Snack: Sirtfood Green Juice
Lunch: Lemon Tuna Steaks with Baby Potatoes
Snack: Chocolate Mousse
Dinner: Sesame Tuna with Artichoke Hearts

Friday
Breakfast: Fluffy Blueberry Pancakes
Snack: Sirtfood Green Juice
Lunch: Baked Salmon with Stir Fried Vegetables
Snack: Chocolate Mousse
Dinner: Lamb, Butternut Squash and Date Tagine

Saturday

Breakfast: Overnight Oats with Strawberries and Chocolate
Snack: Sirtfood Green Juice
Lunch: Chicken and Broccoli Creamy Casserole and Baked Sweet Potato
Snack: Buckwheat Granola and ½ cup plain yoghurt
Dinner: Spinach Quiche

Sunday

Breakfast: Banana Vanilla Pancake
Snack: Sirtfood Green Juice
Lunch: Brussels Sprouts and Ricotta Salad
Snack: Energy Cocoa Balls
Dinner: Mexican Chicken Casserole

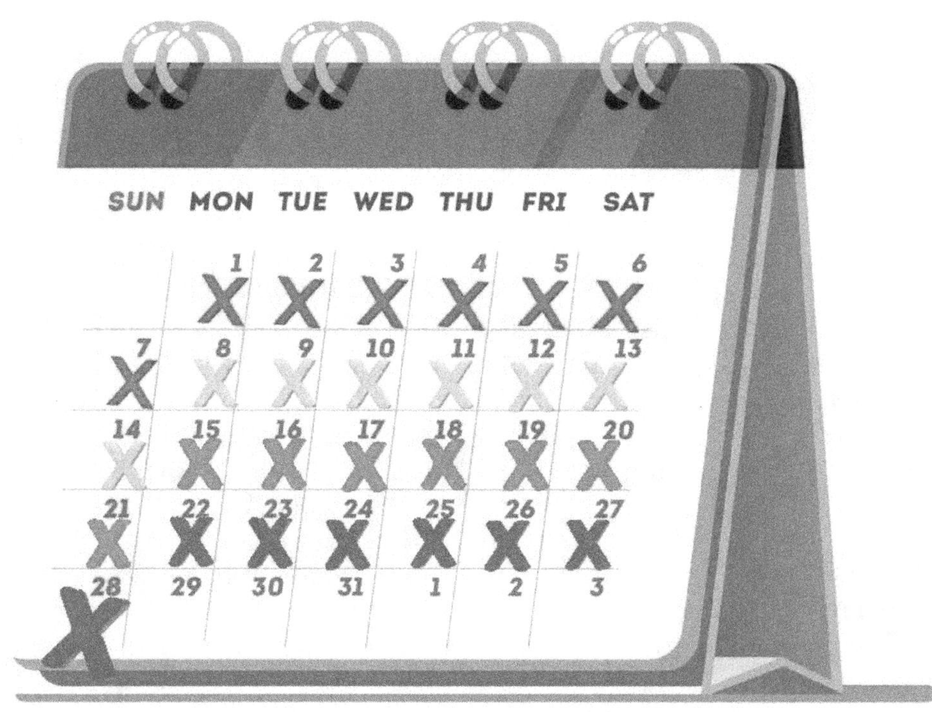

CHAPTER 5:

BREAKFAST RECIPES

Kale Scramble

Preparation Time: 10 minutes
Cooking Time: 6 minutes
Servings: 2
Ingredients:
4 eggs
1/8 tsp ground turmeric
Salt and ground black pepper, to taste 1 tbsp. water
2 teaspoons olive oil
1 cup fresh kale, chopped
Directions:
In a bowl, add the eggs, turmeric, salt, black pepper, and water and with a whisk, beat until foamy. In a skillet, heat the oil over medium heat.
Add the egg mixture and stir to combine.
Reduce the heat to medium-low and cook for about 1–2 minutes, stirring frequently.
Stir in the kale and cook for about 3–4 minutes, stirring frequently. Remove from the heat and serve immediately.
Nutrition Facts:
Calories 183kcal, Fat 13.4 g, Carbohydrate 4.3 g, Protein 12.1 g

Tomato Frittata

Preparation Time: 10 minutes
Cooking Time: 20 minutes
Servings: 2
Ingredients:
¼ cup cheddar cheese, grated
¼ cup kalamata olives halved 8 cherry tomatoes, halved
4 large eggs
1 tbsp. fresh parsley, chopped 1 tbsp. fresh basil, chopped
1 tbsp. olive oil
1 tbsp. tomato paste
Directions:
Whisk eggs together in a large mixing bowl.
Toss in the parsley, basil, olives, tomatoes and cheese, stirring thoroughly. In a small skillet, heat the olive oil over high heat.
Pour in the frittata mixture and cook until firm (around 10 minutes).
Remove the skillet from the hob and place it under the grill for 5 minutes until golden brown.
Divide into portions and serve immediately.
Nutrition Facts:
Calories 269 kcal; Fat: 23.76 g, Carbohydrate: 5.49 g, Protein: 9.23 g

Green Omelet

Preparation Time: 5 Minutes
Cooking Time: 35 Minutes
Servings: 1
Ingredients:
1 tsp of olive oil
1 shallot peeled and finely chopped 2 large eggs
Salt and freshly ground black pepper A handful of parsley, finely chopped A handful of rocket

Directions:

Heat the oil in a large frying pan, over medium low heat. Add the shallot and gently fry for about 5 minutes. Increase the heat and cook for two more minutes.

In a cup or bowl, whisk the eggs; distribute the shallot in the pan then add in the eggs. Evenly distribute the eggs by tipping over the pan on all sides.

Cook for about a minute before lifting the sides and allowing the runny eggs to move to the base of the pan.

Sprinkle rocket leaves and parsley on top and season with pepper and salt to taste.

When the base is just starting to brown, tip it onto a plate and serve right away.

Nutrition Facts:

Calories 221 kcal, Fat 28 g, Carbohydrate 10.6 g, Protein 9.5 g

Apple Blackcurrant Compote Pancakes

Preparation time: 5 minutes

Cooking time: 15 minutes

Servings: 4

Ingredients:

For the compote:

3s of water 2s caster sugar

120 grams blackcurrants, washed and stalks removed For The Apple Pancakes:

2 teaspoons light olive oil 2 egg whites 300 ml semi-skimmed milk 2 apples, cut into small pieces

Pinch of salt

2s of caster sugar

1 teaspoon of baking powder 125 grams plain flour

75 grams porridge oats

Directions:

In a small pan, add the blackcurrants, water and sugar. Bring to a gentle boil and let it cook for 10 to 15 minutes.

In a large bowl, place the flour, oats, baking powder, salt and caster sugar, mix well.

Add in the apple, stir and gently fold in semi-skimmed milk until mixture is smooth.

Beat the egg whites until stiff peaks forms then gently whisk into the flour mixture. Pour batter into a jug.

Heat half teaspoon of oil over medium-high heat in a non-stick frying pan. Add about 1/4 of the batter into the pan. Cook pancake until golden brown on both sides. Drizzle the blackcurrant compote.

Nutrition:

Calories: 337 Net carbs: 40 g Fat: 9.82g Fiber: 6.2 g Protein: 32g

Blueberry Oats Pancakes

Preparation time: 5 minutes

Cooking time: 5 minutes

Servings: 4

Ingredients:

225 grams blueberries

¼ teaspoon salt

2 teaspoon baking powder

150 grams rolled oats

6 eggs

6 bananas

Directions:

Pulse the rolled oats for 1 minute in a (dry) high-speed blender to form oat flour.

Add in the eggs, bananas, salt and baking powder and process for 2 minutes until it forms a smooth batter.

Pour the batter into a large bowl and gently stir in the blueberries. Let sit for at least 10 minutes to activate the baking powder.

Add a large spoonful of butter to the frying pan over a medium high heat.

Scoop the batter and cook until nicely golden underneath. Flip pancake and cook the other side.

Nutrition:

Calories: 494 Net carbs: 68 g Fat: 11.3g Fiber: 6.2 g Protein: 22.23g

Muesli Yoghurt Breakfast

Preparation time: 3 minutes
Cooking time: 0 minutes
Servings: 1

Ingredients:

100g plain Greek, coconut or soya yoghurt
100g hulled and chopped strawberries
10g cocoa nibs
15g chopped walnuts
40g pitted and chopped Medjool dates 15g coconut flakes
10g buckwheat puffs 20g buckwheat flakes

Directions:

Mix together the cocoa nibs, buckwheat flakes, coconut flakes, buckwheat puffs, Medjool dates and walnuts. Add the yoghurt and strawberries.

Nutrition:

Calories: 368 Net carbs: 49g Fat: 11.5g Fiber: 7.4g Protein: 16.54g

Omelette Fold

Preparation time: 3 minutes
Cooking time: 5 minutes
Servings: 1

Ingredients:

1 teaspoon extra virgin olive oil
5 grams thinly sliced parsley 35 grams thinly sliced red chicory 3 medium eggs
50 grams streaky bacon, cut into thin strips

Directions:

Cook the bacon strips in hot non-stick frying pan over high heat until crispy. Remove and drain any excess fat on a kitchen paper.

Beat the eggs in a small bowl and mix with the parsley and chicory. Mix the drained bacon through the egg mixture.

Heat the olive oil in a non-stick pan; add the mixture. Cook until omelette is set. Loose the omelette around the edges with a spatula and fold into half- moon.

Nutrition:

Calories: 471 Net carbs: 3.3g Fat: 38.72g Fiber: 1.5g Protein: 27g

Cherry Tomatoes Red Pesto Porridge

Preparation Time: 10 minutes
Cooking Time: 5 minutes
Servings: 2

Ingredients:

Salt, pepper 1 teaspoon hemp seed 1 teaspoon pumpkin seed 2 teaspoons nutritional yeast ½ cup couscous ½ cup oats
1 teaspoon sun-dried tomato-walnut pesto 1 teaspoon tahini
1 tablespoon callion 1 cup sliced cherry tomatoes 1 cup chopped kale 1 teaspoon dried basil 1.5 teaspoon dried oregano 2 cups veggie stock

Directions:

In a small cooking pot, add oats, oregano, vegetable stock, basil, couscous,
pepper and salt and cook for about 5 minutes on medium heat stirring frequently until porridge is creamy and soft.

Add chopped kale but reserve a bit for garnish, tomatoes and sliced scallion. Cook for additional 1 minute, stir in pesto, tahini, and nutritional yeast. Top with the reserved kale, pumpkin and hemp seeds plus cherry tomatoes.

Nutrition:

Calories: 259 Net carbs: 36g Fat: 7.68g Fiber: 7.4g Protein: 14.26g

Sautéed Veggies Bowl

Preparation time: 5 minutes
Cooking time: 5 minutes
Servings: 1
Ingredients:

For tofu scramble: 1 cup water
Dash of soy sauce Pepper and salt
1 teaspoon turmeric
1 serving medium crumbled firm tofu For the Sautéed Veggies:
1/2 cup red onions, diced 1 cup mushrooms, sliced
1 big handful kale, de-stemmed and chopped For the Bowls
1/2 cup cooked brown rice 1/2 avocado, pitted

Directions:

Mix together the tofu scramble ingredients in a small dish, set aside. Add a splash of water in a skillet over medium-high heat; add the onions, mushrooms and kale. Cook, stirring periodically, for about 5-8 minutes or until it is evenly brown and soft. Set aside in a bowl.
Using the same skillet, pour in the tofu mixture and cook until it starts to brown and heated through for 5 minutes. Transfer tofu scramble into a bowl, add the mushrooms/kale mixture, top with avocado, brown rice and salsa. Serve with flatbreads, buckwheat, basmati rice or couscous.

Nutrition:

Calories: 122g Fats: 6.9g Sodium 867g Net carbs: 8.7g Fiber: 1.7g Sugar: 4.9g Protein: 7.3g

Chocolate Oats Granola

Preparation time: 10 minutes
Cooking time: 20 minutes
Servings: 8
Ingredients:

60 grams good-quality dark chocolate chips (70%) 2 of rice malt syrup or maple syrup
1 tablespoon dark brown sugar 20g roughly chopped butter
3 teaspoons light olive oil 50g roughly chopped pecans
200g of jumbo oats

Directions:

Heat-up your oven to 160°C).
In a large bowl, mix together pecan and oats. Gently heat the butter, olive oil, rice malt syrup and brown sugar in a small non-stick pan until the sugar and syrup is dissolved and butter melted. Do not allow the mixture boil before removing. Spread the mixture on top the oats and stir very well to coat with the oats.
Distribute the oats mixture onto a large parchment lined baking tray, spread out into every corners. You do not need to spread evenly, leave lumps of mixture with spacing.
Place tray in the oven and bake until edges are just tinged golden brown, about 20 minutes. Withdraw from the oven and let completely cool on the tray.
Once cool, use your finger to break up any lager lumps. Add in the chocolate chips and mix. Serve Chocolate granola with cup of green tea.

Nutrition:

Calories: 244 Net carbs: 20.91g Fat: 15.41g Fiber: 4.6 g Protein: 5.24g

Green Chia Spinach Pudding

Preparation Time: 30 minutes
Cooking Time: 0 minutes
Servings: 1
Ingredients:

3 spoons of chia seeds 1 Medjool date, slice in half and remove pit 1 handful fresh spinach 1 cup non-dairy milk Toppings
Banana, berries, etc.

Directions:

Blend the spinach, date and milk in a high speed blender until very smooth.

Pour the mixture in a bowl over the chia seeds. Stir mixture well, and stirring every now and then for about 15 minutes.

Transfer to the fridge and allow to chill at least one hour or overnight. Stir once more, just before serving; top with kiwi, banana, berries,etc.

Nutrition:

Calories: 232g Fats: 9.6g Sodium 86mg Net Carbs: 2.6g Fiber: 9.9g Protein 10.1g

Blackcurrant and Raspberry Breakfast

Preparation time: 5 minutes
Cooking time: 15 minutes
Servings: 2
Ingredients:

300 ml water 2 teaspoons granulated sugar

100 grams blackcurrants, washed and stalks removed 2 leaves gelatin 100 grams raspberries, washed

Directions:

In two serving glasses, add the raspberries and set aside.

Add cold water in a bowl and place the gelatin leaves to soften.

In a small pan, add the blackcurrants with 100 ml of water along with the sugar. Bring to the boil. Let it simmer for five minutes and then turn heat off. Remove and cool for 2 minutes. Remove the gelatin leaves and squeeze out excess water. Place leaves in the saucepan. Stir constantly until completely dissolved, add in the remaining water and stir together. Pour liquid over raspberries in the glasses or dishes. Place in the refrigerator for about 3-4 hours or overnight and allow to set.

Nutrition:

Calories: 76 Net carbs: 13.57g Fat: 0.5g Fiber: 3.3 g Protein: 4g

Kale Mushroom Scramble

Preparation time: 10 minutes
Cooking time: 6 minutes
Servings: 1
Ingredients:

5g of finely chopped parsley

Handful of thinly sliced button mushrooms

½ thinly sliced bird's eye chili 1 teaspoon extra virgin olive oil 20g kale, roughly chopped

1 teaspoon mild curry powder

1 teaspoon ground turmeric 2 eggs

Directions:

Mix together the curry powder, turmeric and a small splash of water to form a light paste. Add the kale to a steamer basket and steam in boiling water for 2– 3 minutes. Heat the oil over medium heat in a frying pan and fry mushrooms and chili for 2 to 3 minutes until soften and starting to brown.

Nutrition:

Calories: 116g Fats: 5.4g Net carbs: 13.2g Fiber: 3.6g Proteins 5.8g

Walnut Medjool Porridge

Preparation time: 10 minutes
Cooking time: 15 minutes
Servings: 1
Ingredients:

50g strawberries, hulled 1 teaspoon walnut butter 35g Buckwheat flakes

1 chopped Medjool date

200 ml almond or coconut milk, unsweetened

Directions:

Add the date and milk into a frying pan over medium low heat, then add in the flakes and cook to your desired consistency.

Add in the walnut butter, stir well. Top porridge with strawberries.

Nutrition:

Calories: 550 Net carbs: 25g Fat: 45g Fiber: 9 g Protein: 6.57g

Avocado Tofu Breakfast Salad

Preparation Time: 5 minutes

Cooking time: 5 minutes

Servings: 1

Ingredients:

Half a lemon juice Half a red onion, chopped 2 tomatoes, chopped One spoon chili sauce 4 handfuls baby spinach

A handful of chopped almonds 1 pink chopped grapefruit

1 Avocado, chopped Half a pack of firm tofu, chopped 2 Tortillas

Directions:

Heat the tortillas in the oven for 8 to 10 minutes.

Combine tomatoes, tofu and onions with some chili sauce in a bowl, place inside the refrigerator to cool.

Add the avocado, grapefruit and almonds. Mix everything together and place into the bowl.

Top with a Squeeze of fresh lemon juice!

Nutrition:

Calories 94g Fats 2.1g Net Carbs 11.3gProtein 3.9g

Buckwheat Coconut Overnight Porridge

Preparation time: 10 minutes

Cooking time: 8 minutes

Servings: 4-6

Ingredients:

1/4 teaspoon of cinnamon 2 teaspoon of vanilla extract 1 cup water 3 cups unsweetened coconut, soy or almond milk 1/4 cup chia seeds 1 cup of buckwheat groats (not kasha) Pinch of salt

For the Toppings:

1 1/2 cup berries 1/2 cup walnuts

Directions:

In a bowl, combine together the buckwheat groats, coconut milk, chia seeds, cinnamon, water, vanilla extract and salt. Cover bowl with stretch film, transfer to the fridge and let sit overnight.

Bring it out in the morning and place it in a pot; cook mixture in the pot for 10-12 minutes, stirring occasionally until your desired thickness is reached. Add the toppings and Serve.

Nutrition:

Calories: 400 Net carbs: 47g Fat: 17.55g Fiber: 3.7g Protein: 11.19g

Strawberry and Cherry Smoothie

Preparation time: 10 minutes

Cooking time: 0 minutes

Servings: 1

Ingredients:

100g strawberries

75g frozen pitted cherries 1 cup plain full-fat yogurt

175mls unsweetened soya milk

Directions:

Place all of the ingredients into a blender and process until smooth.

Nutrition:

Calories: 132 Fats: 1.5g

Net Carbs: 28.4g Fiber: 2.9g Proteins 2.9g

Banana Snap

Preparation time: 10 minutes

Cooking time: 0 minutes

Servings: 1

Ingredients:

2.5cm chunk fresh ginger, peeled 1 banana 1 large carrot

1 apple, cored ½ stick of celery ¼ level teaspoon turmeric powder

Directions:

Place all the ingredients into a blender with just enough water to cover them. Process until smooth

Nutrition:

Calories: 34 Net carbs: 7.8g Fat: 0.1g Fiber: 3.7g Protein: 2g

Green Egg Scramble

Preparation time: 5 minutes

Cooking time: 5 minutes

Servings: 1

Ingredients:

2 eggs, whisked

25g rocket (arugula) leaves 10g chives, chopped

10g teaspoon fresh basil, chopped 10g teaspoon fresh parsley, chopped 1 teaspoon olive oil

Directions:

Mix the eggs together with the rocket (arugula) and herbs. Heat the oil in a frying pan and pour into the egg mixture. Gently stir until it's lightly scrambled. Season and serve.

Nutrition:

Calories: 101 Net carbs: 2.1g Fat: 7g Fiber: 0.5g Protein: 7.1g

Green Sirtfood Smoothie

Preparation time: 10 minutes

Cooking time: 0 minutes

Servings: 1

Ingredients:

100g unsweetened

Greek yoghurt

6 walnut halves

8-10 medium strawberries

A handful of kale leaves

20g dark chocolate (min. 85% cocoa)

1 date

1/2 teaspoon turmeric S

mall piece fresh chili, finely chopped

200ml unsweetened almond milk

Directions:

Put everything into a blender and mix until you get a smoothie.

Nutrition:

Calories: 72 Net carbs: 14g Fat: 0.3g Fiber: 0.8g Protein: 2.8g

Power Cereals

Preparation time: 10 minutes

Cooking time: 0 minutes

Servings: 1

Ingredients:

20g buckwheat flakes 10g puffed buckwheat

15g coconut flakes

40g Medjool dates, seeded and chopped 10g cocoa nibs

100g strawberries

100g Greek natural yoghurt Directions:

Mix all ingredients together.

Nutrition:

Calories: 124g Net carbs: 27.4g Fat: 1.1g Fiber: 1.7g Protein: 2.3g

Berry Yoghurt

Preparation time: 10 minutes

Cooking time: 0 minutes

Servings: 1

Ingredients:

125g mixed berries 150g Greek yoghurt 25g walnuts, chopped 10g dark chocolate (85%)

Directions:

Simply mix all ingredients together.

Nutrition:

Calories: 115 Net carbs: 22.5g Fat: 1.2g Fiber: 1.1g Protein: 3g

Blueberry Frozen Yogurt

Preparation time: 1 hour 10 minutes
Cooking time: 0 minutes
Servings: 4
Ingredients:

1 teaspoon honey
450g plain yogurt 175g blueberries Juice of 1 orange

Directions:

Place the blueberries and orange juice into a food processor or blender and blitz until smooth. Press the mixture through a sieve into a large bowl to remove seeds. Stir in the honey and yogurt. Transfer the mixture to an ice-cream maker and follow the manufacturer's instructions. Alternatively pour the mixture into a container and place in the fridge for 1 hour. Use a fork to whisk it and break up ice crystals and freeze for 2 hours.

Nutrition:

Calories: 66 Net carbs: 8.3g Protein: 8.2g

Vegetable & Nut Loaf

Preparation time: 15 minutes
Cooking time: 1 hour 45 minutes
Servings: 4
Ingredients:

175g mushrooms, finely chopped
100g haricot beans
100g walnuts, finely chopped 100g peanuts, finely chopped 1 carrot, finely chopped
3 sticks celery, finely chopped
1 bird's-eye chili, finely chopped 1 red onion, finely chopped
1 egg, beaten
2 cloves garlic, chopped 2 teaspoons olive oil
2 teaspoons turmeric powder 2teaspoonss soy sauce
4g fresh parsley, chopped 100mls water
60mls red wine

Directions:

Heat the oil in a pan and add the garlic, chili, carrot, celery, onion, mushrooms and turmeric. Cook for 5 minutes. Place the haricot beans in a bowl and stir in the nuts, vegetables, soy sauce, egg, parsley, red wine and water. Grease and line a large loaf tin with greaseproof paper. Spoon the mixture into the loaf tin, cover with foil and bake in the oven at 190C/375F for 60-90 minutes. Let it stand for 10 minutes then turn onto a serving plate.

Nutrition:

Calories: 280 Net carbs: 29.7g Fat: 16.3g Fiber: 1.2g Protein: 4.6g

Dates & Parma Ham

Preparation time: 15 minutes
Cooking time: 0 minutes
Servings: 4
Ingredients:

12 medjool dates
2 slices Parma ham, cut into strips

Directions:

Wrap each date with a strip of Parma ham. Can be served hot or cold.

Nutrition:

Calories: 202 Net carbs: 17.9g Protein: 0.4G

Braised Celery

Preparation time: 15 minutes
Cooking time: 15 minutes
Servings: 4
Ingredients:

250g celery, chopped
100mls warm vegetable stock (broth) 1 red onion, chopped
1 clove of garlic, crushed 1 fresh parsley, chopped 25g butter
Sea salt and freshly ground black pepper

Directions:
Place the celery, onion, stock (broth) and garlic into a saucepan and bring it to the boil, reduce the heat and simmer for 10 minutes. Stir in the parsley and butter and season with salt and pepper. Serve as an accompaniment to roast meat dishes.
Nutrition:
Calories: 367 Net carbs: 5.9g Fat: 0.2g Fiber: 2.4g Protein: 1.2g

Cheesy Buckwheat Cakes

Preparation time: 15 minutes
Cooking time: 10 minutes
Servings: 2
Ingredients:
100g buckwheat, cooked and cooled
1 large egg 25g cheddar cheese, grated (shredded)
25g (1oz) whole meal breadcrumbs
2 shallots, chopped 2 s fresh parsley, chopped
1 olive oil
Directions:
Crack the egg into a bowl, whisk it then set aside. In a separate bowl combine all the buckwheat, cheese, shallots and parsley and mix well.
Pour in the beaten egg to the buckwheat mixture and stir well. Shape the mixture into patties. Scatter the breadcrumbs on a plate and roll the patties in them. Heat the olive oil in a large frying pan and gently place the cakes in the oil. Cook for 3-4 minutes on either side until slightly golden.
Nutrition:
Calories: 358 Net carbs: 121.5g Fat: 5,7g Fiber: 17g Protein: 22.5g

Red Chicory & Stilton Cheese Boats

Preparation time: 5 minutes
Cooking time: 4 minutes
Servings: 4
Ingredients:
200g stilton cheese, crumbled
200g red chicory leaves (or if unavailable, use yellow) 2 fresh parsley, chopped
1 olive oil
Directions:
Place the red chicory leaves onto a baking sheet. Drizzle them with olive oil then sprinkle the cheese inside the leaves. Place them under a hot grill (broiler) for around 4 minutes until the cheese has melted. Sprinkle with chopped parsley and serve straight away.
Nutrition:
Calories: 250 Net carbs: 0.9g Protein: 0.2g

Strawberry, Rocket (Arugula) & Feta Salad

Preparation time: 10 minutes
Cooking time: 0 minutes
Servings: 2
Ingredients:
75g fresh rocket (arugula) leaves 75g feta cheese, crumbled
100g strawberries, halved 8 walnut halves
2 spoons flaxseeds
Directions:
Combine all the ingredients in a bowl then scatter them onto two plates. For
an extra Sirt food boost you can drizzle over some olive oil.
Nutrition:
Calories: 268 Net carbs: 1.1g Fat: 6 Protein: 4g

Diced Seitan and Lentils

Preparation time: 5 minutes
Cooking time: 5 minutes
Servings: 2
Ingredients:
4 slices seitan 1 box lentils Half onion 1spoon soy cream Salt and pepper 1 tablespoon extra-virgin olive oil

A handful of fresh parsley Turmeric (optional)

Directions: Cut the seitan into cubes. Chop the onion and brown it in oil. When it is well colored - but not burnt - add the seitan cubes and, after a few minutes, the lentils drained and well washed. Add salt and pepper and sauté with a little hot water. Finish with the cream, turmeric and chopped parsley, cook a few more minutes and then serve with a nice fresh salad and toasted whole meal bread.

Nutrition:

Calories: 323 Net carbs: 36.7g Fat: 13.2g Fiber: 14.5g Protein: 16.4g

Diced Tofu and Lentils

Preparation time: 15 minutes

Cooking time: 1 hour 20 minutes

Servings: 2

Ingredients:

200g tofu cake Soy sauce (shoyu) Extra virgin olive oil An onion

A sprig of rosemary 2 tablespoons chopped chili pepper 50g red lentils Vegetable stock Breadcrumbs

Directions:

Marinate the diced tofu for half an hour in the soy sauce, adding a little water to cover it. In the meantime, boil the red lentils, previously washed, in the vegetable stock for about 20 minutes, until they are soft enough and the stock has dried a bit.

Then sauté 2 s of chili pepper, the diced onion and rosemary in olive oil until the onion is golden brown and the sauté takes on the smell of spices.

Add the tofu with some of the marinating shoyu and after a few minutes also the lentils with very little broth.

Let everything shrink with the lid and over low heat and to thicken add 2 s of breadcrumbs.

Nutrition:

Calories: 141 Net carbs: 6.5g Fat: 10.8g Fiber: 0.8g Protein: 5.1g

Beans on the Bird

Preparation time: 10 minutes

Cooking time: 25 minutes

Servings: 1

Ingredients:

2 cloves of garlic, minced 2 sage leaves

2 teaspoons extra virgin olive oil Boiled cannellini beans

Fresh well ripe tomatoes Salt and pepper

Directions:

Brown for 2-3 minutes in a pan with oil, garlic and sage. Then add the tomatoes, cut into segments, and let them brown for a couple of minutes. Add the beans, salt and pepper to taste, stir. Cook in a covered pot for 20 minutes, checking and turning occasionally. Serve hot.

Nutrition:

Calories: 153 Net carbs: 6.6g Fiber: 2.8g Protein: 3.4g

White Beans with Lemon

Preparation time: 5 minutes

Cooking time: 10 minutes

Servings: 1

Ingredients:

A jar of white beans from Spain Breadcrumbs Lemons (at least 4 but even more according to taste!) A teaspoon of extra virgin olive oil

A big onion

Directions:

Cut the onion into fillets, put them in a pan with a little water and oil and cook. After a few minutes add the beans (rinse well under the tap). Stir and let it cook for a few minutes. Add salt, oil and breadcrumbs and mix. After a while, pour the lemon juice. Wait a little longer... and the dish is ready. Add more lemon at the end of cooking and eat!

Nutrition:

Calories: 314 Net carbs: 51.6g Fat: 2.5g Fiber: 9.9g Protein: 14.1g

Sponge Beans with Onion

Preparation time: 10 minutes

Cooking time: 3 hours

Servings: 2

Ingredients:

250 g boiled Spanish beans 1 red onion

1 parsley Salt

2 teaspoons oil

1 teaspoon apple vinegar

1 teaspoon dried oregano or 5 fresh oregano leaves

Directions:

Cut the onion into thin slices and cook it for a minute with water in the microwave at full power. Combine all the ingredients in a bowl and leave to rest a couple of hours before serving, stirring a couple of times so that the beans take on the flavor of the seasoning.

Nutrition:

Calories: 832 Net carbs: 23.1g Fat: 11.1g Fiber: 13.9g Protein: 38.1g

Chickling Falafel

Preparation time: 24 hours

Cooking time: 30 minutes

Servings: 2

Ingredients:

Half onion 200 grams Chickling peas already soaked 80g of chickpea flour A teaspoon of cumin seed

A clove of garlic

Paprika

Directions:

Blend the chickling peas (previously soaked for 24 hours) together with the chopped onion, cumin, paprika, and garlic and chickpea flour. Blend until a fairly homogeneous mixture is obtained. Compact in a bowl and leave to rest in the fridge for about an hour. Take the dough and form some meatballs that will be baked in the oven at 180 degrees until golden brown. Notes Cumin can be reduced or eliminated completely.

Nutrition:

Calories: 57 Net carbs: 5.4g Fat: 3g Protein: 2.2g

Chickpeas and Potato Omelette

Preparation time: 10 minutes

Cooking time: 25 minutes

Servings: 2

Ingredients:

4 teaspoons full of chickpea flour Olive oil

Small potatoes

Directions:

This dish is very similar to the traditional 'omelette', but it is better and less heavy. It can be made with any vegetable, as well as potatoes (zucchini, spinach, onion, carrots, etc.).

Put the chickpea flour in a soup plate, add 2 pinches of salt, and a little at a time water, stirring with a fork, until the dough is not too thick.

Cut the potatoes into very thin slices, with the special blade of the grater or potato peeler, and pour them into the batter, stirring well.

Put a little olive oil in a non-stick frying pan and heat over high heat.

When the oil is hot, pour the mixture, quickly distribute it evenly and put the lid on, leaving the heat high.

Both the lid and the lively fire are important to get an omelette cooked to perfection!

After about a minute, you have to turn the omelette: you can do it, if you are not able to turn it all over, by cutting it with a wooden shovel, in four slices, and turning one slice at a time.

Put the lid back on for one more minute, leaving the fire lower.

Then remove the lid, turn the omelette again and cook over high heat for one minute without lid, then turn again and cook for another minute, or until the omelette is golden on both sides.

Nutrition:

Calories: 198 Net carbs: Fat: 4.4g Fiber: 8.4g Protein: 5.3g

Chickpea and Seed Omelette

Preparation time: 10 minutes

Cooking time: 25 minutes

Servings: 4

Ingredients:

5 teaspoons chickpea flour
1 teaspoon salt
Olive oil
1 teaspoon
Sesame seeds 1 teaspoon
Linseed

Directions:

Pour the chickpea flour into a bowl, half a glass of water and mix well with force to remove any lumps of flour. Continue stirring, adding salt and sesame and linseed, for a few minutes until a thick cream is obtained. Heat the olive oil in the non-stick pan and pour the mixture over low heat. Prick the edges and the middle part with the fork and check that the bottom part does not stick to the bottom. It must not have a golden color, so turn it as soon as the cream is absorbed and cook a few more minutes.

Nutrition:

Calories: 209 Net carbs: 36.3g Fat: 0.9g Fiber: 8.9g Protein: 5.6g

Gluten Omelette

Preparation time: 1 hour 25 minutes

Cooking time: 6 minutes

Servings: 2

Ingredients:

1 kg of flour Olive oil
2 pinches of vegetable cube
A handful of parsley
A few drops of lemon
Half a of salt

Directions:

First we have to get the gluten, then we put the flour in a container and knead it with water as if we wanted to make bread. Let the dough rest for about an hour. After the resting period, we take our loaf of bread, tear off a piece not too big and wash it under water until only the gluten remains in our hands (the rinse water must remain almost transparent, no longer white as at the beginning); we repeat the operation for the rest of the pasta. Having finally obtained our gluten, iron it with our hands until it forms a medallion about one cm thick, put it in a pot, cover it with water (not too much, just enough to cover it), add half a of salt and boil it for 6 minutes, being careful not to stick it on the bottom and turn it on the other side halfway through cooking. We take our gluten out of the water and squeeze it with a fork to make it lose the excess liquid, pour the olive oil into a large pan and fry the gluten. While frying, we put a pinch of dice on both sides, chopped parsley and a few drops of lemon. As soon as it's golden and crisp it'll be ready. Place it on blotting paper and serve with a few drops of lemon and a nice salad.

Nutrition:

Calories: 381 Net carbs: 4.6g Fat: 11.8g Fiber: 0.5g Protein: 34.4g

Tomato and Mushroom Omelette

Preparation time: 10 minutes
Cooking time: 15 minutes
Servings: 2
Ingredients:

4 teaspoons of chickpea flour 5 medium tomatoes
One medium onion one Can of mushrooms Baking powder one Glass of water 1/4 of lemon oil for frying to taste

Directions:

Thinly slice the onion and fry it for 5 minutes, then add the chopped tomatoes and drained mushrooms; let it run on medium heat until the water that the tomatoes will tend to release has dried. In a plate, mix the chickpea flour with baking powder, a pinch of salt, a splash of lemon and a glass of water. Make sure the mixture is as velvety as possible and pour it into the pan. Fry for 5 minutes stirring continuously. Dust with a spoonful of yeast and serve.

Nutrition:

Calories: 173 Net carbs: 5.8g Fat: 3.2g Fiber: 1g Protein: 8g

Soy and Zucchini Omelette

Preparation time: 10 minutes
Cooking time: 10 minutes
Servings: 2
Ingredients:

2 teaspoons of olive oil
2 small zucchini (100 g)
3 teaspoons of flour 00 (40 g)
2 pinches of salt
1/3 third glass of soy milk (60 g)

Directions:

Cut the zucchini into very thin slices (with a greater with the appropriate blade, or with a potato peeler, not with a knife). Put the flour and salt in a soup plate, add the soy milk a little at a time and 2 fingers of water, and stir quickly with a fork so as not to form lumps. You have to get a batter that's not too dense, quite liquid. Pour in the zucchini slices and stir well. In a non-stick frying pan put 2 s of oil (so as to cover the bottom just barely) and heat over a high heat. When the oil is hot, pour the batter and level well with a wooden spatula. Put the lid on it and leave the fire high, then after about half a minute lower the fire a little. The omelette must cook in all about 10 minutes, and in this time should be turned a couple of times, so that both sides are browned (you can cut it into 4 slices and turn them one at a time). Hold the lid for the first 5 minutes, for the remaining 5 minutes let it brown without the lid.

Nutrition:

Calories: 115 Net carbs: 24.4g Fat: 0.6g Fiber: 4.6g Protein: 5.6g

Kale Omelette

Preparation time: 5 minutes
Cooking time: 5 minutes
Servings: 1
Ingredients:

Eggs – 3 Garlic – 1 small glove Kale – 2 handfuls
Goat cheese or any cheese of your choice Sliced onion – ¼ cup Extra virgin olive oil – 2 teaspoons

Directions:

Mince the garlic, and finely shred the kale. Break the eggs into a bowl, add a pinch of salt. Beat until well combined. Place a pan to heat over medium heat. Add one teaspoon of olive oil, add the onion and kale, cook for approx. Five minutes, or until the onion has softened and the kale is wilted. Add the garlic and cook for another two minutes.
Add one teaspoon of olive oil into the egg mixture, mix and add into the pan. Use your spatula to move the cooked egg toward the

center and move the pan so that the uncooked egg mixture goes towards the edges. Add the cheese into the pan just before the egg is fully cooked, then leave for a minute.

Nutrition:

Calories: 38 Net carbs: 7.9g Fat: 0.2g Fiber: 2.9g Protein: 2.5g

Turmeric Scrambled Eggs

Preparation time: 10 minutes

Cooking time: 10 minutes

Servings: 3

Ingredients:

Butter

1 tablespoon Large spinach

1 handful Large eggs

6 Salt & pepper to taste Turmeric powder

2 teaspoons

Large tomato

1 (chopped) Coconut oil

1 teaspoon

Directions:

Break the eggs into a medium bowl, whisk and add the pepper, salt, and turmeric. Mix together and set aside. Heat the coconut oil in a small fry pan, add the chopped tomato and cook for about 2 to 3 minutes, until soft. Add the spinach into the pan and cook for another two minutes. Set aside. Add the butter into a small nonstick saucepan to melt under medium-low heat, then add the egg mixture. Use your spatula to push the eggs from side to side across the pan.

Add the tomato and spinach to the pan when the eggs are almost done. Once the egg is cooked, serve immediately.

Nutrition:

Calories: 308 Net carbs: 16.8g Fat: 12.9g Fiber: 1.7g Protein: 20.9g

Parsley Smoothie

Preparation time: 2 minutes

Cooking time: 2 minutes

Servings: 2

Ingredients:

Flat-leaf parsley - 1 cup Juice of two lemons Apple – 1 (core removed) Avocado – 1 Chopped kale - 1 cup Peeled fresh ginger – 1 knob Honey - 1 tablespoon Iced water - 2 cups

Directions:

Add all the ingredients except the avocado into your blender. Blend on high until smooth, then add the avocado, then set your blender to slow speed and blend until creamy. Add a little more iced water if the smoothie is too thick.

Nutrition:

Calories: 5 Net carbs: 1.1g Fiber: 0.2g Protein: 0.2g

Matcha Overnight Oats

Preparation time: 12 hours

Cooking time: 0 minutes

Servings: 2

Ingredients:

For the Oats

Chia seeds - 2 teaspoon Rolled oats – 3 oz.

Matcha powder - 1 teaspoon

Honey - 1 teaspoon Almond milk – 1 ½ cups

Ground cinnamon - 2 pinches For the Topping

Apple – 1 (peeled, cored and chopped) A handful of mixed nuts

Pumpkin seeds – 1 teaspoon

Directions:

Get your oats ready a night before. Place the chia seeds and the oats in a container or bowl. In a different jug or bowl, add the matcha powder and one tablespoon of almond milk and whisk with a hand-held mixer until you get a smooth paste, then add the rest of the milk and mix thoroughly. Pour the milk mixture over the oats, add the honey and cinnamon, and then stir well. Cover the bowl with a lid and place in the fridge overnight. When you want to eat, transfer the oats to two serving bowls, then top with the nuts, pumpkin seeds, and chopped apple.

Nutrition:

Calories: 20 Net carbs: 4.1g Fat: 0.2g Fiber: 1.4g Protein: 1.5g

Dark Chocolate Protein Truffles

Preparation time: 10 minutes

Cooking time: 10 minutes

Servings: 8

Ingredients:

Coconut oil - ¼ cup Vanilla whey protein powder - ¼ cup Medjool dates - ¼ cup (chopped) Almond milk - ¼ cup Honey - 2 tablespoon Steel-cut oats - ⅛ cup

Coconut flour - 1 tablespoon

Dark chocolate bars, minimum 85% cacao – 2

Directions:

Mix the protein powder, honey, almond milk, dates, coconut flour, and oats in a bowl, then mold the mixture into eight balls.

Melt the coconut oil and chocolate over medium heat in a pot.

Turn off the heat once melted and allow the chocolate to cool for about five to ten minutes.

Dip each of the balls into the melted chocolate until well covered.

Place the balls in the freezer to harden.

Nutrition:

Calories: 240 Net carbs: 20g Total fat: 10g

Refreshing Watermelon Juice

Preparation time: 2 minutes

Cooking time: 0 minutes

Servings: 1

Ingredients:

Young kale leaves - 20g (stalks removed)

Cucumber – ½ (peeled, seeds removed and roughly chopped) Watermelon chunks - 250g

Mint leaves - 250g

Directions:

Add all the ingredients into your blender or juicer. Blend and enjoy.

Nutrition:

Calories: 71 Net carbs: 17.9g Fat: 0.3g Fiber: 1g Protein: 1.4g

Matcha Granola with Berries

Preparation Time: 5 minutes

Cooking time: 20 minutes

Servings: 4

Ingredients:

Rolled oats - 1 cup Coconut oil- 2 tablespoon Mixed nuts - ½ cup (chopped) Pumpkin seeds - 1 tablespoon Matcha powder - 1 tablespoon Strawberries - 1 cup (halved or quartered) Sesame seeds - 1 tablespoon

Ground cinnamon - ½ teaspoon Runny honey - 3 tablespoons Blueberries - 2/3 cup

Greek yogurt - 1 ¾ cups

Directions:

Heat your oven to 325 degrees F. place parchment paper on a baking tray. Heat the coconut oil under low heat until it melts. Put off the heat and stir in the seeds, nuts, and oats. Add the cinnamon, matcha powder, and honey, then mix thoroughly. Evenly spread the granola mixture over the lined baking tray and place in the oven to bake for about fifteen minutes, until crisp and toasted – turn it 2 to 3 times. Remove from the oven to cool, then store in an airtight container.

To serve, layer the yogurt in the serving dishes, then add the berries and granola.

Nutrition:

Calories: 133 Net carbs: 18.6g Fat: 5.8g Fiber: 1g Protein: 1.9g

Coffee and Cashew Smoothie

Preparation Time: 5 minutes
Cooking time: 0 minutes
Servings: 1
Ingredients:

Cashew butter - 1 teaspoon Chilled cashew - ½ glass Tahini - 1 teaspoon
Medjool date – 1 (pitted and chopped) Espresso coffee - 1 shot
Ground cinnamon - ½ teaspoon Tiny pinch of salt

Directions:

Add all the ingredients into a high-speed blender. Blend until creamy and smooth.

Nutrition:

Calories: 360 Net carbs: 33.1g Fat: 19.7g Fiber: 5.3g Protein: 14.1g

Buckwheat Pita Bread Sirtfood

Preparation time: 20 minutes
Cooking time: 30 minutes
Servings: 6
Ingredients:

Sea salt - 1 teaspoon Polenta for dusting Packet dried yeast - 1 x 8 gram Lukewarm water - 375ml
Extra virgin olive oil - 3 tablespoon Buckwheat flour - 500 grams

Directions:

Add the yeast in the lukewarm water, mix and set aside for about 10 to 15 minutes to activate. Mix the buckwheat flour, olive oil, salt, and yeast mixture. Work slowly to make a dough. Cover and place in a warm spot for approx. one hour – this is to get the dough to rise. Divide the dough into six parts. Shape one of the pieces into a flat disc and place between two sheets of a baking paper. Gently roll out the dough into a round pita shape that is approximately ¼-inch thick. Use a fork to pierce the dough a few times, then dust lightly with polenta. Heat up your cast iron pan and brush the pan with olive oil. Cook the pita for about 5 minutes on one side, until puffy, then turn to the other side and repeat. Fill the pita with your preferred veggies and meat, then serve immediately.

Nutrition:

Calories: 124 Net carbs: 25g Fat: 0.5g Fiber: 1g Protein: 4.1g

No-Bake Apple Crisp Recipe

Preparation time: 10 minutes
Cooking time: 0 minutes
Servings: 8
Ingredients:

Apples - 8 (peeled, cored and chopped)
Cinnamon - 2 teaspoons (divided) Raisins - 1 cup (soaked and drained) Lemon juice - 2 tablespoons Medjool dates - 1 cup Walnuts - 2 cups Sea salt - ⅛ teaspoon Nutmeg - ¼ teaspoon

Directions:

Add one teaspoon of cinnamon, the raisins, two apples, and the nutmeg into your food processor. Process until smooth. Toss the remaining chopped apples and the lemon juice in a big bowl. Pour the apple puree over the apples in the bowl and mix well. Transfer the mixture into a medium-sized baking dish and keep aside. Add the remaining cinnamon, dates, sea salt, and walnuts into your food processor. Pulse until coarsely grounded. Do not over mix. Sprinkle the mixture over the apples and use your hands to press down lightly. Allow to sit for a few hours for the flavor to marinate or serve immediately.

Nutrition:

Calories: 243 Net carbs: 22g Fat: 8.6g Fiber: 0.5g Protein: 19g

Matcha Latte

Preparation time: 2 minutes
Cooking time: 3 minutes
Servings: 1
Ingredients:
Unsweetened rice milk - 1 mug Date syrup – ½ teaspoon (optional) Matcha powder - 1 teaspoon **Directions:**
Heat the matcha and milk in a pan and froth it until it gets hot, stir in your preferred sweetener.
Pour into your cup and Enjoy!
Nutrition:
Calories: 205Net carbs: 42.4g Fat: 2.5g Fiber: 0.5g Protein: 2.8g

Melon and Grape Juice

Preparation time: 2 minutes
Cooking time: 0 minutes
Servings: 1
Ingredients:
Red seedless grapes – 1 cup
Young spinach leaves – 1 ounce (stalks removed)
Cucumber – ½ (peel if you like, halved, seeds removed and chopped roughly) Cantaloupe melon – 1 cup (peeled, deseeded and chopped into chunks) **Directions:**
Add all the ingredients into your juicer and blend until smooth.
Nutrition:
Calories: 125 Net carbs: 7g Fat: 0.1g Protein: 0.6g

Blackcurrant and Kale Smoothie

Preparation Time: 3 minutes
Cooking time: 0 minutes
Servings: 2
Ingredients:
Ripe banana – 1 Honey - 2 teaspoon
Baby kale leaves - 10 (stalks removed) Freshly made green tea - 1 cup
Blackcurrants – 1/3 cup (washed and stalks removed) Ice cubes – 6
Directions:
Add the honey into the warm green tea. Stir until dissolved. Add all the ingredients into your blender. Blend until smooth. Serve immediately.
Nutrition:
Calories: 18 Net carbs: 4.3g Fat: 0.1g Protein: 0.4g

Pancakes with Apples and Blackcurrants

Preparation Time: 5 Minutes
Cooking Time: 50 Minutes
Servings: 4
Ingredients:
2 apples cut into small chunks 2 cups of quick cooking oats 1 cup flour of your choice
2 egg whites
1 ¼ cups almond milk, unsweetened Cooking spray
1 cup blackcurrants, stalks removed 3 tbsp. water may use less
2 tbsp. raw sugar, or coconut sugar, or honey, or a few stevia drops (optional)
Directions:
Place the ingredients for the topping in a small pot simmer, stirring frequently for about 10 minutes until it cooks down and the juices are released. Take the dry ingredients and mix in a bowl.
After, add the apples and the milk a bit at a time (you may not use it all), until it is a batter. Whisk the egg whites until they are firm and gently mix them into the pancake batter.
Set aside in the refrigerator. Spray a flat pan with cooking spray, and when hot, pour some of the batter into it in a pancake shape. When the pancakes start to have golden brown edges and form air bubbles, they are ready to

be flipped. Repeat for the next pancakes. Top each pancake with the berry topping.

Nutrition Facts:

Calories: 370kcal, Fat: 10.83 g, Carbohydrates: 79 g, Protein: 11.71 g

Flax Waffles

Preparation Time: 5 minutes
Cooking Time: 5 minutes
Servings: 2

Ingredients

½ cup whole-wheat flour
½ tbsp. flaxseed meal
½ tsp baking powder 1 tbsp. olive oil
½ cup almond milk, unsweetened
¼ tsp vanilla extract, unsweetened
2 tbsp. raw sugar, or coconut sugar, or honey, or a few stevia drops (optional)

Directions:

Switch on a mini waffle maker and let it preheat for 5 minutes. Meanwhile, take a medium bowl, place all the ingredients in it, and then mix by using an immersion blender until smooth.

Pour the batter evenly into the waffle maker, shut with lid, and let it cook for 3 to 4 minutes until firm and golden brown.

Serve straight away. Cool the waffles, divide them between two meal prep containers, evenly add berries into the container, and then add maple syrup in mini-meal prep cups.

Cover each container with lid and store in the refrigerator for up to 5 days. When ready to eat, enjoy them cold or reheat them in the microwave for

40 to 60 seconds or more until hot.

Nutrition Facts:

Calories 220kcal, Fat 3.7 g, Carbohydrate 7 g, Protein 21.5g

Raspberries Parfait

Preparation Time: 5 minutes
Cooking Time: 0 minutes
Servings: 2

Ingredients

4 oz. raspberries 3 tbsp. chia seeds
2 ½ tbsp. shredded coconut
3 tbsp. maple syrup
8 oz. almond milk, unsweetened
½ tsp vanilla extract, unsweetened

Directions:

Take a medium bowl, place chia and coconut in it; add maple syrup and vanilla pour in the milk and whisk until well combined. Let the mixture rest for 30 minutes, then stir it and refrigerate for a minimum of 3 hours or overnight.

Assemble the parfait: divide half of the chia mixture into the bottom of serving glass, and then top evenly with three-fourth of raspberries.

Cover berries with remaining chia seed mixture and then place remaining berries on top. Serve straight away.

Use wide-mouth pint jars to layer parfait cover tightly with lids and store jars in the refrigerator for up to 7 days. When ready to eat, enjoy it cold.

Nutrition Facts:

Calories 239kcal, Fat 9.5 g, Carbohydrate 9.9 g, Protein

Blueberries Pancake

Preparation Time: 5 minutes
Cooking Time: 10 minutes;
Servings: 2

Ingredients

1 banana, peeled
4 tbsp. peanut butter
¼ cup whole-wheat flour 2 oz. blueberries
1 tbsp. maple syrup
A pinch of ground cinnamon

½ cup almond milk, unsweetened Cooking spray

Directions:

Add all the ingredients in a blender and then pulse for 2 minutes until smooth. Spray a medium skillet pan with cooking spray, place it over medium heat and until it gets hot.

Pour in some batter into the pan, shape batter to form a pancake, and cook for 2 to 3 minutes per side until golden brown.

Transfer cooked pancakes to a plate and then repeat with the remaining batter. Serve straight away.

Pancakes can be stored up to 3 days in the fridge using a proper container with a lid. When ready to eat, reheat in the microwave oven for 1 to 2 minutes until hot and then serve.

Nutrition Facts:

Calories 408kcal, Fat 14 g, Carbohydrate 53 g, Protein 10.2g

Cashew Biscuits

Preparation Time: 25 minutes

Cooking Time: 14 minutes

Servings: 9

Ingredients

1¼ cups whole wheat flour

⅓ cup toasted whole cashews, unsalted

½ tsp fine sea salt

1½ teaspoons baking powder 1 tbsp. coconut oil

3 tbsp. natural smooth cashew butter

½ cup soft silken tofu or unsweetened plain yogurt

Directions:

Preheat the oven to 425°F. Line a baking sheet with parchment paper. Place the flour and nuts in a food processor.

Pulse until almost all the nuts are chopped: a few larger pieces are okay and add texture to the cookies. Add salt and baking powder and pulse a couple of times.

Add oil and nut butter and pulse to combine. Add tofu or yogurt, and pulse until a crumbly (but not dry) dough forms.

Gather the dough on a piece of parchment and pat it together to shape into a 6-inch square.

Cut into nine 2-inch square biscuits. Transfer the cookies to the baking sheet. Bake for 12 to 14 minutes or until golden brown at the edges cool

on a wire rack and serve.

Nutrition Facts:

Calories 166kcal, Fat 3.7 g, Carbohydrate 27 g, Protein 3.5g

Raspberry Waffles

Preparation Time: 5 minutes

Cooking Time: 5 minutes

Servings: 2

Ingredients:

½ cup whole-wheat flour

1 ½ tbsp. chopped raspberry

½ tsp baking powder 1 tbsp. olive oil

½ cup almond milk, unsweetened

¼ tsp vanilla extract, unsweetened

2 tbsp. coconut sugar or a few drops of stevia (optional)

Directions:

Switch on the waffle maker and let it preheat for 5 minutes. Meanwhile, take a medium bowl, place all the ingredients in it, and then mix by using an immersion blender until smooth. Pour the batter evenly into the waffle maker, shut with lid, and let it cook for 3 to 4 minutes until firm and golden brown. Serve straight away. Cool the waffles, divide them between two meal prep containers, evenly add berries into the container, and then add maple syrup in mini-meal prep cups. Cover each container with lid and store in the refrigerator for up to 5 days. When ready to eat, enjoy them cold or reheat them in the microwave for 40 to 60 seconds or more until hot.

Nutrition Facts:

Calories 229kcal, Fat 3.7 g, Carbohydrate 35.4 g, Protein 3.5g

Cherry Parfait

Preparation Time: 5 minutes
Cooking Time: 0 minutes
Servings: 2

Ingredients

3 oz. cherries, destemmed 3 tbsp. chia seeds
2 ½ tbsp. shredded coconut
3 tbsp. maple syrup
8 oz. almond milk, unsweetened
½ tsp vanilla extract, unsweetened

Directions:

Take a medium bowl, place chia and coconut in it; add maple syrup and vanilla pour in the milk and whisk until well combined.

Let the mixture rest for 30 minutes, then stir it and refrigerate for a minimum of 3 hours or overnight. Assemble the parfait: divide half of the chia mixture into the bottom of serving glass, and then top evenly with three-fourth of cherries.

Cover berries with remaining chia seed mixture and then place remaining cherries on top. Serve straight away.

Nutrition Facts:

Calories 236kcal, Fat 9.2g, Carbohydrate 34.7g, Protein 3.5g

Pancakes with Blackcurrant Compote

Preparation Time: 5 Minutes
Cooking Time: 35 Minutes
Servings: 4

Ingredients:

1 cup plain flour
½ cup porridge oats
2 apples peeled and cut into tiny pieces 1 tsp of baking powder
2 egg whites
1 cup almond milk, unsweetened Cooking spray
Pinch of salt
4 oz. blackcurrants, stalks removed 3 tbsp. of water
2 tbsp. of raw sugar, or coconut sugar, or honey of a few drops of stevia

Directions:

Make the compote first. Place the blackcurrants, water, and sugar in asmall pan. Bring it to a simmer and let it cook for 10 to 15 minutes. Place oats, baking powder, flour, and salt in a large bowl and stir well. Add in the apple then the milk a little at a time as you whisk until you have a smooth batter.

Whisk the egg whites into stiff peaks and fold into the pancake batter. Transfer the ready batter to a jug. Spray a pan with cooking spray, place it
on medium high heat and add in approximately a quarter of the batter. Let it cook on both sides until it turns golden brown.

Remove when ready then repeat to make four pancakes. Drizzle the blackcurrant compote over the pancakes and serve.

Nutrition Facts:

Calories 201kcal, Fat 7 g, Carbohydrate 40g, Protein 5.8g

Strawberry Buckwheat Pancakes

Preparation Time: 5 Minutes
Cooking Time: 45 Minutes
Servings: 4

Ingredients:

3½ oz. strawberries, chopped 3½ oz. buckwheat flour
1 egg
8fl oz. milk

1 tsp olive oil
1 tsp olive oil for frying 1 orange, juiced
Directions:
Pour the milk into a bowl and mix in the egg and a tsp of olive oil. Sift in the flour to the liquid mixture until smooth and creamy.
Allow it to rest for 15 minutes. Heat a little oil in a pan and pour in a quarter of the mixture or to the size you prefer. Sprinkle in a quarter of the strawberries into the batter. Cook for around 2 minutes on each side.
Serve hot with a drizzle of orange juice.
Try this recipe with other berries such as blueberries and blackberries.
Nutrition Facts:
Calories 180kcal, Fat 7.5 g, Carbohydrate 22.5 g, Protein7.4g

Buckwheat Porridge

Preparation Time: 10 minutes
Cooking Time: 15 minutes
Servings: 2
Ingredients:
1 cup buckwheat, rinsed
1 cup almond milk, unsweetened 1 cup water
½ tsp ground cinnamon
½ tsp vanilla extract
¼ cup fresh blueberries
1 tbsp. raw honey (optional)
Directions:
In a pan, add all the ingredients (except honey and blueberries) over medium-high heat and bring to a boil. Now, reduce the heat to low and simmer, covered for about 10 minutes. Stir in the honey and remove from the heat.
Set aside, covered, for about 5 minutes. With a fork, fluff the mixture, and transfer into serving bowls. Top with blueberries and serve.
Nutrition Facts:
Calories 358 kcal; Fat 4.7 g; Carbohydrate 3.7 g; Protein 12

Cherry and Vanilla Protein Shake

Preparation Time: 5 minutes
Cooking Time: 0 minutes **S**
ervings: 1
Ingredients:
2 oz. cherries, destemmed
1 scoop vanilla protein powder
1 cup almond milk, unsweetened
Directions:
Place all the ingredients in the order into a food processor or blender, and then pulse for 1 to 2 minutes until smooth.
Serve immediately.
Nutrition Facts:
Calories 193kcal, Fat 5.2 g, Carbohydrate 38 g, Protein 5.2g

Peanut Butter Cup Protein Shake

Preparation Time: 5 minutes
Cooking Time: 0 minutes
Servings: 2
Ingredients:
1 banana, peeled
1 scoop of chocolate protein powder 1 tbsp. nutritional yeast
2 tbsp. peanut butter
½ cup almond milk, unsweetened
½ tsp turmeric powder
Directions:
Place all the ingredients in the order into a food processor or blender, and then pulse for 1 to 2 minutes until smooth.
Distribute smoothie between two glasses and then serve.
Divide smoothie between two jars or bottles, cover with a lid, and then store the containers in the refrigerator for up to 3 days.
Nutrition Facts:
Calories 233cal, Fat 11 g, Carbohydrate 17 g, Protein 14g

Smoothie-Chocolate-Coconut Muesli

Ingredients:
1 mango
2 apples
150 ml squeezed apple
40 g dull chocolate (at any rate 70% cocoa)
80 g delicate oats
40 g coconut chips
200 g yogurt elective from soy
40 g puffed oats (oat pops, 4 tbsp.)

Arrangement Steps

Peel the mango cut the tissue from the stone and commonly dice. Clean, wash, quarter, middle, and slash apples. Puree the mango, apple pieces, and cuddled apple through a blender to shape a gooey smoothie.

Grate the dim chocolate on a grater and blend with the oat and coconut pieces.

Pour 1 layer of the smoothie into 4 glasses. Include 1 layer of chocolate-coconut muesli, spread soy yogurt on top, and spread with the remainder of the muesli. Pour within the rest of the smoothie and refill the glasses with oat pops.

Mango Banana Drink with fruit crush and Yogurt

Ingredients:
5 juice oranges
1 little ready mango
1 ready banana
150 g yogurt (3.5% fat)

Planning Steps

Halve and press oranges.

Peel the mango. Cut the mash into cuts from the stone and typically dice.

Peel the banana and disruption it into pieces. Puree with squeezed orange, mango pieces, and yogurt during a blender (or with a hand blender). Fill in 2 glasses (300 ml each).

Yogurt with Berries, Chocolate and Brazil Nuts

Ingredients:
400 g yogurt (3.5% fat)
150 g strawberries
100 g blueberries
40 g dull chocolate (in any event 70% cocoa)
50 g Brazil nut piece
2 tsp. linseed oil

Arrangement Steps

Stir yogurt until smooth and partition into two dishes. Clean, wash and slash strawberries. Wash and touch the blueberries. Roughly cut dim chocolate and Brazil nuts. Put the berries on the yogurt. Sprinkle with chocolate and nuts and shower with the linseed oil.

Ricotta Pancakes with Apricots

Ingredients:
80 g ricotta
1 egg
3 tbsp. juice
1 tsp. nectar
40 g buckwheat flour
½ tsp. preparing powder
1 tsp. copra oil
2 apricots
3 tbsp. yogurt (3.5% fat)
1 stem mint

Arrangement Steps

Mix the ricotta with the egg, lemon squeeze, and nectar until smooth. Include buckwheat flour and preparing powder and blend it into a thick mixture. Warmth coconut oil during a skillet and

include a huge tablespoon of a player to the dish, steel oneself against 1 moment over medium warmth, divert, and keep heating from the opposite side. Do likewise for around 5 hotcakes.

within the interim, wash, divide, and cut apricots. Blend the yogurt until smooth. Wash mint, shake dry, and pluck leaves. Stack the flapjacks on a plate, including the yogurt and apricot wedges, and serve adorned with mint.

Vanilla Curd with Strawberries

Ingredients:

100 g strawberries
150 g low-fat quark
2 tbsp. yogurt (3.5% fat)
1 tbsp. milk (3.5% fat)
1 tsp. vanilla powder
1 tsp. entire pure sweetener
1 tbsp. almond pieces

Directions:

Clean, wash pat dry strawberries, and dig pieces.
Mix the lean quark with yogurt, milk, vanilla powder, and sugar until rich with a whisk, at that fact overlay in 3/4 of the strawberries.
Roughly cleave the almonds. Shake the vanilla curd with the rest of the strawberries and almonds and serve.

Honey Skyr with Nuts

Ingredients:

400 g skyr
1 tbsp. nectar (on the other hand maple syrup)
1 tsp. vanilla powder
1 bunch pecan parts (25 g)
1 bunch almond parts (25 g; unpeeled)
2 tsp. linseed oil

Planning Steps

Mix Skier with nectar and vanilla. Generally, hack pecans and
almonds.
Divide the Skier into two dishes, pour the nuts over it, and shower with 1 teaspoon of linseed oil. Serve and appreciate Skyr.

Soy Quark with Apple, Kiwi, and Oatmeal

Ingredients:

300 g soy quark
1 apple
2 kiwi natural products
3 tbsp. flaxseed dinner
4 tbsp. succinct cereal

Arrangement Steps

Stir soy quark until smooth and appropriate in two dishes. Clean, divide, center, and cut apples into little pieces. Strip and hack the kiwi.
Put the apple and kiwi blocks on the soy curd. Serve sprinkled with flax seeds and oats.

Blueberry and Coconut Rolls

Ingredients:

150 g whole meal flour
150 g spelled flour
1½ tsp. heating powder
1 squeeze salt
50 g crude unadulterated sweetener
4 tbsp. rape oil
250 g low-fat quark
1 egg
5 tbsp. milk (3.5% fat)
120 g blueberries
4 tbsp. ground coconut

Planning Steps

Put the flour with heating powder and salt during a bowl. Include sugar and blend. Include rapeseed oil, quark, egg and 4 tablespoons of milk and utilize a hand blender to ply into a
smooth mixture.
Wash the blueberries, pat dry, and overlay in in conjunction with rock bottom coconut under the batter.
Line a preparing sheet with material paper. Structure 9 round moves with floured hands and spot them on the preparing sheet. Brush

the blueberry and coconut moves with the rest of the milk and heat during a preheated stove at 200 ° C (fan broiler 180 ° C; gas: setting 3) for 12–15 minutes.

Chia Pudding with Yogurt and Strawberry Puree

Fixing

200 g strawberries (new or solidified)
2 tbsp. chia seeds
350 g yogurt (3.5% fat)
1 tsp. nectar
1 squeeze Tonka bean
50 g almond bits
20 g dim chocolate (at any rate 70% cocoa)

Directions:

Put the strawberries during a pan with slightly water and cook delicately on medium warmth in around 7 minutes and crush them if essential. Meanwhile, blend the chia seeds well with yogurt and nectar and season with Tonka beans.

Roughly cleave the almonds and chocolate. But layer chia yogurt and strawberry puree in glasses and serve sprinkled with almonds and chocolate.

Coconut Soy Yogurt with Pineapple and Sesame

Ingredients:

300 g soy yogurt
3 tbsp. coconut milk (45 g)
200 g pineapple mash
3 tsp. sesame
3 tsp. syrup
2 tbsp. delicate oats

Directions:

Mix the soy yogurt with coconut milk. Cut the pineapple mash into pieces.

Fry the pineapple pieces during a hot dish with 1 teaspoon syrup and 1 teaspoon sesame over medium-high warmth for 4-5 minutes, letting them caramelize marginally. At that point expel the skillet from the oven and let it cool.

Fill coconut soy yogurt in two dishes, orchestrate pineapple on top, sprinkle with residual sesame and cereal, and shower with 1 teaspoon syrup.

Savvy Whole meal Spelled Rolls

Ingredients:

350 g whole meal spelled flour
150 g spelled flour type 1050
1 tsp. salt
1 parcel dried yeast or 1/2 3D square of latest yeast
½ tsp. crude genuine sweetener
355 ml oat drink (oat milk)
1 tbsp. cereal
1 tsp. poppy seeds

Directions:

Mix flour with salt, include yeast and sugar and manipulate with
350 ml oat drink to a smooth and versatile batter. Leave it shrouded during a warm spot for thirty minutes to hour.

Then manipulate once more. Split the batter into two long frankfurters and gap it into five pieces. Shape the pieces into balls and spot on a preparing sheet secured with heating paper. Somewhat cut within the middle with a blade, brush with the rest of the oat drink and sprinkle with cereal and poppy seeds.

Let the mixture pieces rest during a warm spot for an extra half- hour. Preheat the broiler to 200 degrees (fan stove 180 degrees). At that point slide the sheet into the broiler and spot a flame- resistant holder with some water on rock bottom of the stove. Heat the moves for around 20 minutes until they're brilliant yellow. At that point expel from the stove and let cool.

Chocolate Banana Spread

Ingredients:

50 g dull chocolate
250 g without lactose curd cheddar (20% fat)
2 tbsp. oat drink (oat milk)
1 banana
4 cuts oat bread

Directions:

Grate dull chocolate. Put around 1 tbsp. of the grate.
Mix the curd cheddar with the oat drink until smooth. Crease within the bottom chocolate.
Peel the banana and cut it at an edge.
Brush the bread with the chocolate curd, organize the banana cuts on the very best and sprinkle with the rest of the chocolate shavings.

Chocolate Curd with Banana

Ingredients:

50 g dim chocolate
1 banana
250 g sans lactose low-fat curd
2 tbsp. sans lactose milk (3.5% fat)

Planning Steps

Grate dim chocolate. Put around 1 tbsp. of the scratch.
Peel the banana and finely dice the substance. Put 1–2 tbsp. for the enhancement.
Stir the curd with milk until smooth. Overlay within the bottom chocolate and thus the banana solid shapes.
Spread the chocolate quark in two little dishes and embellishment with the remaining ground chocolate and banana solid shapes.

Spring Cloud bread

Fixing

3 eggs
200 g cream cheddar (60% fat in dry issue)
1 tsp. heating powder
5 g salt
Milk (3.5% fat) ½ tsp.
Medium-hot mustard pepper
½ group chives (10 g)
100 g sheep's lettuce
½ group radish
1 bunch red radish cress

Planning Steps

Separate the eggs and blend the egg yolks in with 100 g cream cheddar and preparing powder. Beat the egg whites with slightly of salt until solid and overlap in divides under the cream cheddar cream.
Spread the mixture in 8 level bits on a heating sheet secured with preparing paper and heat during a preheated stove at 150 ° C (convection 130 ° C; gas: setting 1-2) for around 20 minutes. Remove and let cool for around 10 minutes.
Mix the rest of the cream cheddar with milk, mustard, somewhat salt, and pepper. Wash the chives, shake dry, dig folds and blend into the cream.
Clean sheep's lettuce, wash and shake dry. Clean, wash and cut radishes into slim cuts. Wash the cress and channel well. Spread some cream on the underside of 4 cloud bits of bread each, orchestrate sheep's lettuce, radish cuts, remaining cream and cress on top, and spot 1 cloud bread each on top as a top.

Pea Protein Sandwiches

Ingredients:

370 g solidified peas
225 g cereal
75 g stripped hemp seeds
1½ tsp. fennel seeds
1 tsp. coriander seeds
1 tsp. caraway seeds
2 tsp. heating powder
2 tsp. prepared salt
3 eggs
2 carrots

250 g quark (20% fat in dry issue)
Salt pepper
½ pack chives (10 g)

Directions:

Let the peas defrost. Pound cereal and hemp seeds to flour during a blender. Finely grind the fennel, coriander seeds, and caraway seeds during a mortar and increase the flour. Include heating powder and salt and blend.

Put the peas and eggs within the blender and slash until you get a smooth mixture. Line a heating tin with preparing paper and include the batter.

Peel the carrots, quarter them lengthways and place them on the batter. Heat during a preheated stove at 180 ° C (fan broiler 160 ° C; gas: levels 2–3) for 55–an hour. At that point let it chill off for around half-hour.

Within the interim blend the curd in with salt, pepper, and a few of tablespoons of water. Wash chives, shake dry, and dig rings. Cut bread into cuts, brush with the curd cheddar, and enhancement with chives.

Bircher Muesli within the Caribbean Style

Ingredients:

90 g terse cereal
1 tbsp. squashed linseed
270 g pineapple (1/4 pineapple)
25 g hazelnuts (2 tbsp.)
60 g coconut drink
1 tbsp. ground coconut

Directions:

Mix cereal and flaxseed with 250 ml of water and spread and let swell within the cooler short-term.

Peel the pineapple and cut or mesh the mash into extremely fine strips. Slash hazelnuts and include a couple of portion of the cereal in conjunction with the pineapple pieces and coconut drink.

Spread the Bircher muesli in two dishes and serve decorated with staying nuts and coconut pieces.

Buckwheat Groats with Banana and Chocolate Topping

Ingredients:

400 ml oat drink (oat milk)
½ flavorer
1 tsp. ground cardamom
1 tsp. cinnamon powder
3 tsp. chocolate
1 tbsp. crude genuine sweetener
125 g buckwheat groats
1 banana
1 tbsp. cocoa nibs
1 tsp. chia seeds

Planning Steps

Heat the oat drink a pan. Split the length of the vanilla case lengthways and cut out the mash with a blade. Include the vanilla mash, the scratched out the vanilla unit, cardamom, cinnamon, cocoa, and crude genuine sweetener to the oat drink, mix and convey to the bubble.

Stir within the buckwheat, bring back the bubble quickly and let it swell for 10 minutes over medium warmth, mixing once during a short time.

Meanwhile, strip the banana and cut the mash. Warmth the spread during a skillet and daintily earthy colored the cuts of banana over medium warmth.

Fill buckwheat groats in little dishes and serve embellished with bananas, cocoa nibs, and chia seeds.

Sweet Millet Casserole with Clementine's

Ingredients:

150 g brilliant millet
1 flavored
½ natural lemon
½ tsp. cinnamon powder
2 tbsp. crude natural sweetener
380 ml oat drink (oat milk)
2 tangerines
3 eggs
1 squeeze salt
300 g without lactose curd cheddar (20% fat)
1 tbsp. spread
2 tbsp. cut almonds

Arrangement Steps

Wash millet hot. Split the vanilla unit lengthways and cut out the mash with a blade. Flush 50% of the lemon hot, pat dry and rub the pizzazz finely. Crush out the juice.

Put millet, vanilla mash, cinnamon, sugar, and oat drink a pot. Bring back the bubble and stew over medium-high warmth for around 7-10 minutes, mixing periodically. Expel from the warmth and let douse for 10 minutes without a top.

Meanwhile, strip the tangerines and cut them into thick cuts. Separate eggs. Beat egg whites with 1 spot of salt until egg whites are hardened. Blend the egg yolks in with lemon get-up- and-go, juice, and quark and increase the millet mass. Cautiously crease within the egg whites.

Butter the preparing dish. Pour within the millet curd blend, smooth and top with the mandarins. Prepare during a preheated stove at 180 ° C (fan broiler 160 ° C; gas: levels 2–3) for 40–50 minutes. Sprinkle millet goulash with ground almonds to serve.

Spread with Tomatoes

Ingredients:

100 g dried tomato in oil
100 g sunflower seeds
3 tbsp. rapeseed oil salt pepper
3 stems basil
4 cuts oat bread

Arrangement Steps

Let the tomatoes channel marginally and cut generally. At that point put during a tall holder and puree in conjunction with 90 g sunflower seeds, rape oil, and 3-4 tablespoons of water. At that point season with salt and pepper.

Wash the basil, shake dry and finely slash the leaves. Include 3/4 of the basil to the tomato spread and blend in.

Spread the spread with tomatoes on four cuts of oat bread. Sprinkle with residual sunflower seeds and basil and serve.

Vegan Overnight Oats with Blueberries and Coconut

Ingredients:

5 tbsp. cereal (75 g)
3 tbsp. coconut pieces (30 g)
150 g yogurt elective from soy
150 ml coconut drink
1 tbsp. syrup (for example coconut bloom syrup; 15 g)
100 g blueberries (new or solidified)
2 tbsp. pumpkin seeds (30 g)

Directions:

Mix the oats with 2 tablespoons of coconut pieces, yogurt elective, coconut drink, and coconut bloom syrup. Include half the blueberries and refrigerate for at any rate 2 hours, better for the nonce.

Subsequent morning, include vegetarian short-term oats with blueberries and coconut to 2 dishes or closable glasses. Sprinkle with pumpkin seeds and remaining blueberries and coconut chips.

Overnight Oats with Apple and Walnuts

Ingredients:

75 g buckwheat chip
1 tsp cinnamon
Salt
250 ml milk (3.5% fat)
1 tbsp. fruit purée (15 g; no added sugar)
2 tbsp. chia seeds (10 g)
1 apple
1 tbsp. syrup (15 g)
2 tbsp. pecan pieces (30 g)

Arrangement Steps

Mix the buckwheat drops with slightly cinnamon and a spot of salt. Include milk, fruit purée, and 1 tablespoon of chia seeds, mix well, and put within the cooler for in any event 2 hours, better for the nonce.

Subsequent morning, wash, quarter, and center the apple. Half- cut into fine cuts, the other half into blocks. Put the apple 3D shapes with syrup and thus the rest of the cinnamon during a pot, warmth, and permit them to caramelize.

Roughly cleave pecan pieces. Put for the nonce oats in two dishes or closable glasses.

Spread apple cuts, caramelized apple 3D shapes, and pecan pieces over them and serve the overnight oats with apple and pecans with the remaining chia seeds.

Overnight Oats with Banana and spread

Ingredients:

5 tbsp. cereal (75 g)
2 tbsp. squashed linseed (15 g)
200 ml almond drink (almond milk)
2 tbsp. nutty spread (30 g)
1 tsp agave syrup (5 g)
1 banana
1 tbsp. salted nut part (15 g)

Planning Steps

Mix cereal and 1 tablespoon of flax seeds. Include almond milk,

1 tablespoon of nutty spread, and agave syrup and blend all directly. A spot within the cooler for in any event 2 hours, ideally overnight.

Subsequent morning, strip the banana and cut it into reduced down pieces. Generally, cleave nut parts as wanted.

Place short-term oats in two little dishes or closable glasses and spread the staying nutty spread and bananas on top. Sprinkle for the nonce oats with nutty spread and banana with residual flaxseed and nut parts.

Overnight Oats with Chocolate and Figs

Ingredients:

1 pc dull chocolate (30 g; in any event 70% cocoa)
5 tbsp. spelled pieces (75 g)
1 tbsp. chocolate (10 g; intensely oiled)
200 ml oat drink (oat milk)
2 tbsp. pistachio portions (30 g)
2 figs
2 stems mint
1 tbsp. cocoa nibs (10 g)

Directions:

Chop the chocolate and blend in with spelled drops, chocolate, and oat milk and put within the refrigerator for at any rate 2 hours, better for the nonce.

Subsequent morning, generally slash the pistachio nuts. Wash the figs, pat dry, and quarter them. Wash mint, shake dry and pluck the leaves.

Put short-term oats in two dishes or closable glasses. Spread figs and mint leaves on top. Sprinkle for the nonce oats with chocolate and figs with hacked pistachio nuts and cocoa nibs.

Overnight Oats with Coffee and Blackberries

Ingredients:

5 tbsp multigrain chips (75 g; as an example grain, oats, rye, rice)
1 tsp vanilla powder
1 tsp entire pure sweetener (5 g)
100 ml espresso (cooled)
100 ml milk (3.5% fat)
100 g blackberry (new or solidified)
1 PC dull chocolate (15 g; in any event 70% cocoa)
2 tbsp walnut half (30 g)

Arrangement Steps

Mix the multigrain chips with vanilla powder and full natural sweetener. Include espresso and milk and blend all directly. Include blackberries and refrigerate for at any rate 2 hours, better for the nonce.

Subsequent morning, generally slash chocolate and walnuts. Put for the nonce oats with espresso and blackberries in two dishes or closable glasses and sprinkle with chocolate and nuts.

Oriental Porridge with Oranges and Figs

Ingredients:

400 ml oat drink (oat milk)
75 g pointed oats
25 g delicate cereal
2 tbsp syrup
2 cardamom containers
1 tsp cinnamon
¼ tsp vanilla powder
1 squeeze salt
1 orange
1 defeatist
2 tbsp white almond margarine
1 tbsp squashed gold flax seeds (10 g)
1 tbsp hacked pistachio nuts (15 g)

Arrangement Steps

Heat the oat drink a pot. Mix in cereal, syrup, cardamom, cinnamon, vanilla, and slightly of salt and stew over medium warmth for 2-3 minutes. At that point permit growing for around 5 minutes over low warmth.

Meanwhile, strip the orange so all white is evacuated. Cut out natural product filets between the fingernail skins while getting the juice. Wash the fig, pat dry, and dig eighths. Blend the
almond margarine with squeezed orange.

Fill the oriental porridge in little dishes and present with orange filets, fig cuts, linseed, and pistachios. Shower the almond margarine over the porridge before serving.

Sweet Pumpkin Buns

Ingredients:

300 g Hokkaido pumpkin
50 ml squeezed orange
450 g spelled flour type 1050
1 3D shape yeast
70 g entire natural sweetener
150 ml tepid milk (3.5% fat)
1 flavored
1 egg (m)
80 groom temperature spread
½ tsp cinnamon
1 MSP. Cardamom powder
1 squeeze salt
1 ingredient

Directions:

Wash, center, and bones the pumpkin. Spot during a pot with squeezed orange and cook delicately on low warmth for approx. quarter-hour. Puree and let cool.

Within the interim, put the flour during a bowl and press an empty within the middle. Disintegrate the yeast and include 1 tsp entire pure sweetener and milk to the well. Spread and let ascend for 10 minutes.

Slit the vanilla case lengthways and cut out the mash. Include the vanilla mash, remaining sugar, egg, spread, cinnamon, cardamom, 1 spot of salt, and cooled pumpkin puree to the hitter. Massage everything into a smooth batter and spread and let ascend for hour.

Divide the batter into 8 equivalent pieces and shape them into rolls. Spot on a heating sheet secured with preparing the paper. Whisk the ingredient with water and brush the makes due.

Bake the moves during a preheated stove at 180 ° C (constrained air 160 ° C, gas: level 2–3) in 20–30 minutes until brilliant earthy colored.

CHAPTER 6:

Snacks

Lemongrass Green Tea

Preparation time: 3 minutes
Cooking time: 12 min
Servings: 1
Ingredients:

Two teaspoons cleaved lemongrass One teaspoon green tea leaves
1 cup of water
One teaspoon nectar

Directions:

Move the water to a treated steel pot.
Hurl in the lemongrass and heat the water to the point of boiling. Let it bubble for 5 minutes.
Expel the pot from the fire and let the water cool till the temperature is 80-85 degrees C.
Presently, include the green tea and let it soak for 3 minutes. Strain the tea into your cup.
Include nectar and mix a long time before drinking.

Nutrition:

Calories: 2.5 Calcium: 3mg Potassium: 34mg Magnesium: 2.9g

Grape and Melon Juice

Preparation time: 10 minutes
Cooking time: 0 minutes
Servings: 1
Ingredients:

½ cucumber, stripped whenever liked, split, seeds evacuated and generally slashed
30g youthful spinach leaves stalks expelled 100g red seedless grapes
100g melon, stripped, deseeded

Directions:

Cut into pieces. Blend in a juicer or blender until smooth.

Nutrition:

Calories: 125 Net carbs: 31.7g Fat: 0.24g Protein: 0.63g

Kale and Blackcurrant Smoothie

Preparation time: 10 minutes
Cooking time: 0 minutes
Servings: 2
Ingredients:

2 teaspoon nectar
1 cup crisply made green tea
Ten infant kale leaves stalk expelled One ready banana
40 g blackcurrants, washed and stalks evacuated Six ice blocks

Directions:

Mix the nectar into the warm green tea until disintegrated. Master all the **Ingredients:** together in a blender until smooth. Serve right away.

Nutrition:

Calories: 86 Net carbs: 32.9g Protein: 4.5g

Kale, Edamame and Tofu Curry

Preparation time: 5 minutes
Cooking time: 8 minutes
Servings: 4
Ingredients:

1 teaspoon rapeseed oil One huge onion, cleaved

Four cloves garlic stripped and ground
One massive thumb (7cm) crisp ginger, stripped and ground One red bean stew, deseeded and meagerly cut
1/2 teaspoon ground turmeric 1/4 teaspoon cayenne pepper
1 teaspoon paprika 1 teaspoon salt 1/2 teaspoon ground cumin
250g dried red lentils 1-litre bubbling water
50g solidified soy edamame beans
200g firm tofu, cleaved into solid shapes Two tomatoes, generally cleaved
Juice of 1 lime
200g kale leaves stalks expelled and torn

Directions:

Put the oil in an overwhelming bottomed container over a low-medium warmth. Include the onion and cook for 5 minutes before including the garlic, ginger and stew and preparing for a further 2 minutes. Include the turmeric, cayenne, paprika, cumin and salt. Mix through before including the red lentils and blending once more.

pour in the bubbling water and bring to a generous stew for 10 minutes, at that point decrease the warmth and cook for a further 20-30 minutes until the curry has a thick '•porridge' consistency. Add the soya beans, tofu and tomatoes and cook for a further 5 minutes. Include the lime juice and kale leaves and cook until the kale merely is delicate.

Nutrition:

Protein: 12.6g Calories: 342 Net carbs: 8.4g Fat: 17g

Green Tea Smoothie

Preparation time: 10 minutes
Cooking time: 0 minutes
Servings: 2
Ingredients:

Two ready bananas 250 ml of milk 2 teaspoon matcha green tea powder
1/2 teaspoon vanilla bean glue (not separate) or a little scratch of the seeds from a vanilla unit
Six ice blocks 2 teaspoon nectar

Directions:

Just mix all the **Ingredients:** in a blender and serve in two glasses.

Nutrition:

Calories: 183 Net carbs: 33g Fat: 0.6g Fiber: 3.8g Protein: 2.1g

Sirt Muesli

Preparation time: 10 minutes
Cooking time: 0 minutes
Servings: 2
Ingredients:

20g buckwheat flakes sirtfood plans 10g buckwheat puffs
15g parched coconut
40g Medjool dates, hollowed and cleaved 15g pecans, cleaved
10g cocoa nibs
100g strawberries, hulled and cleaved
100g plain Greek yoghurt (or veggie lover elective, for example, soya or coconut yoghurt)

Directions:

Blend the entirety of the above **Ingredients:**, possibly including the yoghurt and strawberries before serving on the off chance that you are making it in mass.

Nutrition:

Calories: 25 Net carbs: 43.3g Fat: 7.2g Fiber: 6.5g Protein: 9.0g

Fruit Salad

Preparation time: 10 min
Cooking time: 0 minutes
Servings: 1
Ingredients:

½ cup crisply made green tea

1 teaspoon nectar One orange, split One apple, cored and generally cleaved Ten red seedless grapes
Ten blueberries
Directions:
Stir the nectar into a large portion of some green tea. At the point when broken up, include the juice of a large part of the orange. Leave to cool. Chop the other portion of the orange and spot in a bowl together with the hacked apple, grapes and blueberries. Pour over the cooled tea and leave to soak for a couple of moments before serving.
Nutrition:
Calories: 157 Net carbs: 13g Fiber: 1g Protein: 0.5g

Golden Turmeric Latte

Preparation time: 3 minutes
Cooking time: 7 minutes
Servings: 3
Ingredients:
3 cups of coconut milk
One teaspoon turmeric powder One teaspoon cinnamon powder One teaspoon crude nectar
Directions:
Spot of dark pepper (expands retention) Modest bit of new stripped ginger root
Place of cayenne pepper (discretionary)
Mix all **Ingredients:** in a fast blender until smooth.
Fill a little container and warmth for 4 minutes over medium heat until hot however not bubbling.
Nutrition:
Calories: 50 Net carbs: 98g Fat: 2.7g

The Sirt Juice

Preparation time: 7-8 min
Cooking time: 0 minutes
Servings: 2

Ingredients: Two huge bunches (75g) kale A huge bunch (30g) rocket
A tiny bunch (5g) level leaf parsley
A small bunch (5g) lovage leaves (discretionary)
2–3 huge stalks (150g) green celery, including its leaves
½ medium green apple Juice of ½ lemon
½ level teaspoon matcha green tea
Directions:
Blend the greens (kale, rocket, parsley and lovage, on the off chance that was utilizing), at that point juice them. We discover juicers can indeed vary in their effectiveness at squeezing verdant vegetables, and you may need to re- squeeze the leftovers before proceeding onward to different **Ingredients:**. The objective is to wind up with about 50ml of juice from the greens. Presently squeeze the celery and apple. You can strip the lemon and put it through the juicer also, however, we think that it's a lot simpler just to crush the lemon by hand into the juice. By this stage, you ought to have around 250ml of milk altogether, maybe marginally more. It is just when the sauce is made and prepared to serve that you include the matcha green tea. Pour a limited quantity of the juice into a glass, at that point include the matcha and mix enthusiastically with a fork or teaspoon. We just use matcha in the first two beverages of the day as it contains reasonable measures of caffeine (a similar substance as a typical cup of tea). For individuals not accustomed to it, it might keep them wakeful whenever alcoholic late once the match is broken up, including the rest of the juice. Give it a last mix; at that point, your juice is prepared to drink. Don't hesitate to top up with plain water, as indicated by taste.
Nutrition: Calories: 75 Net carbs: 3.8g Fat: 0.6g Fiber: 2.9g Protein: 0.4g

Kale Pesto Hummus

Preparation time: 10 minutes
Cooking time: 7 minutes
Servings: 12
Ingredients:

Chickpeas, drained and liquid reserved – 15 ounces Reserved chickpea liquid - .25 cup
Sea salt - .5 teaspoon Tahini paste - .5 cup Garlic, minced – 2 cloves Lemon juice – 2.5 s
Extra virgin olive oil - .33 cup Black pepper, ground - .5 teaspoon
Kale, chopped and leaves packed – 2 cups Pine nuts – 2 s
Basil leaves, packed – 1.25 cups
Garlic, minced – 4 cloves Extra virgin olive oil - .25 cup

Directions:

Into a food processor add the basil, kale, pine nuts, and four cloves of minced garlic. Pulse until the leaves and garlic are finely chopped. Pour in the olive oil, and once again pulse until smooth. Remove the pesto from the bowl of the food processor and set aside.

Into the empty food processor add the remaining ingredients to assemble the hummus, pulsing until creamy. Add in the prepared pesto, and pulse just until the two are combined.

Transfer the pesto hummus to a serving bowl or store in the fridge.

Nutrition:

Calories: 194 Net carbs: 3.8g Fat: 2.2g Fiber: 1.8g Protein: 5.6g

Parsley Hummus

Preparation time: 5 minutes
Cooking time: 7 minutes
Servings: 6
Ingredients:

Chickpeas, drained and rinsed – 15 ounces Curly parsley, stems removed – 1 cup
Sea salt – .5 teaspoon
Soy milk, unsweetened - .5 cup Extra virgin olive oil – 3 teaspoons Lime juice – 1 s
Red pepper flakes -.5 teaspoons Black pepper, ground - .25 teaspoon
Pine nuts – 2 s
Sesame seeds, toasted – 2 s

Directions:

In the food processor pulse the parsley and toasted sesame seeds until it forms a fine powdery texture. Drizzle in the extra virgin olive oil in while you continue to pulse, until it is smooth.

Add the chickpeas, lime juice, and seasonings to the food processor and pulse while slowly adding in the soy milk. Continue to pulse the parsley hummus until it is smooth and creamy.

Adjust the seasonings to your preference and then serve or refrigerate the hummus.

Nutrition:

Calories: 107 Net carbs: 7.7g Fat: 4.5g Fiber: 0.2g Protein: 8.6g

Edamame Hummus

Preparation time: 7 minutes
Cooking time: 0 minutes
Servings: 10
Ingredients:

Edamame, cooked and shelled – 2 cups Sea salt – 1 teaspoon
Extra virgin olive oil – 1 Tahini paste - .25 cup Lemon juice - .25 cup Garlic, minced – 3 cloves
Black pepper, ground - .25 teaspoon

Directions:

Add the cooked edamame and remaining ingredients to a blender or food processor and mix on high until it forms a creamy and completely smooth
mixture. Taste it and adjust the seasonings to your preference.

Serve the hummus immediately with your favorite vegetables or store in the fridge.

Nutrition:

Calories: 88 Net carbs: 3.8g Protein: 2.6g

Edamame Guacamole

Preparation time: 7 minutes

Cooking time: 0 minutes

Servings: 6

Ingredients:

Edamame, cooked and shelled – 1 cup Avocado, pitted and halved – 1

Red onion, diced - .5 cup Cilantro, chopped - .25 cup Jalapeno, minced – 1 Garlic, minced – 2 cloves

Lime juice – 2 s Water – 3 s Lime zest - .5 teaspoon Roma tomato, diced – 2 Cumin - .125 teaspoon

Sea salt - .5 teaspoon

Directions:

Into a blender or food processor add all of the ingredients, except for the diced tomato, onion, and jalapeno. Blend the tomato mixture on high speed until it is smooth and creamy, making sure that the edamame has been

completely blended.

Adjust the seasoning to your preference and then transfer the guacamole to a serving bowl. Stir in the tomato, onion, and jalapeno. Place the bowl in the fridge, allowing it to chill for at least thirty minutes before serving.

Nutrition:

Calories: 100 Net carbs: 13g Fat: 6.6g Fiber: 6.2g Protein: 45g

Eggplant Fries with Fresh Aioli

Preparation time: 10 minutes

Cooking time: 25 minutes

Servings: 4

Ingredients:

Eggplants – 2

Black pepper, ground - .25 teaspoon Extra virgin olive oil – 2 s Cornstarch – 1

Basil, dried – 1 teaspoon Garlic powder - .25 teaspoon Sea salt - .5 teaspoon

Mayonnaise, made with olive oil - .5 cup Garlic, minced – 1 teaspoon

Basil, fresh, chopped – 1 Lemon juice – 1 teaspoon Chipotle, ground - .5 teaspoon Sea salt - .25 teaspoon

Directions:

Begin by preheating your oven to Fahrenheit four-hundred and twenty-five degrees. Place a wire cooking/cooling rack on a baking sheet.

Remove the peel from the eggplants and then slice them into rounds, each about three-quarters of an inch thick. Slice the rounds into wedges one inch in width.

Add the eggplant wedges to a large bowl and toss them with the olive oil. Once coated, add the pepper, cornstarch, dried basil, garlic powder, and sea salt, tossing until evenly coated.

Arrange the eggplant wedges on top of the wire rack and set the baking sheet in the oven, allowing the fries to cook for fifteen to twenty minutes.

Meanwhile, prepare the aioli. To do this, add the remaining ingredients into a small bowl and whisk them together to combine. Cover the bowl of aioli and allow it to chill it in the fridge until the fries are ready to be served.

Remove the fries from the oven immediately upon baking, or allow them to cook under the broiler for an additional three to four minutes for extra crispy fries. Serve immediately with the aioli.

Nutrition:

Calories: 243 Net carbs: 12.6g Fat: 0.5g Fiber: 13.2g Protein: 5.3g

Eggplant Caponata

Preparation time: 10 minutes
Cooking time: 25 minutes
Servings: 4

Ingredients: Eggplant, sliced into 1.5-inch cubes – 1 pound Bell pepper, diced – 1
Green and black olives, chopped - .5 cup
Capers - .25 cup
Sea salt – 1 teaspoon Garlic, minced – 4 Red onion, diced – 1
Diced tomatoes – 15 ounces
Extra virgin olive oil – 4 s, divided Black pepper, ground - .25 teaspoon Parsley, chopped - .25 cup

Directions:

Preheat your oven to Fahrenheit four-hundred degrees and line a baking sheet with kitchen parchment. Toss the eggplant cubes in half of the olive oil and then arrange them on the baking sheet, sprinkling the sea salt over the top. Allow the eggplant to roast until tender, about twenty minutes. Meanwhile, add the remaining olive oil into a large skillet along with the red onions, bell pepper, diced tomatoes, and garlic. Sautee the vegetables until tender, about ten minutes. Add the roasted eggplant, capers, olives, and black pepper to the skillet, continuing to cook together for five minutes so that the flavors meld. Remove the skillet from the heat, top it off with parsley, and serve it with crusty toast.

Nutrition:

Calories: 209 Net carbs: 1.6g Fat: 2.3g Fiber: 5.4g Protein: 0.3g

Buckwheat Crackers

Preparation time: 10 minutes
Cooking time: 1 hour
Servings: 12
Ingredients:

Buckwheat groats – 2 cups Flaxseeds, ground - .75 cup Sesame seeds - .33 cup
Sweet potatoes, medium, grated – 2 Extra virgin olive oil – .33 cup Water – 1 cup
Sea salt – 1 teaspoon

Directions:

Soak the buckwheat groats in water for at least four hours before preparing the crackers. Once done soaking, drain off the water.

Preheat the oven to a temperature of Fahrenheit three-hundred and fifty degrees, prepare a baking sheet, and set aside some kitchen parchment and plastic wrap.

In a kitchen bowl, combine the ground flaxseeds with the warm water, allowing the seeds to absorb the water and form a substance similar to gelatin. Add the buckwheat groats and other remaining ingredients.

Spread the cracker dough onto a sheet of kitchen parchment and cover it with a sheet of plastic wrap. Use a rolling pen on top of the plastic wrap (so that it doesn't stick) and roll out the buckwheat cracker dough until it is thin.

Peel the plastic wrap off of the crackers and transfer the dough-coasted sheet of kitchen parchment to the prepared baking sheet. Allow it to partially bake for fifteen minutes and then remove the tray from the oven.

Reduce the oven temperature to Fahrenheit three-hundred degrees. Use a pizza cutter and slice the crackers into squares, approximately two inches in width. Return the crackers to the oven until they are crispy and dry, about thirty-five to forty minutes.

Remove the crackers from the oven, allowing them to cool completely before storing them in an air-tight container.

Nutrition:

Calories: 158 Net carbs: 6.6g Fat: 3.8g Fiber: 2.6g Protein: 3.4g

Matcha Protein Bites

Preparation time: 15 minutes
Cooking time: 70 minutes
Servings: 12
Ingredients:

Almond butter - .25 cup Matcha powder – 2 teaspoons Soy protein isolate – 1 ounce Rolled oats - .5 cup
Chia seeds – 1
Coconut oil – 2 teaspoons Honey – 1
Sea salt - .125 teaspoon

Directions:

In a food processor combine all of the matcha protein bite ingredients until it forms a mixture similar to wet sand, that will stick together when squished between your fingers. Divide the mixture into twelve equal portions. You can do this by eye while estimating, or you can use a digital kitchen scale if you want the portions to be exact. Roll each portion between the palms of your hands to form balls.

Chill the bites in the fridge for up to two weeks.

Nutrition:

Calories: 164 Net carbs: 13.3g Fat: 4.7g Fiber: 1.2g Protein: 4.5g

Chocolate-Covered Strawberry Trail Mix

Preparation time: 5 minutes
Cooking time: 0 minutes
Servings: 10
Ingredients:

Freeze-dried strawberries – 1 cup Dark chocolate chunks - .66 cup Walnuts, roasted – 1 cup Almonds, roasted - .25 cup Cashews, roasted - .25 cup

Directions:

Mix together all of the trail mix ingredients in a bowl, and then store it in a large glass jar or divide each serving into its own transportable plastic bag. Store for up to one month.

Nutrition:

Calories: 164 Net carbs: 17.2g Fat: 3.2g Fiber: 6.7g Protein: 2.2g

Moroccan Spiced Eggs

Preparation time: 1 hour 10 minutes
Cooking time: 45 minutes
Servings: 2
Ingredients:

1 tablespoon olive oil
One shallot, stripped and finely hacked
One red (chime) pepper, deseeded and finely hacked One garlic clove, stripped and finely hacked
One courgette (zucchini), stripped and finely hacked 1 tablespoon tomato puree (glue)
½ teaspoon gentle stew powder
¼ teaspoon ground cinnamon
¼ teaspoon ground cumin
½ teaspoon salt
400g can hacked tomatoes 400g may chickpeas in water
A little bunch of level leaf parsley cleaved
Four medium eggs at room temperature

Directions:

Heat the oil in a pan, include the shallot and red (ringer) pepper and fry delicately for 5 minutes. At that point include the garlic and courgette (zucchini) and cook for one more moment or two. Include the tomato puree (glue), flavors and salt and mix through.

Add the cleaved tomatoes and chickpeas (dousing alcohol and all) and increment the warmth to medium. With the top of the dish, stew the sauce for 30 minutes – ensure it is delicately rising all through and permit it to lessen in volume by around 33%.

Remove from the warmth and mix in the cleaved parsley. Preheat the grill to 200C/180C fan/350F.

When you are prepared to cook the eggs, bring the tomato sauce up to a delicate stew and move to a little broiler confirmation dish. Crack the eggs on the dish and lower them delicately into the stew. Spread with thwart and prepare in the grill for 10-15 minutes. Serve the blend in

unique dishes with the eggs coasting on the top.

Nutrition:

Calorie: 116 Protein: 6.97 g

Fat: 5.22 g

Carbohydrates: 13.14 g

Exquisite Turmeric Pancakes with Lemon Yogurt Sauce

Preparation time: 45 minutes

Cooking time: 15 minutes

Servings: 8 hotcakes

Ingredients:

For The Yogurt Sauce

1 cup plain Greek yogurt 1 garlic clove, minced

1 to 2 tablespoons lemon juice (from 1 lemon), to taste

¼ teaspoon ground turmeric 10 crisp mint leaves, minced

2 teaspoons lemon pizzazz (from 1 lemon)

For The Pancakes

2 teaspoons ground turmeric 1½ teaspoons ground cumin 1 teaspoon salt

1 teaspoon ground coriander

½ teaspoon garlic powder

½ teaspoon naturally ground dark pepper 1 head broccoli, cut into florets

3 enormous eggs, gently beaten

2 tablespoons plain unsweetened almond milk 1 cup almond flour

4 teaspoons coconut oil

Directions:

Make the yogurt sauce. Join the yogurt, garlic, lemon juice, turmeric, mint and pizzazz in a bowl. Taste and enjoy with more lemon juice, if possible. Keep in a safe spot or freeze until prepared to serve.

Make the flapjacks. In a little bowl, join the turmeric, cumin, salt, coriander, garlic and pepper.

Spot the broccoli in a nourishment processor, and heartbeat until the florets are separated into little pieces. Move the broccoli to an enormous bowl and include the eggs, almond milk, and almond flour. Mix in the flavor blend and consolidate well.

Heat 1 teaspoon of the coconut oil in a nonstick dish over medium-low heat. Empty ¼ cup player into the skillet. Cook the hotcake until little air pockets start to show up superficially and the base is brilliant darker, 2 to 3 minutes. Flip over and cook the hotcake for 2 to 3 minutes more. To keep warm, move the cooked hotcakes to a stove safe dish and spot in a 200°F oven.

Keep making the staying 3 hotcakes, utilizing the rest of the oil and player.

Nutrition:

Calories: 262

Protein: 11.68 g

Fat: 19.28 g

Carbohydrates: 12.06 g

Sirt Chili Con Carne

Preparation time: 1 hour 20 minutes

Cooking time: 1 hour 3 minutes

Servings: 4

Ingredients:

1 red onion, finely cleaved

3 garlic cloves, finely cleaved

2 10,000 foot chilies, finely hacked

1 tablespoon additional virgin olive oil 1 tablespoon ground cumin

1 tablespoon ground turmeric
400g lean minced hamburger (5 percent fat) 150ml red wine
1 red pepper, cored, seeds evacuated and cut into reduced down pieces 2 x 400g tins cleaved tomatoes
1 tablespoon tomato purée 1 tablespoon cocoa powder 150g tinned kidney beans 300ml hamburger stock
5g coriander, cleaved 5g parsley, cleaved 160g buckwheat

Directions:

In a meal, fry the onion, garlic and bean stew in the oil over a medium heat for 2-3 minutes, at that point include the flavors and cook for a moment.

Include the minced hamburger and dark colored over a high heat. Include the red wine and permit it to rise to decrease it considerably.

Include the red pepper, tomatoes, tomato purée, cocoa, kidney beans and stock and leave to stew for 60 minutes.

You may need to add a little water to accomplish a thick, clingy consistency. Just before serving, mix in the hacked herbs.

In the interim, cook the buckwheat as indicated by the bundle guidelines and present with the stew.

Nutrition:

Calories: 346 kcal
Protein: 14.11 g
Fat: 11.37 g
Carbohydrates: 49.25 g

Salmon and Spinach Quiche

Preparation time: 55 minutes
Cooking time: 45 minutes
Servings: 2
Ingredients:

600g frozen leaf spinach 1 clove of garlic
1 onion
150g frozen salmon fillets 200g smoked salmon
1 small Bunch of dill 1 untreated lemon
50 g butter
200 g sour cream 3 eggs
Salt, pepper, nutmeg 1 pack of puff pastry

Directions:

Let the spinach thaw and squeeze well.

Peel the garlic and onion and cut into fine cubes. Cut the salmon fillet into cubes 1-1.5 cm thick. Cut the smoked salmon into strips. Wash the dill, pat dry and chop.

Wash the lemon with hot water, dry, rub the zest finely with a kitchen grater and squeeze the lemon.

Heat the butter in a pan. Sweat the garlic and onion cubes in it for approx. 2-3 minutes.

Add spinach and sweat briefly.

Add sour cream, lemon juice and zest, eggs and dill and mix well. Season with salt, pepper and nutmeg.

Preheat the oven to 200 degrees top / bottom heat (180 degrees convection).

Grease a spring form pan and roll out the puff pastry in it and pull up on edge. Prick the dough with a fork (so that it doesn't rise too much).

Pour in the spinach and egg mixture and smooth out. Spread salmon cubes and smoked salmon strips on top.

The quiche in the oven (grid, middle inset) about 30-40 min. Yellow gold bake.

Nutrition:

Calories: 903 Protein: 65.28 g
Fat: 59.79 g Carbohydrates: 30.79 g

Choc Chip Granola

Preparation time: 55 minutes
Cooking time: 20 minutes
Servings: 2
Ingredients:

200g large oat flakes

Roughly 50 g pecan nuts chopped 3 tablespoons of light olive oil 20g butter
1 tablespoon of dark brown sugar 2 tablespoon rice syrup
60 g of good quality (70%) Dark chocolate shavings

Directions:

Oven preheats to 160 ° C (140 ° C fan / Gas 3). Line a large baking tray with a sheet of silicone or parchment for baking.

In a large bowl, combine the oats and pecans. Heat the olive oil, butter, brown sugar, and rice malt syrup gently in a small non-stick pan until the butter has melted, and the sugar and syrup dissolve. Do not let boil. Pour the syrup over the oats and stir thoroughly until fully covered with the oats.

Spread the granola over the baking tray and spread right into the corners. Leave the mixture clumps with spacing, instead of even spreading. Bake for 20 minutes in the oven until golden brown is just tinged at the edges. Remove from the oven, and leave completely to cool on the tray.

When cold, split with your fingers any larger lumps on the tray and then mix them in the chocolate chips. Put the granola in an airtight tub or jar, or pour it. The granola is to last for at least 2 weeks.

Nutrition:

Calories: 914 Protein: 40.19 g
Fat: 63.05 g Carbohydrates: 88.74 g

Aromatic Chicken Breast, Kale, Red Onion, and Salsa

Preparation time: 55 minutes C
ooking time: 30 minutes
Servings: 2
Ingredients:

120g skinless, boneless chicken breast 2 teaspoons ground turmeric
¼ lemon
1 tablespoon extra-virgin olive oil 50g kale, chopped
20g red onion, sliced
1 teaspoon fresh ginger, chopped 50g buckwheat

Directions:

To prepare the salsa, remove the tomato eye and finely chop. Add the chili, parsley, capers, lemon juice and mix.

Preheat the oven to 220°C. Pour 1 teaspoon of the turmeric, the lemon juice and a little oil on the chicken breast and marinate. Allow to stay for 5–10 minutes.

Place an ovenproof frying pan on the heat and cook the marinated chicken for a minute on each side to achieve a pale golden color. Then transfer the pan containing the chicken to the oven and allow to stay for 8–10 minutes or until it is done. Remove from the oven and cover with foil, set aside for 5 minutes before serving.

Put the kale in a steamer and cook for 5 minutes. Pour a little oil in a frying pan and fry the red onions and the ginger to become soft but not colored. Add the cooked kale and continue to fry for another minute.

Cook the buckwheat following the packet's instructions using the remaining turmeric. Serve alongside the chicken, salsa, and vegetables.

Nutrition:

Calories: 149
Protein: 15.85 g
Fat: 5.09 g
Carbohydrates: 10.53 g

Braised Leek With Pine Nuts

Preparation time: 45 minutes
Cooking time: 15 minutes
Servings: 2
Ingredients:

20g Ghee

2 teaspoon Olive oil 2 pieces Leek
150 ml Vegetable broth Fresh parsley
1 tablespoon fresh oregano
1 tablespoon Pine nuts (roasted)

Directions:

Cut the leek into thin rings and finely chop the herbs. Roast the pine nuts in a dry pan over medium heat.

Melt the ghee together with the olive oil in a large pan.

Cook the leek until golden brown for 5 minutes, stirring constantly.

Add the vegetable broth and cook for another 10 minutes until the leek is tender.

Stir in the herbs and sprinkle the pine nuts on the dish just before serving.

Nutrition:

Calories: 95
Protein: 1.35 g
Fat: 4.84 g
Carbohydrates: 12.61 g

Sweet and Sour Pan with Cashew Nuts

Preparation time: 30 minutes
Cooking time: 0 minutes
Servings: 2
Ingredients:

2 tablespoon Coconut oil 2 pieces Red onion
2 pieces yellow bell pepper 250 g White cabbage
150 g Pak choi
50 g Mung bean sprouts 4 pieces Pineapple slices 50 g Cashew nuts
For the sweet and sour sauce: 60 ml Apple cider vinegar
4 tablespoon Coconut blossom sugar 11⁄2 tablespoon Tomato paste
1 teaspoon Coconut-Amines 2 teaspoon Arrowroot powder 75 ml Water

Directions:

Roughly cut the vegetables.

Mix the arrow root with five tablespoons of cold water into a paste.

Then put all the other ingredients for the sauce in a saucepan and add the arrowroot paste for binding.

Melt the coconut oil in a pan and fry the onion.

Add the bell pepper, cabbage, pak choi and bean sprouts and stir-fry until the vegetables become a little softer.

Add the pineapple and cashew nuts and stir a few more times. Pour a little sauce over the wok dish and serve.

Nutrition:

Calories: 573
Protein: 15.25 g
Fat: 27.81 g
Carbohydrates: 77.91 g

Vegetarian Paleo Ratatouille

Preparation time: 1 hour 10 minutes
Cooking time: 55 minutes
Servings: 2
Ingredients:

200 g Tomato cubes (can) 1/2 pieces Onion
2 cloves Garlic
1/4 teaspoon dried oregano
1 / 4 TL Chili flakes 2 tablespoon Olive oil 1 piece Eggplant
1 piece Zucchini
1 piece hot peppers
1 teaspoon dried thyme

Directions:

Preheat the oven to 180 ° C and lightly grease a round or oval shape. Finely chop the onion and garlic.

Mix the tomato cubes with garlic, onion, oregano and chili flakes, season with salt and pepper and put on the bottom of the baking dish.

Use a mandolin, a cheese slicer or a sharp knife to cut the eggplant, zucchini and hot pepper into very thin slices.
Put the vegetables in a bowl (make circles, start at the edge and work inside).
Drizzle the remaining olive oil on the vegetables and sprinkle with thyme, salt and pepper.
Cover the baking dish with a piece of parchment paper and bake in the oven for 45 to 55 minutes.

Nutrition:

Calories: 273
Protein: 5.66 g
Fat: 14.49 g
Carbohydrates: 35.81 g

Frittata with Spring Onions and Asparagus:

Preparation time: 15 minutes
Cooking time: 10 minutes
Servings: 2
Ingredients:

5 pieces Egg
80 ml Almond milk
2 tablespoon Coconut oil 1 clove Garlic
100 g Asparagus tips 4 pieces Spring onions 1 teaspoon Tarragon
1 pinch Chili flakes

Directions:

Preheat the oven to 220 ° C.
Squeeze the garlic and finely chop the spring onions.
Whisk the eggs with the almond milk and season with salt and pepper.
Melt 1 tablespoon of coconut oil in a medium-sized cast iron pan and briefly fry the onion and garlic with the asparagus.
Remove the vegetables from the pan and melt the remaining coconut oil in the pan.
Pour in the egg mixture and half of the entire vegetable.
Place the pan in the oven for 15 minutes until the egg has solidified.
Then take the pan out of the oven and pour the rest of the egg with the vegetables into the pan. Place the pan in the oven again for 15 minutes until the egg is nice and loose. Sprinkle the tarragon and chili flakes on the dish before serving.

Nutrition:

Calories: 464 kcal Protein: 24.23 g Fat: 37.84 g Carbohydrates: 7.33 g

Apple Pastry

Preparation time: 15 minutes
Cooking time: 30 minutes
Servings: 1
Ingredients:

Three cups all-purpose flour Dash of salt
Two teaspoons margarine One plain low-fat yogurt One small apple
Dash each ground nutmeg and ground cinnamon
Two teaspoons reduced-calorie apricot spread (16 calories per 2 teaspoons)

Directions:

In a small mixing bowl, combine flour and salt; with a pastry blender, or two knives used scissors-fashion, cut in margarine until the mixture resembles a coarse meal. Add yogurt and mix thoroughly. Form dough into a ball; wrap in plastic wrap and refrigerate for at least 1 hour (maybe kept in the refrigerator for up to 3 days).
Between 2 sheets of a wax paper roll dough, forming a 4/2-inch circle about 1/2. Inch thick. Carefully remove wax paper and place dough on foil or small cookie sheet—Preheat oven to 350°F.
Core, pare, and thinly slice apple; arrange slices decoratively over the dough and sprinkle with nutmeg and cinnamon. Bake until crust is golden, 20 to 30 minutes.

During the last few minutes, that pastry is baking, in a small metal measuring cup or other small flameproof container heat apricot spread; as soon as the pie is done, brush with a warm space.

Nutrition:

238 calories; 4 g protein; 8 g fat; 38 g carbohydrate; 228 mg sodium; 1 mg cholesterol.

Baked Maple Apple

Preparation time: 10 minutes

Cooking time: 30 minutes

Servings: 2

Ingredients:

Two small apples

Two teaspoons reduced-calorie apricot Spread

One teaspoon reduced-calorie maple-flavored syrup

Directions:

Remove the core from each apple to 1/2 inch from the bottom. Remove a thin strip of peel from around the center of each apple (this helps keep skin from bursting). Fill each apple with one teaspoon apricot spread and 1/2 teaspoon maple syrup. Place each apple upright in individual baking dish; cover dishes with foil and bake at 400°F until apples are tender, 25 to 30 minutes.

Nutrition:

75 calories; 0.2 g protein; 1 g fat; 19 g carbohydrate; 0.3 mg sodium;

Apple-Raisin Cake

Preparation time: 20 minutes

Cooking time: 50 minutes

Servings: 12

Ingredients:

One teaspoon baking soda 1/2 cups applesauce (no sugar added)

Two small Golden Delicious apples, cored, pared, and shredded 1 cup less 2 s raisins

2/4 cups self-rising flour

1 teaspoon ground cinnamon

1/2 teaspoon ground cloves 1/3 cup plus 2 teaspoons unsalted margarine 1/4 cup granulated sugar

Directions:

Spray an 8 x 8 x 2-inch baking pan with nonstick cooking spray and set aside. Into a medium bowl sift together flour, cinnamon, and cloves; set aside.Preheat oven to 350°F. In a medium mixing bowl, using an electric mixer, cream margarine, add sugar and stir to combine. Stir baking soda into applesauce, then add to margarine mixture and stir to combine; add sifted ingredients and, using an electric mixer on medium speed, beat until thoroughly combined. Fold in apples and raisins; pour batter into the sprayed pan and bake for 45 to 50 minutes (until cake is browned and a cake tester or toothpick, inserted in center, comes out dry). Remove cake from pan and cool on wire rack.

Nutrition: 151 calories; 2 g protein;

4 g fat; 28 g carbohydrate; 96 mg sodium;

Cinnamon-Apricot Bananas

Preparation time: 45 minutes

Cooking time: 0 minutes

Servings: 2

Ingredients:

4 graham crackers 2x2-inch 1 medium banana, peeled and cut in squares),

made into crumbs half lengthwise 2 teaspoons shredded coconut

1/4 teaspoon ground cinnamon

1 plus 1 teaspoon reduced-calorie apricot spread (16 calories per 2 teaspoons)

Directions:

In small skillet combine crumbs, coconut, and cinnamon and toast lightly, being careful not to burn; transfer to a sheet of wax paper or a paper plate and set aside.

In the same skillet heat apricot spread until melted; remove from heat. Roll each banana half in a spread, then quickly roll in crumb mixture, pressing crumbs so that they adhere to the banana; place coated halves on a plate, cover lightly, and refrigerate until chilled.

Variation: Coconut-Strawberry Bananas — Omit cinnamon and substitute reduced-calorie strawberry spread (16 calories per 2 teaspoons) for the apricot spread.

Nutrition:

130 calories; 2g protein; 2g fat; 29g carbohydrate; 95mg sodium;

Meringue Crepes with Blueberry Custard Filling

Preparation time: 10 minutes

Cooking time: 20 minutes

Servings: 4

Ingredients:

2 cups blueberries (reserve 8 berries for garnish) 1 cup evaporated skimmed milk

2 large eggs, separated

1 plus 1 teaspoon granulated sugar, divided

2 teaspoons each cornstarch Lemon juice

Directions:

In 1-quart saucepan, combine milk, egg yolks, and one sugar; cook over low heat, continually stirring, until slightly thickened and bubbles form around sides of the mixture. In a cup or small bowl dissolve cornstarch in lemon juice; gradually stir into milk mixture and cook, constantly stirring, until thick. Remove from heat and fold in blueberries; let cool.

Spoon Vs. of custard onto the center of each crepe and fold sides over filling to enclose; arrange crepes, seam-side down, in an 8 x 8 x 2-inch baking pan. In a small bowl, using an electric mixer on high speed, beat egg whites until soft peaks form; add remaining teaspoon sugar, and continue beating until stiff peaks form.

Fill the pastry bag with egg whites and pipe an equal amount over each crepe (if pastry bag is not available, spoon egg whites over crepes); top each with a reserved blueberry and broil until meringue is lightly browned, 10 to 15 seconds. Serve immediately.

Nutrition:

300 calories; 16g protein; 6g fat; 45g carbohydrate; 180mg sodium; 278mg cholesterol

Chilled Cherry Soup

Preparation time: 5 minutes

Cooking time: 5 minutes

Servings: 2

Ingredients:

20 large frozen pitted cherries (no sugar added) 1/2 cup water

1/2 teaspoons granulated sugar 2-inch cinnamon stick

1 strip lemon peel 2 s rose wine

1 teaspoon cornstarch

1/4 cup plain low-fat yogurt

Directions:

In a small saucepan, combine cherries, water, sugar, cinnamon stick, and lemon peel; bring to a boil. Reduce heat, cover, and let simmer for 20 minutes.

Remove and discard the cinnamon stick and lemon peel from a cherry mixture. In measuring cup or small bowl combine wine and cornstarch, stirring to dissolve cornstarch; add to cherry mixture and, constantly stirring, bring to a boil. Reduce heat and let simmer until the mixture thickens.

In a heatproof bowl, stir yogurt until smooth; add cherry mixture and stir to combine.

Cover with plastic wrap and refrigerate until well chilled

Nutrition:

98 calories; 2 g protein; 1 g fat; 19 g carbohydrate; 21 mg sodium; 2 mg cholesterol

Iced Orange Punch

Preparation time: 20 minutes
Cooking time: 0 minutes
Servings: 8
Ingredients:

Ice Mold Club soda
1 lemon, sliced 1 lime, sliced Punch
1 quart each chilled orange juice (no sugar added), club soda, and diet ginger ale)

Directions:

To Prepare Ice Mold: Pour enough club soda into a 10- or 12-cup ring mold to fill mold; add lemon and lime slices, arranging them in an alternating pattern. Cover the mold and carefully transfer to freezer; freeze until solid. To Prepare Punch: In a large punch bowl, combine juice and sodas. Remove
ice mold from ring mold and float ice mold in a punch.

Nutrition:

56 calories; 1g protein; 0.1 g fat; 14 g carbohydrate; 35 mg sodium;

Meatless Borscht

Preparation time: 15 minutes
Cooking time: 45 minutes
Servings: 2
Ingredients:

1 teaspoon margarine 1 cup shredded green cabbage
1/4 cup chopped onion 1/4 cup sliced carrot
1 cup coarsely shredded pared
2 s tomato paste beets 1 lemon juice 2 cups of water
1/2 teaspoon granulated sugar
2 packets instant beef broth and 1 teaspoon pepper Seasoning mix 1/2 bay leaf
1/4 cup plain low-fat yogurt

Directions:

In 1 1/2-quart saucepan heat margarine until bubbly and hot; add onion and sauté until softened, 1 to 2 minutes. Add beets and toss to combine; add water, broth mix, and bay leaf and bring to a boil. Cover pan and cook over medium heat for 10 minutes; stir in remaining ingredients except for yogurt, cover, and let simmer until vegetables are tender about 25 minutes. Remove and discard bay leaf. Pour borscht into 2 soup bowls and top each portion with 2 s yogurt.

Nutrition:

120 calories; 5g protein; 3g fat; 21g carbohydrate; 982mg sodium; 2mg cholesterol

Sautéed Sweet 'N' Sour Beets

Preparation time: 10 minutes
Cooking time: 10 minutes
Servings: 2
Ingredients:

Serve hot or chilled.
2 teaspoons margarine
1 diced onion
1 cup drained canned small whole beets, cut into quarters 1 each lemon juice and water
1 teaspoon each salt and pepper Dash granulated sugar substitute **Directions:**

In small nonstick skillet heat margarine over medium-high heat until bubbly and hot; add onion and sauté until softened, 1 to 2 minutes. Reduce heat to low and add remaining ingredients; cover pan and cook, stirring once, for 5 minutes longer.

Nutrition:

70 calories; 1g protein; 4g fat; 9g carbohydrate; 385 mg sodium;

Orange Beets

Preparation time: 10 minutes
Cooking time: 10 minutes
Servings: 2
Ingredients:

1 /2 teaspoons lemon juice
1 teaspoon cornstarch Dash salt 1 teaspoon orange marmalade
1 cup peeled and sliced cooked beets 2 teaspoons margarine
1 teaspoon firmly packed brown
Sugar 1/4 cup orange juice (no sugar added)

Directions:

In a 1-quart saucepan (not aluminum or cast-iron), combine beets, margarine, and sugar; cook over low heat, continually stirring until margarine and sugar are melted.
In 1-cup measure or small bowl combine juices, cornstarch, and salt, stirring to dissolve cornstarch; pour over beet mixture and, constantly stirring, bring to a boil. Continue cooking and stirring
Until the mixture thickens.
Reduce heat, add marmalade, and stir until combined. Remove from heat and let cool slightly; cover and refrigerate for at least 1 hour. Reheat before serving.

Nutrition:

99 calories; 1g protein; 4g fat; 16g carbohydrate; 146mg sodium;

Cabbage 'N' Potato Soup

Preparation time: 10 minutes
Cooking time: 40 minutes Servings: 4
Chokolate cupcakes (Matcha icing)
Ingredients:

6 oz castor sugar 2 oz cocoa
½ tsp salt
½ tsp fine espresso coffee, decaf if preferred
½ cup milk
½ tsp vanilla 3 tbsp oil
1 egg
½ cup boiling water Ingredients for the icing:
2 oz butter, at temperature 2 oz powdered sugar
1 tbsp matcha tea powder
½ tsp flavorer paste 2 oz soft cheese

Directions:

Preheat the oven to 340 °F. Line a cupcake tin with paper or silicone cake cases.
Place the flour, sugar, cocoa, salt and espresso powder during a large bowl and blend thoroughly.
Add the milk, vanilla, vegetable oil and egg to the dry ingredients and use an electrical mixer to beat until well combined. Carefully pour in the boiling water slowly and beat on a coffee speed until fully combined. Use a high speed to beat for a further minute to add air to the batter. The batter is far more liquid than a traditional cake mix. Have faith, it'll taste amazing!
Spoon the batter evenly between the cake cases. Each cake case should be no quite ¾ full. Bake in the oven for 15-18 minutes, until the mixture bounces back when tapped. Remove from the oven and allow to chill completely before icing.
To make the icing, cream the butter and powdered sugar together until its pale and smooth. Add the matcha powder and vanilla and stir again. Finally add the cheese and beat until smooth. Pipe or spread over the cakes.

Sirt Muesli

Ingredients:

1 oz buckwheat flakes
0.3 oz buckwheat puffs
0.5 oz coconut flakes or desiccated coconut
About 1 oz Medjool dates, pitted and chopped
0.5 oz walnuts, chopped
0.3 oz cocoa nibs
4 oz strawberries, hulled and chopped

4 oz plain Greek yoghurt (or vegan alternative, like soya or coconut yoghurt)

Directions:

Mix all of the above ingredients together (leave out the strawberries and yoghurt if not serving straight away).

Apricot Bread with Fresh chevron

Ingredients:

4 apricots
½ favorer
1 tsp nectar
2 cuts entire bread
30 g goat cream cheddar
Salt
Pepper
1 branch rosemary

Planning Steps

Wash, divide, expel the seeds and cut the apricot parts into wedges. Cut an open portion of the vanilla case and cut out the mash. Spot during a pot with the nectar and apricots and braise on low warmth for 3 minutes.

Within the interim spread the two cuts of bread with new goat cheddar and season with somewhat salt and pepper. Wash the rosemary, shake dry and pluck the needles. Spread the apricot cuts on the bread cuts, sprinkle with rosemary needles and serve.

Tomato and Zucchini Salad with Feta

Ingredients:

2 zucchini
4 tbsp oil
Salt
Pepper
400 g tomatoes
200 g cherry tomatoes
3 spring onions
1 pack basil (20 g)
2 tbsp fruit crush vinegar
100 g feta (45% fat in dry issue)

Planning Steps

Clean, wash, and cut zucchini. Warmth 1 tablespoon of oil during a dish, fry the zucchini in it over medium warmth for five minutes. Season with salt and pepper.

Clean, wash and hack tomatoes. Wash and split cherry tomatoes.

Mix zucchini, tomatoes, cherry tomatoes, and basil. Include the rest of the oil and fruit crush vinegar, blend, and season with salt and pepper. Disintegrate the feta. Serve the plate of mixed greens sprinkled with feta.

Vanilla Curd with Strawberries

Ingredients:

100 g strawberries
150 g low-fat quark
2 tbsp yogurt (3.5% fat)
1 tbsp milk (3.5% fat)
1 MSP. Vanilla powder
1 tsp entire natural sweetener
1 tbsp almond portions

Directions:

Clean, wash pat dry strawberries, and dig pieces.

Mix the lean quark with yogurt, milk, vanilla powder, and sugar until velvety with a whisk, at that point overlay in 3/4 of the strawberries.

Roughly slash the almonds. Sprinkle the vanilla curd with the rest of the strawberries and almonds and serve.

Blueberry and Coconut Rolls

Ingredients:

150 g whole meal flour
150 g spelled flour
1½ tsp preparing powder
1 squeeze salt
50 g crude natural sweetener

4 tbsp rapeseed oil
250 g low-fat quark
1 egg
5 tbsp milk (3.5% fat)
120 g blueberries
4 tbsp ground coconut

Directions:

Put the flour with preparing powder and salt during a bowl. Include sugar and blend. Include rapeseed oil, quark, egg and 4 tablespoons of milk and utilize a hand blender to regulate into a smooth batter.

Wash the blueberries, pat dry, and overlay in alongside rock bottom coconut under the batter.

Line a preparing sheet with material paper. Structure 9 round moves with floured hands and spot them on the preparing sheet. Brush the blueberry and coconut moves with the rest of the milk

and heat during a preheated stove at 200 ° C (fan broiler 180 ° C; gas: setting 3) for 12–15 minutes.

Vanilla Energy Balls with Coconut Shell

Ingredients:

100 g almond pieces
200 g dried date (pitted)
½ tsp vanilla powder
20 g ground coconut (approx. 2 tbsp)

Arrangement Steps

Put almonds, dates, and vanilla powder during a home appliance or solid blender and hack into clingy mush.

Form bundles of equivalent size from the mass.

Put coconut chips on A level plate. Roll the vanilla vitality balls within the coconut drops and press them down gently.

Place the vanilla vitality balls during a hermetically sealed sealable box and confine the cooler.

Wake-up Energy Balls

Ingredients:

120 g dried dates (without stone)
120 g pecans
6 tsp chocolate (18 g; intensely oiled)
1 squeeze salt
1 squeeze vanilla powder
2 tbsp espresso bean (30 g)
2 tsp ground espresso (10 g)
Chili pieces

Directions:

Put the dates alongside the nuts, 4 teaspoons of chocolate, 1 spot of salt, and vanilla powder during a blender and puree until you get a homogeneous batter.

Add the espresso beans and blend quickly. Cut 16 bits of batter with a tablespoon and shape into balls.

Mix the rest of the chocolate with espresso powder and bean stew

drops and roll the vitality balls in it.

Brain Food Cookies

Ingredients:

150 g spelled flour type 1050
1 tsp preparing powder
100 g entire pure sweetener
1 squeeze salt
120 groom temperature spread
3 ready bananas
1 egg
150 g succinct cereal
60 g gave almonds
1 tbsp cocoa nibs
2 tbsp chocolate drop (produced using dim chocolate; 15 g)

Arrangement Steps

and blend. Strip the bananas, squash them with a fork and add them to the batter alongside the egg and blend well with a hand blender.

Overlay within the cereal, almonds, cocoa nibs, and half the chocolate drops.

Line a heating sheet with material paper. Spot the batter on the preparing sheet with a tablespoon, leaving enough space between the treats. Sprinkle with the rest of the chocolate drops and heat during a preheated stove at 200 ° C (fan broiler 180 ° C; gas: setting 3) for 10–15 minutes.

Moon milk with Lavender

Ingredients:

500 ml milk (3.5% fat)
1 tsp dried lavender blossoms
¼ tsp cinnamon
¼ tsp ashwagandha powder flavor
2 tsp nectar
2 tsp dried cornflower (blossoms)

Arrangement Steps

Put the milk, lavender blossoms, cinnamon, and ashwagandha during a pan and warmth. Bring back the bubble quickly, expel from the warmth and let cool somewhat. Include nectar and blend in.

Foam with a hand blender spread quite 2 glasses and serve sprinkled with cornflowers.

Cucumber and Radish Salad with Feta

Ingredients:

1½ cucumbers
1 pack radish
1 pack rocket (80 g)
4 gherkins
200 g feta
4 tbsp oil
3 tbsp juice
1 tsp mustard
1 tsp nectar salt pepper

Planning Steps

Clean, wash and cut cucumber and radishes into dainty cuts. Wash the rocket and shake it dry. Divide the cured gherkins lengthways and dig cuts. Disintegrate the feta.

Whisk for the dressing oil with juice, mustard, and nectar, season with salt and pepper. Blend the cucumber, radish, and cured cucumber cuts and blend in with the dressing. Spot on a plate and sprinkle with the feta and rocket.

Tacos with Cauliflower Bean Mole and sour cream

Ingredients:

1 little cauliflower (800 g)
2 tbsp oil
2 red onions
1 clove of garlic
2 tbsp vinegar
800 g thick tomato (glass)
½ group parsley (10 g)
100 g low-fat quark
50 g acrid cream
1 sprinkle juice
Salt
Pepper
240 g dark beans (glass; depleted weight)
1 PC dim chocolate (30 g; at any rate 85% cocoa)
1 tsp smoked paprika powder
8 little wholegrain tortilla shops

Planning Steps

Wash, clean, and partition the cauliflower into little florets. Warmth the oil during a dish and fry the cauliflower over medium warmth for five minutes.

Peel the onions and garlic. 1 onion in solid shapes, the other dig rings. Hack garlic. Include the onion 3D shapes and garlic to the cauliflower and sauté for 2–3 minutes.

Include the vinegar and tomatoes and stew secured over low warmth for around quarter-hour.
Within the interim, wash the parsley, shake dry and pluck the leaves. For the sharp cream, finely slash half the parsley leaves and blend in with the quark, acrid cream, and juice. Season with salt and pepper.
Drain the beans and permit them to channel. Include the cauliflower with chocolate and paprika powder, mix, and warmth the cauliflower bean mole for an extra 5 minutes. Season with salt and pepper.
within the interim, a warm tortilla during a container or within the broiler. Fill the tortilla with the cauliflower bean mole, pour a dab of harsh cream over it and sprinkle with onion rings and remaining parsley leaves.

Spring Cloud bread

Ingredients:
3 eggs
200 g cream cheddar (60% fat in dry issue)
1 tsp preparing powder
Salt
50 ml milk (3.5% fat)
½ tsp medium-hot mustard
Pepper
½ pack chives (10 g)
100 g sheep's lettuce
½ pack radish
1 bunch red radish cress

Arrangement Steps

Separate the eggs and blend the egg yolks in with 100 g cream cheddar and preparing powder. Beat the egg whites with slightly of salt until solid and overlay in divides under the cream cheddar cream.
Spread the mixture in 8 level parts on a preparing sheet secured with heating paper and heat during a preheated stove at 150 ° C (convection 130 ° C; gas: setting 1-2) for around 20 minutes. Remove and let cool for around 10 minutes.
Mix the rest of the cream cheddar with milk, mustard, somewhat salt, and pepper. Wash the chives, shake dry, dig folds and blend into the cream.
Clean sheep's lettuce, wash and shake dry. Clean, wash and cut radishes into meager cuts. Wash the cress and channel well. Spread some cream on the underside of 4 cloud bread each, mastermind sheep's lettuce, radish cuts, remaining cream and cress on top, and spot 1 cloud bread each on top as a cover.

Vegan Wontons

Ingredients:
10 g dried mu-fail mushroom (on the other hand clam mushrooms)
60 g solidified sugar snap peas
2 carrots
70 g Chinese cabbage
60 g bamboo shoots (glass)
60 g mung seedling
1 clove of garlic
2 tbsp cashew nuts (30 g)
1 tbsp rapeseed oil
Soy
5-zest blend
¾ to sambal oelek
26 wonton leaves (9 x 9 cm)

Planning Steps

Pour boiling water over the mushrooms and permit them to drench for 2-3 hours. At that point cut the mushrooms into fine strips.
Within the interim, let the sugar snap peas defrost and afterward dig meager strips. Clean, strip, and cut the carrots into little 3D shapes. Clean, wash and cut Chinese cabbage into fine strips. Channel the sprouts and slash finely. Wash the mung seedlings, shake dry, strip the garlic, and cleave both.

Chop the cashew nuts, cook them during a skillet without fat for 3 minutes over medium warmth, and put during a secure spot. Warmth the oil within the container. Braise all vegetables in it for around 5 minutes over medium warmth. Include with soy, 5-zest powder, 1–2 tbsp water, and Sambal Oelek and stew for 3–5 minutes. At that point include the seeds.

Brush the wonton leaves with water on each of the four edges, place 1-2 teaspoons of vegetable filling within the middle and press the edges together. Heat salt water to the aim of boiling during a liner. Put the wontons on top (don't contact) and cook for 5–7 minutes.

Chocolate Granola Bars

Ingredients:

50 g dried date (without stone)
100 g nut blend
20 g vigorously deoiled chocolate
250 g concise cereal
30 g linseed
200 g dim chocolate (at any rate 70% cocoa)
50 g hazelnut margarine
300 g fruit purée or marrow
20 g unsweetened spelled drops
20 g puffed amaranth
2 tsp cinnamon
1 tsp vanilla powder
½ tsp ground cardamom
1 tsp natural orange strip

Planning Steps

Roughly slash dates, nuts, chocolate, oats, and flaxseed during a home appliance or a ground-breaking blender.

Chop 100 g chocolate and blend into the date combine with hazelnut margarine, apple mash, spelled chips, amaranth, and flavors.

Pour the blend into a heating tin fixed with preparing paper and press well. Prepare during a preheated stove at 200 ° C (fan broiler 180 ° C, gas: setting 3) for 20–25 minutes until the surface is seared. At that point let cool within the shape.

Remove the chocolate muesli bar from the shape and thus the preparing paper, dig 16 bars. Dissolve the rest of the chocolate, brighten the bar with it and let it cool.

Kale Avocado and Chili Dip with Keto Crackers

Ingredients:

75 g linseed
75 g pumpkin seeds
50 g sesame seeds
40 g almond flour (4 fl. el)
2 tbsp marginally fluid coconut oil
Salt
3 avocados
200 g kale
1 little green bean stew pepper
4 tbsp oil
1 natural lemon (pizzazz and juice)
Pepper
1 bunch watercress (5 g)

Directions:

Place seeds and parts with almond flour during a bowl, pour 125 ml of boiling water over them and permit them too steep for 10 minutes. At that point include coconut oil, season with salt, and blend everything.

Spread the blend meagerly on a heating sheet secured with preparing the paper, around 5 mm slim. Prepare wafers during a preheated stove at 175 ° C top and base warmth (gas: level 2–3) for 25–30 minutes. At that point expel, let cool for 10 minutes and break the wafers into pieces.

Within the interim, divide the avocados for the plunge, evacuate the stones, lift the mash out of the bowl with a spoon, and typically dice. Clean kale, pluck the green from the stems, wash, shake dry and dig little pieces.

Divide, hack, wash, and cleave lengthways. Put the avocado, kale, and bean stew alongside oil during a blender and coarsely puree. Season everything with salt, lemon strip and squeeze, and pepper. Fill the plunge into a bowl, embellish with watercress, and present with the wafers.

Grilled Eggplant Rolls with Walnut and Feta Filling

Ingredients:

2 eggplants
Salt
100 g moment couscous
1 clove of garlic
1 bundle parsley (20 g)
5 dried dates
10 g ginger root
60 g pecan parts
200 g feta (45% fat in dry issue)
3 tbsp juice
½ tsp rose hot paprika powder
Pepper
2 tbsp oil

Directions:

Clean and wash the eggplants, cut lengthways into 1/2 cm cuts, sprinkle with somewhat salt, and put during a secure spot for 10 minutes.
Pour 250 ml of bubbling water over the couscous and let it douse for 10 minutes. Meanwhile, strip the garlic, wash the parsley and shake dry, forgot 1 bunch. Center the dates. Strip the ginger. Finely cleave garlic, remaining parsley, dates, ginger, and pecans.
Put the feta during a bowl and disintegrate finely. Include the couscous, 2 tablespoons of juice, garlic, slashed parsley, dates, ginger, and cleaved pecans and massage everything great alongside your hands. Season with paprika powder and pepper.
Dab eggplant cuts with a perfect fabric and brush with oil on the two sides.
Heat the flame broil dish. Fry the aborigine cuts on all sides for 1-2 minutes over medium warmth, at that point, let cool for around 5 minutes. Put a number of the feta mass on each cut, move it up and place it on a plate or plate with the highest down and set the parsley aside.

Berry Ice-cream with Mint

Ingredients:

4 ready bananas
50 ml oat drink (oat milk)
½ flavorer
50 g blackberry (solidified)
50 g blueberries (solidified)
50 g blueberries (new)
Mint for enhancement

Directions:

Peel the bananas and cut them into finger-thick pieces. Put everything during a freeze-evidence pack and put it within the cooler for at any rate 4 hours.
Halve portion of the vanilla unit lengthways and cut out the vanilla mash with a blade.
Put solidified banana cuts with goat milk, vanilla mash, and solidified berries during a ground-breaking blender. Puree to a velvety mass and include somewhat fluid as wanted.
Wash and dry the blueberries and a couple of mint leaves. Put Ice-cream in two glasses, finish with new blueberries and mint leaves and serve.

Chocolate Bark

Fixing

1 slight strip orange
¾ cup pistachio nuts, cooked, chilled and cleaved into huge pieces
¼ cup hazelnuts, toasted, chilled, stripped and cleaved into enormous pieces
¼ cup pumpkin seeds, toasted and chilled
1 tablespoon chia seeds

1 tablespoon sesame seeds, toasted and cooled
1 teaspoon ground orange strip
1 cardamom case, finely squashed and sieved
12 ounces (340 g) tempered, sans dairy dim chocolate (65% cocoa content)
2 teaspoons flaky ocean salt
Candy or thermometer

Planning Steps

Preheat the stove to 100-150 ° F (66 ° C). Line a preparing sheet with material paper.

Finely cut the orange across and place it on the readied preparing sheet. Heat for 2 to 3 hours until dry yet somewhat clingy. Expel it from the stove and let it cool.

Once they sufficiently cool to affect them, cut the orange cuts into sections; put them during a secure spot.

During an enormous bowl, blend the nuts, seeds, and ground orange strip until totally consolidated. Spot the blend during a solitary layer on a heating sheet fixed with kitchen material. Put it during a secure spot.

Melt the chocolate during a water shower until it arrives at 88 to 90 ° F (32 to 33 ° C) and pours it over the nut blend to cover it totally.

When the chocolate is semi-cold yet at the same time clingy, sprinkle the surface with ocean salt and bits of orange.

Place the blend during a cold zone of your kitchen or refrigerate until the surface cools totally, and cut it into reduced down pieces.

Choc Chip Granola

Ingredients:

200 g huge oat chips
Roughly 50 g walnut nuts hacked
3 tablespoons of sunshine oil
20g spread
1 tablespoon of lifeless earthy colored sugar
2 tbsp rice syrup
60 g of fantastic quality (70%)
Bittersweet chocolate shavings

Arrangement Steps

Oven preheats to 160 ° C (140 ° C fan/Gas 3). Line a huge preparing plate with a sheet of silicone or material for heating.

During a huge bowl, join the oats and walnuts. Warmth the oil, spread, earthy colored sugar, and rice malt syrup tenderly during a touch non-stick skillet until the margarine has liquefied, and thus the sugar and syrup hack. Attempt to not let bubble. Pour the syrup over the oats and blend completely until completely secured with the oats. Spread the granola over the heating plate and spread directly into the corners. Leave the blend bunches with dividing, rather than spreading. Heat for 20 minutes within the stove until brilliant earthy colored is simply touched at the edges. Expel from the stove, and leave totally to relax on the plate.

When cool, split alongside your fingers any bigger knots on the plate and afterward blend them within the chocolate chips. Put the granola during a water/air proof tub or container, or pour it. The granola is to remain going for at any rate fourteen days.

Homemade cooked Celery Hummus:

Ingredients::

One inexperienced serrano bean stew, minced (discretionary)
one cup grilled chickpeas
1/3 cup spread
A pair of tablespoons new lime or juice
Four stems of celery, cut and dig
one cm items (around one cup)
five tablespoons edible fat (ideally EV)
A pair of cases of garlic
one teaspoon salt or to style
one tablespoon minced parsley

Guidelines:
Place the celery into a heating platter.
High with a pair of spoonful's of oil
Place the two garlic cases throughout a plate corner, and disperse with the bean stew.
Bake for forty five minutes inside the broiler.
Delivery the chickpeas into the liquidizer.
Add with any lingering oil into the liquidizer, inside the recent grilled celery and completely different vegetables.
Add the spread, lime or lemon squeeze, salt and mix well for 3-4 minutes till sleek and sweet.
Take away from the liquidizer into a bowl, combine inside the staying 3 tablespoons of edible fat, and hacked parsley.

Dish Kale Chips

Ingredients::
one tsp dried oregano
one tsp dried Marjoram
one tsp Garlic Powder
one tsp Onion Powder
eight cups Kale
one cup crude Cashews
1/2 cup ingredient
1/2 tsp Salt
1/4 tsp Red Pepper Flakes
a pair of Tbsp biological process Yeast
one tsp dried basil
1/2 tsp dried Rosemary
Directions:
Place the cashews throughout a pot, unfold with separated water, and allow the cashews, ideally nightlong, to douse cold for in any event a pair of hours.
Drain out the cashew water. Place the cashews throughout a household appliance or liquidizer.
To simply unfold the cashews, embrace sifted water, and procedure till wealthy sleek.
Stir along the cashew cream in a very Brobdingnagian mixing bowl in with the rest of the Ingredients: with the exception of the kale. Combine till the mixture is even.
Rinse the kale and take the leaves off the stringy roots. Tear the items into "chip" size.
Toss the kale with the cashew cream ready with "pizza." you may ought to do this directly, making certain even inclusion is ensured.
Dehydrate the kale chips for twelve hours, at that point cook at 105-115 degrees.

Basil and Walnut Pesto

Ingredients::
Zest and juice of one lemon
1/4 teaspoon red pepper drops
1/2 cup extra virgin edible fat
1/2 teaspoon new split dark pepper
one teaspoon match salt
four cups basil leaves
Three cloves garlic stripped
1/2 cup pecans cooked
1/2 cup parmesan-
Reggiano Guidelines:
Add basil, lemon oomph, juice, garlic, pecans, parmesan, and red pepper items to the bowl of a household appliance or Vitamix liquidizer.
Pulse the basil to half some of times.
Apply edible fat throughout a continual current, beating till the edible fat is mixed with completely different Ingredients:, and creating a free glue. On the off likelihood that the pesto is too thick, gift every tablespoon of extra edible fat in turn before you've an ideal quality.
Season with pepper and salt, and appreciate.

Turmeric and Lemon Dressing

Ingredients::
A pair of tsp ground turmeric
One lump new stripped ginger (or one tsp ground ginger)
five tbsp Ellyndale Naturals Avocado Oil
Juice of 3 very little lemons (simply over ¼ c of a replacement squeeze)
½ tsp garlic powder
one tbsp currently secretion in Honey
Salt to style

Directions:
Place everything of the Ingredients: throughout a liquidizer, at that point combine well. do not hesitate to vary your seasonings as per want.
Pour over the flame-broiled vegetables, greens, which is simply the beginning. Keep extras inside the cooler.

Walnut Vinaigrette

Ingredients::
A pair of tablespoons minced shallots
A pair of teaspoons fine ocean salt
1/4 teaspoon new ground dark pepper
one cup pecans, daintily cooked (see Note underneath)
one cup of water
1/2 cup fortified wine vinegar
1/2 cup foreign pecan oil
1/2 cup edible fat

Directions:
Insert everything of the Ingredients: throughout a liquidizer, exclusion the oils and procedure at a high pace. With the machine running, together with the olive and pecan oils step by step, around one moment, till the French dressing is blended. Refrigerate to arrange for serving. (The French dressing might be stuffed, wrapped, and cooled as long as multi-week before time.)

Mushroom Buckwheat Pancakes:

Ingredients::
55g cereal flour
55g buckwheat flour
275ml Alpro Almond Milk
One fenceless egg
30g marge, for searing
For the filling:
50g flour
50g marge
100g cut chestnut mushrooms
3 huge bunches of child spinach
Vegetable oil

Guidelines:
Soften marge throughout a pot of fifty g. Addition the flour to form a glue. Begin cookery for thirty seconds.
Bit by bit embrace the milk, mixing energetically till the white sauce is swish. (Make some extent to mix suitably with the goal that bumps do not form.)
Fry the mushrooms among the oil till the spinach is earthy colored and wither. Drop the mushrooms into the white sauce, apply the cheese and nutmeg to style, and at that point season.
Among the meanwhile, add the two flour structures to a pot, and build somewhat well.
Whisk the egg into the milk, gently. Pour many of the egg mix
into the flour and begin whisking. Begin embedding's the fluid and speeding till the hitter is swish.
Soften the marge and apply a spoon of the hitter throughout a non-stick griddle. Whirl for covering rock bottom of the dish equally, and flip it once the griddlecake gets able to shake. Rehash till all the hitter has been eaten up, and subsequently fill it with mushroom and spinach stuffing.

Chicory and Nut Salad:

Ingredients::

1/2 teaspoon metropolis mustard
Salt and fresh ground dark pepper
1/2 pound chicory, or different abundant inexperienced
1/4 cup smooth-shaven cheese
1/2 cup coarsely cleaved pecans
one tablespoon fortified wine vinegar
three tablespoons pecan oil

Directions:

You'd wish to toast the loco throughout a dry fry pan over medium-high heat till they are sweet, around two minutes.
Put to relax off.
Whisk the vinegar, oil, mustardsalt, and pepper along throughout a little cup, to taste.
Place the chicory throughout a large bowl with the covering. Place pecans on the serving plates and prime, and grate cheese.

Honey, Garlic and chilly Oven-Roasted Squash:

Ingredients::

one kilo organized squash and pumpkin (at any rate 5 distinctive sorts), cut in medium size items
Four red or inexperienced chilies
2 branches thyme
three Tbsp (15 ml) nectar
three Tbsp (15 ml) edible fat
3 entire garlic cloves, softly press
One branch rosemary
Salt and pepper to style

Guidelines:

Heat your broiler to a hundred and fifty ° C.
Place all the enhancements throughout a large bowl and wish to represent 30 minutes, admixture intermittently.
Throughout a boiling plate, place the squash and unfold with foil.
Roast secured at a hundred and fifty ° C for ten minutes.
Increase the temperature of the broiler to a hundred and eighty ° C, expel the foil, and dish for an additional ten minutes allowing the squash to caramelize softly.

Vegetable and Nut Loaf:

Ingredients::

One medium onion, cleaved
one teaspoon dried thyme
one cup cashews or almonds, cleaved
Vino or fortified wine
one teaspoon dried tarragon
one tablespoon unfold or oil
3/4 pound ground cheese (any mix)
1/2 cup integrated new cleaved herbs (parsley, oregano, thyme)
Salt and pepper
two cups finely cleaved mushrooms
Two cloves garlic, finely cleaved
one teaspoon dried marjoram
one teaspoon dried sage
one cup curds
two cups medium earthy colored rice
one teaspoon dried basil
two cups pecans, cleaved finely
5 eggs

Guidelines:

Heat broiler to degrees F of 350.
In marge or oil, mix the onion till it begins to soften. At that point embrace the mushrooms and a spot of pepper and salt, and cook till the mushrooms discharge and relax their juices. Mix the dried herbs and garlic, and subsequently, keep cookery. At the aim once your instrumentation begins drying out all over again, embrace Associate in Nursing honest sprinkle of fortified wine or wine and cook till it gets littler. The items have to be compelled to be soggy nonetheless they are

doing not glide among the oil. Cut the fireplace and let it cool a touch.

Whereas mushroom combine chills off, do oil your 9-inch portion dish and line it with foil or material paper.

Toss the loco and earthy colored rice each along throughout an enormous bowl. The eggs with the curds were overwhelmed throughout a unique bowl. Embrace the cheese and egg mix to your mix of rice and nut, at that point combine among the bottom cheese, cooled mushrooms, and new herbs. Mix well. Style to vary and season. (You will likewise broil)

At this stage, your mix area unit typically mounted, in your icebox for not over at some purpose.

Refill your portion dish with the mix of loco, rap on the counter many of times to evacuate air bubbles if there exists any, and clean the sting with a spatula. At that point adorn with mushroom cuts, chime pepper cuts, or pecans, if necessary. Spot the portion fry pan into you're getting ready plate.

Bake it for on the brink of hour, or till the portion gets firm (a very little longer once the mix is cooled). At that point expel from your stove. At that point lay on a cooling rack for 10 minutes and utilizing the extra foil or material paper to urge eliminate the portion from the stove. Strip the foil or material and serve adorned it with new herbs on your platter.

Serve along with your most popular vegetables joined by a sauce.

Sirtfood Granola

Preparation Time: 1 hour 10 minutes
Cooking Time: 50 minutes
Servings: 12
Ingredients:

7 oz. oats
9 oz. buckwheat flakes
3 ½ oz. walnuts, chopped 3 ½ oz. almonds, chopped 3 ½ oz. dried strawberries 1 ½ tsp. ground ginger
1 ½ tsp. ground cinnamon
4 fl. oz. extra virgin olive oil 2 tbsp. honey (optional)

Directions:

Preheat oven to 300°F. Line a tray with parchment paper. Stir together walnuts, almonds, buckwheat flakes and oats with ginger and cinnamon. In a large pan, warm olive oil and honey, heating until the honey has dissolved.

Pour the honey-oil over the other ingredients, stirring to ensuring an even coating. Distribute the granola evenly over the lined baking tray and roast for 50 minutes, or until golden.

Remove from the oven and leave to cool. Once cooled add the berries and store in an airtight container. Eat dry or with milk and yogurt. It stays fresh for up to 1 week.

Nutrition Facts:

Calories: 178 kcal Fat: 10.9 g Carbohydrates: 22 g Protein: 6.7 g

Choc Chip Granola

Preparation Time: 45 minutes
Cooking Time: 30 minutes
Servings: 8
Ingredients

8oz jumbo oats 2oz pecans
3 tbsp. olive oil
1oz butter
1 tbsp. brown sugar
2 tbsp. rice malt syrup 2oz 70% chocolate chips

Directions

Preheat the oven to 325°.Line a large baking tray with parchment paper.

Mix the oats and pecans together in a huge bowl. In a small skillet, gently warm the olive oil, butter, brown sugar and rice malt butter till the butter has melted and the sugar and butter have simmer. Pour the syrup over the mix and stir thoroughly until the oats are fully covered.

Put the mix in baking tray and bake it in the oven for about 30 minutes until gold brown at the edges. Remove from the oven and leave to cool entirely.

Once cool, divide any larger lumps with your hands and mix in the chocolate chips. Put the granola in an airtight jar or tub. It will last around two weeks.

Nutrition Facts:

Calories 220kcal Fat 8g Carbohydrates 35g Protein 6g

Rosemary & Garlic Kale Chips

Preparation Time: 10 minutes
Cooking Time: 15 minutes
Servings: 6
Ingredients:

9oz kale chips, chopped 2 sprigs of rosemary
2 cloves of garlic
2 tbsp. olive oil Sea salt
Freshly ground black pepper

Directions:

Gently warm the olive oil, rosemary and garlic over a low heat for 10 minutes. Remove it from the heat and set aside to cool.

Take the rosemary and garlic out of the oil and discard them.

Toss the kale leaves in the oil making sure they are well coated. Season with salt and pepper. Spread the kale leaves onto 2 baking sheets and bake them in the oven at 325F for 10 minutes, until crispy.

Nutrition Facts:

Calories: 187kcal Fat: 13g Carbohydrates: 14g Protein: 6g

Honey Chili Nuts

Preparation Time: 25 minutes
Cooking Time: 10 minutes
Servings: 20
Ingredients:

5oz walnuts 5oz pecan nuts
2oz butter, softened
1 tbsp. honey
½ bird's-eye chili, very finely chopped

Directions:

Preheat the oven to 360F. Combine butter, honey and chili in a bowl then add the nuts and stir them well.

Spread the nuts onto a lined baking sheet and roast them in the oven for 10 minutes, stirring once halfway through. Remove from the oven and allow them to cool before eating.

Nutrition Facts:

Calories: 260kcal Fat: 15g Carbohydrates: 20g Protein: 6g

Crunchy And Chewy Granola

Preparation Time: 45 minutes
Cooking Time: 60 minutes
Servings: 20
Ingredients:

1 tbsp. flax seeds 1/4 tsp. salt
1/2 tsp. cinnamon
1/2 cup honey
2 tbsp. brown-sugar 3/4 cup rolled oats
1/2 cup almonds, slivered 1/2 cup golden raisins 1/2 cup dried cranberries

Directions:

Pre-heat oven to 300°F. Line baking tray with parchment paper.

Mix flax seeds, cinnamon, honey, sugar oats and almonds. Insert 1 cup hot water, then mix together with hands. Spread into a thin layer over the baking tray.

Bake for 50-60 minutes, until gold brown. Remove from the oven and let cool.

Stir in dried fruit. Put the granola in an airtight jar or tub. It will last around two weeks.

Nutrition Facts:

Calories: 233 Fat: 13g Carbohydrates: 31g Protein: 5g

Power Balls

Preparation Time: 15 minutes

Cooking Time: 2 minutes

Servings: 20

Ingredients:

1 cup old fashion oats

1/4 cup quinoa cooked using 3/4 cup orange juice 1/4 cup shredded unsweetened coconut

1/3 cup dried cranberry/raisin blend 1/3 cup dark chocolate chips

1/4 cup slivered almonds

1 tbsp. peanut butter

Directions:

Cook quinoa in orange juice. Bring to boil and simmer for approximately 15 minutes. Let cool. Combine quinoa and the remaining ingredients into a bowl.

With wet hands and combine ingredients and roll in ball sized chunks. Put in a container and let cool in the fridge for at least 2 hours before eating them.

Nutrition Facts:

Calories: 189 Fat: 11g Carbohydrates: 22g Protein: 5g

Sirt Muesli

Preparation Time: 15 minutes

Cooking Time: 0 minutes

Servings: 1

Ingredients:

½ oz. buckwheat flakes

½ oz. buckwheat puffs

½ oz. shredded coconut

2 Medjool dates, pitted and chopped 4 walnuts, chopped

1tbsp cocoa nibs

4 oz. strawberries, hulled and chopped 4 oz. plain Greek yogurt

Directions:

Simply mix the dry ingredients and place them in an airtight container so that they are ready to eat. If you want, you can make it in bulk by multiplying the quantities.

To enjoy the sirt muesli, put the yogurt in bowl, put strawberries on top and then add the muesli.

Nutrition Facts:

Calories: 368 Fat: 16g Carbohydrates: 54g Protein: 26g

Sirtfood Bites

Preparation Time: 35 minutes

Cooking Time: 0 minutes

Servings: 12

Ingredients:

4 oz. walnuts

1 oz. 85% dark chocolate 8 oz. Medjool dates, pitted 1 tbsp. cocoa powder

1 tbsp. ground turmeric

1 tbsp. extra virgin olive oil

1 tsp. vanilla extract, unsweetened 2 tbsp. water

Directions:

Put the walnuts and chocolate in a food processor and process until you have an even mixture. Add all the remaining ingredients except water and combine until the mixture forms a disc. Depending on the consistency of the mixture, you may or may not have to add the water; you don't want it to be too sticky. Shape the mixture into bite-sized balls using your wet hands and roll them in cocoa powder. Refrigerate for at least 1 hour in an airtight container before eating them.

They last up to 1 week in the fridge.

Nutrition Facts:

Calories: 127kcal Fat: 6g Carbohydrates: 14g Protein: 4g

Dark Chocolate Pretzel Cookies

Preparation Time: 40 minutes
Cooking Time: 17 minutes
Servings: 4
Ingredients:
1 cup yogurt
1/2 tsp. baking soda 1/4 tsp salt
1/4 tsp. cinnamon
4 Tbsp. butter, softened 1/3 cup brown sugar
1 egg
1/2 tsp. vanilla
1/2 cup dark chocolate chips 1/2 cup pretzels chopped
Directions:
Pre Heat oven to 350°F.In a bowl, whisk together sugar, butter, vanilla, and egg. In another bowl, stir together the flour, baking soda, and salt.
Pour the liquid mix over the flour mix along with the chocolate chips and pretzels and stir until just blended.
Drop large spoonfuls of dough on a baking tray lined with parchment paper.
Bake for 15-17 minutes, or until the bottoms are crispy. Allow cooling on
a wire rack.
Nutrition Facts:
Calories: 290 Fat: 15g Carbohydrates: 36g Protein: 3g

Pear, Cranberry And Chocolate Crisp

Preparation Time: 40 minutes
Cooking Time: 45 minutes
Servings: 8
Ingredients:
1/2 cup flour
1/2 cup brown sugar 1 tsp. cinnamon
⅛ tsp. salt
3/4 cup yogurt 1/4 cup apples
1/3 cup butter, melted 1 tsp vanilla
1 tbsp. brown sugar
1/4 cup dried cranberries 1 tsp lemon juice
1 pear, diced
2 handfuls of dark chocolate chips
Directions:
Pre-heat oven to 375°F. Spray a casserole dish with a cooking spray. Put flour, sugar, cinnamon, salt, apple, yogurt and butter into a bowl and mix. Pour it on a baking tray lined with parchment paper.
In a large bowl, combine sugar, lemon juice, vanilla, pear, and cranberries. Pour this fruit mix along with chocolate chips over the baking tray. Bake for 45 minutes. until golden. Cool before serving.
Nutrition Facts:
Calories: 239kcal Fat: 5g Carbohydrates: 46g Protein: 3g

Potato Bites

Preparation Time: 10 minutes
Cooking Time: 20 minutes
Servings: 3
Ingredients:
1 potato, sliced
2 bacon slices,
cooked and crumbled
1 small avocado, pitted and cubed Cooking spray
Directions:
Spread potato slices on a lined baking sheet, spray with cooking oil, introduce in the oven at 350°F, bake for 20 minutes, arrange on a platter, top each slice with avocado, and crumbled bacon and serve as a snack.
Nutrition Facts:
Calories 180 kcal, Fat 4g, Carbohydrates 8g, Protein 6g

Dill Bell Pepper Snack Bowls

Preparation Time: 10 minutes
Cooking Time: 0 minutes
Servings: 4
Ingredients:
2 tbsp. dill, chopped
1 yellow onion, chopped
1 lb. bell peppers, cut into thin strips 3 tbsp. olive oil
2 and ½ tbsp. white vinegar Black pepper to the taste
Directions:
In a salad bowl, mix bell peppers with onion, dill, pepper, oil, and vinegar, toss to coat, divide into small bowls and serve as a snack.
Nutrition Facts:
Calories 120 kcal, fat 3g, fiber 4g, carbs 2g, Protein 3g

Cocoa Bars

Preparation Time: 10min + 12 hours
Cooking Time: 0 minutes
Servings: 12
Ingredients:
1 cup unsweetened cocoa chips 2 cups rolled oats
1 cup low-fat peanut butter
½ cup chia seeds
½ cup raisins
¼ cup of coconut sugar
½ cup of coconut milk
Directions:
Put 1 cup oats in the blender, pulse and transfer to a bow.
Add the rest of the oats, cocoa chips, chia seeds, raisins, sugar and milk, stir well, spread into a square pan, press well, keep in the fridge for 12 hours, slice into 12 bars and serve. Bars can also be put in the freezer.
Nutrition Facts:
Calories 198 kcal Fat 5g, Carbohydrates 10g, Protein 89g

Cinnamon Apple Chips

Preparation Time: 10 minutes
Cooking Time: 2 hours
Servings: 4
Ingredients:
Cooking spray
2 teaspoons cinnamon powder 2 apples, cored and thinly sliced
Directions:
Arrange apple slices on a lined baking sheet, spray them with cooking oil, sprinkle cinnamon, introduce in the oven and bake at 300°F for 2 hours. Divide into bowls and serve as a snack.
Nutrition Facts:
Calories 80kcal, Fat 0.5g, Carbohydrates 7g, Protein 4g

Cinnamon-Scented Quinoa

Preparation Time: 5 minutes
Cooking Time: 0 minutes
Servings: 4
Ingredients:
Chopped walnuts 1
½ cup water Maple syrup
2 cinnamon sticks
1 cup quinoa
Directions:
Add the quinoa to a bowl and wash it until the water is clear. Use a fine- mesh sieve to drain it.
Prepare your pressure cooker with a trivet and steaming basket. Place the quinoa and the cinnamon sticks in the basket and pour the water.
Close and lock the lid. Cook at high pressure for 6 minutes. When the cooking time is up, release the pressure using the quick release method.
Fluff the quinoa with a fork and remove the cinnamon sticks. Divide the cooked quinoa

among serving bowls and top with maple syrup and chopped walnuts.

Nutrition Facts:

Calories: 160, Fat: 3 g, Carbohydrates: 28 g, Protein: 6 g

No-Bake Choco Cashew Cheesecake

Preparation Time: 25 minutes
Cooking Time: 0 minutes
Servings: 8

Ingredients

2 cups raw cashews
¼ cup coconut cream
¼ cup unsweetened cocoa powder
¼ cup pure maple syrup 1 tsp vanilla extract
1¼ cups walnuts
¼ cup chopped dates
¼ tsp ground cinnamon
¼ cup almond meal

Directions:

Line the bottom of four 4-inch spring-form pans with a parchment paper circle.

Place cashews, coconut cream, cocoa powder, maple syrup and vanilla in a high-speed food processor. Repeat the process until it is entirely smooth, occasionally scraping the pieces with a rubber spatula. Transfer the mixture to a medium bowl and set aside. Clean the food processor or blender with a paper towel. This is the cream.

Place walnuts, dates, and cinnamon in the same food processor and blend quickly. This is the base.

Put the base mix in a baking tin. Create an even layer by pressing well. Pour in the cream and put in the fridge for 12 hours before enjoying it.

Nutrition Facts:

Calories: 168kcal Fat: 11g Carbohydrates: 11g Protein: 7g

Cacao-Coated Almonds

Preparation Time: 10 minutes
Cooking Time: 15 minutes
Servings: 10

Ingredients:

¼ cup cocoa nibs
¼ cup light brown sugar
1 tsp instant espresso powder Pinch of salt
2 teaspoons cornstarch 2 teaspoons warm water
1 tbsp. pure maple syrup
1 tsp pure vanilla extract, unsweetened 2 cups roasted whole almonds

Direction:

Preheat the oven to 325°F. Line a large baking tray with parchment paper.

Place the cocoa nibs, sugar, espresso powder, and salt in a coffee grinder. Grind to turn into a fine powder.

In a large bowl, whisk the cornstarch with the warm water until thoroughly combined. Stir the maple syrup and vanilla into the mixture. Add the almonds on top and fold until thoroughly coated.

Add the ground cacao mixture and combine until the almonds are thoroughly coated.

Place the almonds evenly on the baking tray. Toast for 10 minutes remove from the oven and stir gently. Toast for another 5 minutes or until the coating looks mostly dry. Be careful not to burn them! Let cool on the sheet. The coating will further harden once cooled. Store in an airtight container in the refrigerator for up to 2 weeks.

Nutrition Facts:

Calories 132kcal, Fat 1g, Carbohydrate 6g, Protein 5g

Seed Crackers

Preparation Time: 30 minutes
Cooking Time: 8 minutes
Servings: 20
Ingredients
3 tbsp. white chia seeds
⅓ cup water
⅓ cup amaranth, cooked
⅓ cup whole wheat flour, 3 tbsp. shelled hemp seeds
3 tbsp. golden roasted flaxseeds
2 tbsp. almond flour
1½ teaspoons nutritional yeast
⅓ tsp fine sea salt 2 tbsp. olive oil
Direction:
Combine the chia seeds with the water in a small bowl. Let stand 2 minutes to thicken.
Add flour, amaranth, hemp seeds, flaxseed, almond flour, yeast, and salt. Add the thick mixture of chia and oil on top. Use a stand mixer with flat blades to mix perfectly and form a very sticky dough.
Wrap it tightly in a plastic wrap and refrigerate for 2 hours or (better) overnight.
Heat the oven to 400°F. Line two large baking trays with parchment paper.
Divide the dough into 4 parts. Roll out a quarter super thin (0.5 inch) directly onto the baking tray. Use a cutter to cut the dough in rectangles. Put the tray in the oven and cook for 8 minutes Repeat until you cooked all the dough. Allow cooling on a rack before stacking in an airtight container at room temperature. They will last for 5 days.
Nutrition Facts:
Calories: 150kcal Fat: 8g Carbohydrates: 15g Protein: 4g

Spelt And Seed Rolls

Preparation Time: 20 minutes
Cooking Time: 2.5 hours +30 minutes
Servings: 9
Ingredients
1 cup almond milk, unsweetened, 2 tsp apple cider vinegar
⅓ cup water, lukewarm
2 tbsp. neutral-flavored oil 2 tbsp. agave nectar
⅓ cup whole spelt flour
¼ cup oat flour or finely ground oats
¼ cup vital wheat gluten
3 tbsp. shelled hemp seeds 3 tbsp. sunflower seeds
2 tbsp. golden roasted flaxseeds 2 tbsp. chia seeds
1 tbsp. poppy seeds 1 tsp fine sea salt
2 tsp instant yeast
Directions:
Combine milk and vinegar in a measuring cup. Allow 5 minutes to curdle. Filter curd, add water, oil and agave and set aside. In a bowl, place a flours, wheat gluten, seeds, salt, and yeast.
Mix them and the pour the wet mixture made with curd over.
Knead the dough with a stand mixer for 10 minutes until the dough becomes soft and not too dry or too sticky. If necessary, gently add 1 tbsp. of water until you get the desired result.
Cover and let it rest for 2 hours until doubled.
Divide the dough in 9 parts and give them the form of a roll and put them on a tray to rest for 25 minutes.
While the rolls rise, heat the oven to 400°F .
When hot, cook the rolls for 20-22 minutes.
Let cool on a rack.
Store the rest in an airtight container at room temperature. They are best enjoyed fresh, but they will last up to 2 days.
Nutrition Facts:
Calories: 140kcal Fat: 6g Carbohydrates: 14g Protein: 10g

CHAPTER 7:

MAIN DISHES

Colorful Vegetable Noodles

Ingredients:

200 g little carrots (3 little carrots)
200 g little zucchini (1 little zucchini)
125 g leek (1 stick)
150 g linguine wholegrain pasta
2 tbsp oil
Salt
Pepper
125 ml exemplary vegetable stock
150 ml soy cream
1 squeeze saffron strings
Chervil freely

Arrangement Steps

Peel and clean carrots, wash zucchini, rub dry, and clean. Cut both lengthways into slim strips utilizing a peeler or a vegetable slicer.

Clean the leek, split lengthways, wash, and separate the individual leaves.

Within the interim, heat oil during a dish. Braise the carrots and zucchini in it over medium warmth for 1 moment, blending.

Add the leek and braise for an extra 1 moment. Season everything with salt and pepper.

Add the vegetable stock, soy cream, and thus the saffron strings and convey them to the bubble. Cook until gloss over medium warmth for 2-3 minutes.

Drain the pasta during a strainer, channel well, and increase the dish.

Mix the pasta with the vegetables. Season once more. Placed on plates and serve sprinkled with chervil as you would like.

Buckwheat Noodles and King Prawn

Ingredients:

400 g buckwheat noodles
Two red onions (thinly sliced)
Three stalks of fresh celery (chopped)
Three tbsps. Vegetable oil
150 g of every
Chopped kale
Chopped green beans
Two garlic cloves (grated or chopped)
Two cm fresh ginger (sliced or grated)
Two tbsps. Fresh parsley (chopped)
Two tsp. tamari sauce
600 g king prawn
One red chili (chopped, no seeds)

Method:

Heat a fry pan and add noodles thereto. Cook the noodles for five minutes.

Wash the noodles under running water. Drain the noodles and add vegetable oil thereto.

Because the noodles cook within the pan, arrange the opposite ingredients.

Take a fry pan and add vegetable oil thereto. Add purple onion and celery to the oil and cook for five minutes or until soft.

Add kale and beans to the pan and blend the ingredients properly.

Reduce the warmth and add the remainder of the ingredients to the pan. Add garlic, ginger, chili, and prawns. Cook the prawns until browned.

Add noodles to the pan and toss everything properly. Add tamari sauce to the noodles and blend well.
Serve the prawn noodles and garnish with chopped parsley from the highest.

Chicken Sesame Salad

Ingredients:
One pound thighs of chicken (boneless)
One cup shredded carrot
Half cup sliced almond
Four green onions (cubed)
Half cup fresh cilantro (roughly chopped)
One tbsp. sesame seeds (white)
One tin of orange (mandarin, no syrup)
Half small green cabbage (thinly sliced)
Half small red cabbage (thinly sliced)
Two tbsps. Sesame seeds (black)
For dressing
Two tbsps. Avocado oil
Half cup coconut amino
Three tsps. Salt
Two tsps. Ground pepper
Half tsp. onion powder
Two tbsps. Ginger (minced)
One and a half cup of vinegar (red wine)
Method:
1. Prepare the salad during a large bowl.
2. Mix all the ingredients of the dressing and keep it aside.
3. Coat the chicken thighs during a bowl with three tbsps. Of the dressing.
4. Let the chicken marinate for 2 hours.
5. Take a fry pan and begin grilling the marinated chicken. You'll add a touch of oil to the pan. Grill each side of the chicken properly.
6. Remove the chicken and let it cool at normal temperature. Chop the chicken in small cubes to combine with the salad.
7. Add the chicken pieces to the bowl of salad and toss.
8. Add the remaining dressing to the salad and blend well.
9. Serve during a plate with dressing from the highest.

Baked Potatoes and Spicy Chickpea Stew

Ingredients:
Two tins of every
Tomatoes (chopped)
Chickpeas (kidney beans also can be used)
Six large baking potatoes (the potatoes are required to be pricked)
Three red onions (large, finely chopped)
Two tbsps. Of each
Cumin seeds
Cocoa (powdered, unsweetened)
Four tbsps. Of vegetable oil (preferably extra-virgin)
Three fresh garlic cloves (grated or minced)
- Three tsps. Chili flakes (the quantity are often adjusted consistent with your need)
Two cups of water
One cm ginger (fresh, grated)
Four tbsps. Fresh parsley (chopped)
One tbsp. ground turmeric
One large pepper (yellow, chopped)
- Salt and pepper (for seasoning)

Method:
Preheat the oven to a temperature of 300 degrees Celsius. While the oven gets heated, you'll start preparing the opposite ingredients. After the oven gets hot, start adding the pricked potatoes to the oven. Cook the potatoes for one hour or until you think that they're cooked perfectly. If you are doing not have an oven, an equivalent are often done by using the normal method.
Take a skillet and place it over medium flame. Add oil to the skillet and permit the oil to urge hot.

Start adding onions to the oil and stir it gently. You'll got to sauté the onions for four to 5 minutes or until soft. Make sure that the onions don't get browned.

Add garlic, chili, ginger, and cumin to the onions. Cook for one to 2 minutes and reduce the flame.

Add turmeric to the mixture of onions and add a splash of water to the pan.

Confirm that the pan doesn't get dried out. Keep cooking the onion mixture for 2 more minutes.

Add tomatoes, pepper, chocolate, and chickpeas to the onion mixture. Add some water to the pan and convey the mixture to a boil. Simmer the mixture for 40 minutes on a reduced flame. You'll cover the pan with a lid. Confirm that the sauce turns thick.

Add parsley to the stew and provides it a pleasant stir. Add the seasonings consistent with your taste.

Start plating by placing the baked potat oes because the base. Serve the potatoes with the stew from the highest. You'll add a mix of straightforward salad also.

Prawn Arrabbiata

Ingredients:

One yellow pepper (chopped)
Five tbsps. Vegetable oil (preferably extra-virgin)
One purple onion (finely chopped)
One tsp. of chili flakes (you can use chili paste)
Two fresh garlic cloves (minced)
Two tins of tomato (chopped)
One large zucchini (noodles or shaped like ribbons)
Two tsps. Salt
Half cup cheese (parmesan)
250 g prawn or shrimp (large, raw, peeled)
Parsley or basil (chopped, optional)

Method:

Start by making spirals of zucchini. You'll use a peeler or vegetable spiralizer for creating the zucchini noodles. If you are doing not have a spiralizer or peeler, the zucchini are often dig fine

Take a fry pan and add one tbsp. oil to it. Allow the oil to urge hot. Start adding prawns to the oil and cook an equivalent for five minutes. Confirm to stir the prawns occasionally; otherwise, they could grind to a halt to the recent pan.

Take another pan and add some oil thereto. Heat the oil over medium flame and add pepper and onions thereto. Sauté the mixture for 3 to four minutes. Sauté until the onions get soft.

Add garlic, salt, and chili to the mixture of onions and stir.

Now it's time to feature the chopped tomatoes to the pan. Reduce the flame and cook the tomatoes with the onions for 3 minutes.

If the pan gets dry, you'll add a splash of water.

Add zucchini noodles and cooked prawns to the mixture and provides it a pleasant mix.

Mix the noodles for a few time. You'll got to make sure that the noodles don't get tender. If the noodles are tender, the dish will get soggy.

Serve the noodles during a bowl. Garnish with cheese from the highest. You'll also add parsley and basil. Serve hot.

Plaice Rolls on Pointed Cabbage

Ingredients:

3 stems dill
2 stems parsley
½ pack chives
320 g plaice filet (without skin;
8 place filets)

100 g brilliant, seedless grapes
325 g cabbage
1 onion
1 tbsp rapeseed oil
Salt
Pepper
Nutmeg
150 ml wine or light fruit crush
5 tbsp soy cream
½ lemon

Directions:

Wash and shake all herbs. Pluck and hack the leaves of dill and parsley, cut chives into little rolls.

Rinse the spot filets, pat them dry and spot them on the surface with the dim side looking up. Sprinkle with the hacked herbs.

Roll up the plaice filets immovably towards the sharp end and pin them with toothpicks.

Wash the grapes, channel well, and hamper the middle. Clean, wash, and cut pointed cabbage into thin strips.

Peel the onion and dig fine strips.

Heat oil during a container. Braise the onions during a refined warmth for 2-3 minutes. Include pointed cabbage and braise for an additional 2 minutes while blending. Season with salt, pepper, and a couple of new ground nutmeg.

Put the grapes within the container and pour within the wine or squeeze.

Lightly salt the plaice rolls and spread them over the cabbage. Spread and cook over medium warmth for 7-8 minutes.

Remove the very best, including the soy cream, and let it cook open for a further 1-2 minutes. Crush lemon. Season the cabbage with salt, pepper, and lemon squeeze and serve directly.

May Beet Salad with Cucumber

Ingredients:

3 May turnips
1 cucumber
1 onion
2 stems parsley
150 g greek yogurt
1 tbsp fruit crush vinegar
1 tsp nectar
1 tsp mustard
Sea-salt
Cayenne pepper
Pepper

Arrangement Steps

Clean, strip, and cut the turnips. Clean and wash the cucumber and furthermore slicer. Clean, wash and cut the spring onions into rings. Put everything during a serving of mixed greens bowl and blend.

Wash parsley, shake dry and slash finely. Combine dressing with yogurt, fruit crush vinegar, nectar, mustard, and 2–3 tbsp water. Season with salt and cayenne pepper.

Mix the plate of mixed greens dressing with the mayonnaise and cucumber and let it steep for around 10 minutes, at that point crush it with pepper and serve.

Sweet Potatoes with Asparagus, Eggplant and Halloumi

Ingredients:

1 aubergine
9 tbsp oil
Chili drops
Salt
Pepper
2 yams
1 red bean stew pepper
2 tbsp sunflower seeds
1 bundle green asparagus
4 tbsp juice
200 g chickpeas (can; dribble weight)

½ pack basil
½ pack lemon demulcent
1 tsp mustard
½ tsp turmeric powder
1 tsp nectar
300 g halloumi

Arrangement Steps

Clean, wash and cut the eggplant. Warmth 2 tablespoons of oil during a dish and sauté the aubergine cuts in medium warmth on the two sides for 5–7 minutes until brilliant earthy colored and season with bean stew chips, salt, and pepper. Expel from the dish and put it during a secure spot.

Within the interim, strip the yam and cut it into 3D shapes. Split the bean stew lengthways, expel the stones, wash and dig cuts. Warmth 1 tablespoon of oil within the dish, fry the yam solid shapes in it for 10 minutes. Include 1 tbsp sunflower seeds and bean stew cuts and season with salt and pepper.

Wash asparagus as an afterthought, remove the woody finishes, and strip the lower third of the stalks if vital. Warmth 1 tablespoon of oil within the dish, fry the asparagus in it for five minutes over medium warmth. Deglaze with 1 tablespoon of juice, pour in 2 tablespoons of water and spread and cook for an extra 3 minutes.

Rinse the chickpeas and permit them to channel. Wash the basil and lemon medicine, shake dry and slash. Blend chickpeas in with half the herbs and 1 tablespoon of oil and season with salt and pepper.

Whisk the rest of the oil with the remainder of juice, mustard, turmeric and nectar, season with salt and pepper, and blend within the rest of the herbs.

Cut the halloumi and cut during a hot skillet on the two sides for five minutes over medium warmth until brilliant yellow.

Arrange yams, aubergine cuts on plates, present with chickpeas, asparagus, and halloumi and sprinkle with the dressing. Sprinkle with the rest of the sunflower seeds.

Lentil Salad with Spinach, Rhubarb, and Asparagus

Ingredients:

100 g beluga lentils
2 tbsp oil
Salt
250 g white asparagus
100 g rhubarb
1 tsp nectar
50 g child spinach (2 bunches)
20 g pumpkin seeds

Directions:

Bring the beluga lentils to the overflow with multiple times the measure of water. Cook over medium warmth for around 25 minutes. Channel, flush, and channel. Blend in with 1 tablespoon of oil and a spot of salt. Meanwhile, wash, clean, strip, and cut asparagus into pieces. Wash, clean, and cut the rhubarb into pieces.

Heat 1 tablespoon of oil during a container and fry the asparagus in it for around 8 minutes over medium warmth, turning every so often. At that point include rhubarb and nectar and fry and salt for an extra 5 minutes. Wash spinach and switch dry. Generally slash the pumpkin seeds.

Arrange spinach with lentils, asparagus, and rhubarb on two plates and serve sprinkled with pumpkin seeds.

Strawberry and Avocado Salad with Chicken Nuggets

Ingredients:

350 g chicken bosom
1 tbsp soy
Pepper

1 tsp sweet paprika powder
2 tsp tomato glue
4 bunches blended serving of mixed greens (arugula, lollo rosso, lettuce)
150 g strawberries
1 lemon
1 avocado
1 egg
2 tbsp whole meal flour
70 g cornflakes (without sugar)
3 tbsp rapeseed oil
1 tbsp nectar
Salt
½ red onion
5 g ginger
2 tsp sunflower seeds
2 tsp pine nuts

Planning Steps

Rinse the chicken bosom, pat dry, and dig 6 pieces. Blend during a bowl with soy, pepper, paprika powder, and tomato glue and let marinate for around 10 minutes.

Within the interim, clean, wash and switch dry lettuce. Clean, wash pat dry strawberries and dig little pieces. Crush lemon. Divide the avocado, evacuate the stone, expel the mash from the skin, shakers and blend in with half the juice.

Place the egg during a plate and race with a fork. Put the flour on a subsequent plate. Disintegrate the cornflakes and put them on another plate. Bread chicken pieces first in flour, at that point in egg, and afterward within the chips. Warmth the oil during a dish and fry the chicken on all sides over medium warmth.

Mix a dressing out of nectar, remaining lemon squeeze, salt, and pepper. Strip the onion and ginger, dice the onion and mesh the ginger, add both to the dressing. Blend sunflower and pine nuts and dish during a hot skillet without fat on low warmth for around 4 minutes.

Spread the serving of mixed greens on two plates, pour the strawberries and avocado over it and sprinkle with the dressing. Present with chicken tenders and sprinkle the serving of mixed greens with the seeds.

Carrot Risotto with Eggplant and Pesto Sauce

Ingredients:

2 carrots
1 clove of garlic
1 branch rosemary
4 tbsp oil
100 g risotto rice
500 ml vegetable stock
3 tbsp soy cream
1 tsp juice
Salt
Pepper
1 aubergine
1 tbsp rosemary
1 squeeze cayenne pepper
1 tsp wholemeal spelled flour
100 ml oat drink (oat milk)
1 tbsp pesto

Directions:

Clean, strip, and cut the carrots into little blocks. Strip and cleave garlic. Wash the rosemary, shake it dry, pluck the needles, and cut them into little pieces.

Heat 1 tablespoon of oil during a pan, braise the carrots and garlic for five minutes over medium warmth, at that point include the rice and braise for an extra 2 minutes. At that point pour during a touch stock with the goal that everything is delicately secured, continually mixing. Step by step pours within the stock while blending until the stock is spent. At that point let swell on low warmth for 10 minutes. At that point mix in 1 tablespoon of soy cream and season with salt, pepper, half the rosemary, and juice.

Alongside, clean, wash, and cut the eggplant into little 3D shapes. Warmth 2 tablespoons of oil during a container, braise eggplant 3D shapes, and raisins in them for 8 minutes. Season with salt, pepper, remaining rosemary, and cayenne pepper.

Heat 1 tablespoon of oil during a pan, dust with flour, pour within the oat drink with a whisk while mixing and stew for 3 minutes until a light-weight bond is made. Blend within the pesto and remaining soy cream and season with salt and pepper.

Tofu and Vegetable Curry with Rice and Nuts

Ingredients:

1 aubergine
2 carrots
1 parsnip
1 clove of garlic
3 tbsp coconut oil
1 tbsp tomato glue
2 tbsp yellow curry glue (somewhat fiery)
400 ml of coconut milk
250 g parboiled rice
Salt
½ tsp turmeric powder
200 g cherry tomatoes
1 red stew pepper
Pepper
300 g smoked tofu
70 g nut blend (salted)
1 bunch basil leaves

Arrangement Steps

Clean the eggplant, carrots, parsnips, strip, wash, and dig 3D squares if important. Strip and cleave garlic.

Heat 2 tablespoons of coconut oil during a wok or huge dish, include vegetables and sauté for five minutes over high warmth. Include tomato glue and curry glue and fry for an extra 3 minutes. At that point pour in coconut milk and stew for five minutes over low warmth. Within the interim, stew the rice in bubbling salted water with turmeric for around 10-15 minutes and let it douse for five minutes until secured.

Wash and split tomatoes as an afterthought. Wash the bean stew pepper, dig dainty cuts, and add both to the curry. Season the curry with salt and pepper.

Meanwhile, cut the tofu into 3D shapes. Warmth the rest of the oil during a skillet, sauté the tofu and nuts in it over medium warmth for five minutes and season with pepper. Wash the basil and shake dry.

Arrange rice with curry, tofu in bowls and serve sprinkled with basil.

Jackfruit Fricassee with Pea Rice

Ingredients:

250 g earthy colored rice
Salt
250 g solidified peas
400 g jackfruit (can; depleted weight)
1 little onion (40 g)
200 g mushrooms
3 carrots
2 tbsp rapeseed oil
25 g whole meal spelled flour (2 tbsp)
400 ml vegetable stock
250 ml of soy cream
Pepper
½ natural lemon (pizzazz and juice)
Nutmeg
½ group chervil

Directions:

Put earthy colored rice in 500 ml of bubbling salted water, mix once, and let cook during a shut pan over low warmth for 25–30 minutes until the rice has consumed the water. Include the peas over the foremost recent 5 minutes and acquire through with cooking. At that point quickly relax up the rice within the pot and let it swell for a couple of moments within the stopped pan on the exchanged the hob.

While the rice is cooking, flush bits of jackfruit, channel well, and pluck into little pieces. Strip the onion and dig fine strips. Clean the mushrooms and cut them in cuts. Strip the carrots, divide lengthways and dig cuts.

Heat oil during a pot. Include the onion and braise for 2 minutes over medium warmth. Include bits of jackfruit and sauté for five minutes. At that point include mushrooms and carrots and braise for 3 minutes. Residue everything with flour and pour within the vegetable stock while blending and stew on low warmth for 10 minutes, including slightly water if vital.

Then mix within the soy cream, season with salt, pepper, lemon pizzazz and juice, and newly ground nutmeg. Warmth rice over low warmth. Wash chervil, shake dry, and cleave. Serve fricassee sprinkled with rice and chervil.

Red Chicory, Pear and Hazelnut dish

Ingredients::

Two red chicory, or white if not accessible

Two a good handful of rocket leaves

25g hazelnuts, cooked and chopped

For the dressing

one tsp green peppercorns in H2O, discretionary

two tbsp hazelnut or olive oil

Two tbsp mild salad oil, such as sunflower oil sunflower oil oil

One fortified wine or cider vinegar

Instructions:

Make the dressing. At intervals the event that using green peppercorns, daintily crush them in a bowl with a wood spoon, or utilize a pestle and mortar. Mix in the oils and vinegar and add salt to style.

Trim away the chicory tail ends and discard any limp or tired outer leaves. Carefully separate the leaves and arrange 5-6 on four plates – if they are massive, cut or tear all into items.

Remove the stalks from the two and quarter the two lengthways. Cut out the cores, then thinly slice the organic product. Mastermind the pear cuts on high of the high leaves and high over half the dressing. Pour the remaining dressing over the rocket and season with salt and pepper. Give the leaves a brisk toss and pile on top of each plate of mixed greens. Sprinkle with the nuts and serve.

Italian Kale

Ingredients:

three tbsp olive oil

Three garlic cloves, finely sliced

Three tbsp red wine vinegar

300g cavolo Nero or kale, roughlyshredded

Instructions:

Heat the oil in a dish with AN lid and sizzle the garlic, at that point that point that point a sprinkle of water.

Tip the kale into the pan, unfold and unfold in the unfold for 4-5 mins, adding a sprinkle additional water if the dish gets too dry. Once wilted, season cajan pea an embrace sea salt.

Broccoli and Kale

Ingredients:

500ml stock, made by mixing one tbsp broth broth and broth water in a instrumentation

One tbsp sunflower oil

Two garlic cloves, sliced

Thumb-sized piece ginger, sliced ½ tsp ground coriander

3cm/1in piece fresh turmeric root, stripped and grated, or ½ tsp ground turmeric squeeze of pink chain salt

200g courgettes, roughly sliced

85g broccoli100g kale, chopped
1 lime, zested and juiced
Small pack parsley, roughly cleaved, reserving a couple of a couple of a couple of

Guidelines

place the oil place a profound AN, embrace the garlic, ginger, coriander, turmeric and salt, fry on a medium heat preparation two mins, then add three tbsp water cajan pea give bit embrace moistness to the flavors.

Add the courgettes, making certain you mix certain to coat the slices altogether the spices, and continue cooking for three mins. Embrace 400ml stock and leave cajan pea simmer for three mins.

Add the broccoli, kale and lime juice with the rest of the stock. Leave to cook again preparation another 3-4 minutes.

Take off the heat and embrace the slashed parsley. Pour everything into a blender and blend on high speed till till. It will be a beautiful green with bits of dark speckled through (which is the kale). Garnish cajan pea lime zest and parsley.

Kale with Lemon spread Dressing

Ingredients::

Juice one lemon (about three tbsp juice)
One garlic clove, crushed
50g go
one tbsp olive oil
200g kale

Instructions:

First, make embrace dressing. Place the lemon juice, garlic, spread and 50ml cold water in barely bowl. Mix well to frame a free dressing and season cajan pea taste. 2. Heat the oil throughout a throughout throughout A and pan sear the kale for three minutes. Add 0.5 the dressing to the dish and cook for a further thirty secs. Move to a serving bowl and shower over the remaining dressing.

The Sirt Food Diet's cooked Puy Lentils

Ingredients::

Eight Cherry tomatoes, halved
2 tsp. Extra virgin olive oil
forty g Red onion, daintily cut
One Garlic clove, finely chopped
forty g Celery, thinly sliced
forty g Carrots, stripped and thinly sliced
1 tsp. Paprika
1 tsp. Thyme (dry or fresh)
Seventy five g seventy five lentils
220 milliliter Vegetable stock
fifty g fifty, roughly hacked
1 tbsp. Parsley, hacked
twenty g Rocket

Instructions:

Heat your oven to 120°C/gas ½.

Place the tomatoes into barely barely and broil in the oven for 35–45 minutes.

Heat a pot over a low–medium heat. Embrace one teaspoon of the oil with oil embrace, garlic, celery and carrot and fry for 1–2 minutes, minutes mellowed. Combine place the paprika and thyme and embrace for a further minute.

Rinse the lentils throughout a throughout filter and add them to the pan along with the stock. Bring to the boil, at that point reduce the heat and stew gently for twenty minutes with a high on the pan. Provide the a combination a combination a combination provide, 5 barely water if the level drops too much.

Add the kale and cook for a further ten thirty. When the lentils are sauteed, combine in embrace parsley and roasted tomatoes. Serve with the rocket showered with the remaining teaspoon two olive oil.

Baked Potatoes with Spicy Chickpea Stew

Ingredients::
4-6 baking potatoes pricked all over
Two tablespoons olive oil
Two very little onions finely cleaved
Four cloves garlic grated or four
two cm ginger grated
½ - two teaspoons chilli flakes depending on how hot you like things
Two tablespoons cumin seeds
two tablespoons turmeric
Splash of water
Two x 400g tins chopped tomatoes
Two tablespoons sugarless cocoa powder or flowering tree
Two x 400g tins chickpeas or kidney beans if you prefer together with embrace chickpea water don't drain!!
Two yellow peppers or whatever colour you like! Cleaved into bitesize items
two tablespoons parsley in addition to in addition for in addition
Salt and pepper cajan pea style discretionary
Side facet discretionary

Guidelines:
Heat up the broiler to 200C; meanwhile you will prepare all your ingredients.
When the broiler is hot enough put your baking potatoes at intervals the oven and cook for one hour or until they square measure done square measure however however them.
Once the potatoes square measure in the oven, place the olive oil and chopped red onion in a large wide saucepan and cook finely, with embrace lid on preparation five minutes, till the onions square measure soft nevertheless not earthy coloured.
Take away the best the best the best, ginger, cumin and stew. Cook preparation a preparation minute on a occasional heat, then add the turmeric and a flavoursome small sprinkle of water and cook preparation another minute, taking care to not thought embrace thought get too dry.
Next, embrace in embrace tomatoes, chocolate (or cacao), and chickpeas (including the chickpea water) and yellow pepper. Bring to the boil, at that point simmer on a occasional heat for forty five minutes until the forty five is options and unctuous (however don't forty five it consume!). The stew ought to ought to ought to ought to ought to the potatoes.
Finally stir in the two tablespoons of parsley, and some salt and pepper if you wish, and serve the stew on top of embrace baked potatoes, perhaps with a simple side salad.

Vegan Raw Meatballs

Ingredients:
250 g fine bulgur
1 clove of garlic
2 meat tomatoes
1 tsp salt
½ tsp cayenne pepper
1 tsp cumin
1 tsp paprika powder
1 squeeze bean stew chips
40 g paprika showcase (3 tbsp)
25 g tomato glue (2 level tablespoons)
2 spring onions
½ group parsley (10 g)
½ group mint (10 g)
2 lettuce hearts
1 natural lemon
5 radish

Directions:
Pour 250 ml of high temp water over the bulgur, mix and permit expanding for 10 minutes.
Peel and finely cleave the garlic. Singe the tomatoes with bubbling water, extinguish,

and skin. Evacuate the seeds and cut the mash into fine 3D shapes.

Add garlic, tomatoes, salt, and flavors whilst paprika and tomato glue to the bulgur and ply energetically for around 5 minutes (ideally with gloves). Let it rest for 20 minutes.

Within the interim, clean, wash and cut the spring onions into exceptionally fine rings. Wash parsley and mint, shake dry, and cleave finely. Separate lettuce leaves from the lettuce head, wash and shake dry. Wash the lemon hot, grind dry, hamper the middle, and cut. Clean, wash, and cut radishes into little solid shapes.

Knead parsley, half the mint and spring onions under the mixture. Stop around 30 pecans estimated pieces and pound them in your grasp with the goal that lengthened rolls (köfte) are made.

Place the kofte during a leaf of lettuce, sprinkle with the staying mint and radishes, and present with lemon.

Pide with Eggplant and Bell Pepper Filling

Ingredients:

½ shape yeast
½ tsp fluid nectar
200 g yogurt (3.5% fat)
2½ tbsp oil
200 g spelled flour type 630
230 g spelled flour type 1050
1 tsp salt
1 shallot
1 clove of garlic
1 enormous eggplant (400 g)
2 red peppers
1 tsp ground cumin
1 tsp rose hot paprika powder
½ tsp cinnamon
½ tsp sumac (oriental zest)
2 tbsp tomato glue (30 g)
½ group mint (10 g)
20 g pistachios (1 stored tablespoon)
½ pomegranate

Planning Steps

Dissolve yeast in 150 ml of heated water. Include the nectar, 2 tablespoons of yogurt and a few of tablespoons of oil , mix and put during a secure spot. Blend the two sorts of flour in with the salt during a subsequent bowl. Add the yeast blend to the flour and manipulate well for 5-10 minutes. Shape the mixture into a ball and spread and leave to ascend during a warm spot for hour.

Within the interim, strip the shallot and clove of garlic and cleave finely. Clean, wash, and cut the eggplant and peppers into little pieces. Warmth the staying oil during an enormous skillet. Braise shallot and garlic in it over low warmth for 2 minutes. Include flavors and stew for 1 moment.

Put the vegetables and tomato glue within the container and sauté for 10 minutes over medium warmth, salt. Take it from the oven and let it chill. Meanwhile, wash the mint, shake it dry, pluck the leaves, dig fine strips, and put half under the container vegetables.

Knead the yeast batter again on a floured surface and partition it into 6 equivalent segments. Reveal the bits lengthened and shape them into vessels. Top every batter with vegetable filling, forgetting about the edges of the mixture and afterward collapsing them inside. Heat during a preheated stove at 240 ° C (fan broiler 220 ° C; gas: level 4) for 10 minutes.

Meanwhile, generally slash the pistachios and expel the pomegranate seeds from the organic product. Remove the pide from the broiler and let it chill off a touch. Orchestrate pide with pistachios, staying mint, outstanding yogurt, and pomegranate seeds.

Vegetarian Asparagus Baked with Grilled Eggplant

Ingredients:

24 sticks white asparagus
2 eggplants
Salt
2 tbsp spread (30 g)
2 tbsp wholemeal spelled flour
500 ml milk (3.5% fat)
Pepper
Nutmeg
1 tbsp juice
1 pack chervil
1 tbsp oil
100 g veggie-lover mountain cheddar (45% fat in dry issue)

Planning Steps

Peel the asparagus, remove the woody finishes, and cook the asparagus in bubbling salted water for 10 minutes. At that point pour and put during a secure spot. Clean, wash and cut the eggplants lengthways into 1/2 cm cuts. Sprinkle with salt and put it during a secure spot.

Heat the margarine during a pan. Residue with flour, mix with a whisk, pour within the milk, and convey to the bubble while blending. Expel from the warmth, season with salt, pepper, nutmeg, and juice. Wash chervil, shake dry, cleave and blend half into the sauce.

Pat the eggplant cuts dry and brush with oil. Warmth a flame broil container and burn the cuts on the two sides for 1 moment over high warmth. Mesh mountain cheddar.

Bundle 3 stalks of asparagus, wrap with 1 eggplant cut, and a spot during a preparing dish. Pour sauce over, pour cheddar over it. Prepare during a preheated broiler at 200 ° C (fan stove: 180 ° C; gas: speed 3) for 15–20 minutes. Remove from the broiler and sprinkle with the rest of the chervil.

Vegan Mushroom Ragout with Broccoli

Ingredients:

500 g blended mushrooms (white mushrooms, clam, and shitake mushrooms)
1 carrot
1 clove of garlic
2 branches marjoram
2 tbsp oil
200 ml oat cream (or soy cream)
Pepper
1 squeeze ground cumin
¼ natural lemon
300 g broccoli

Planning Steps

Clean mushrooms, wash and split if important. Clean, strip, and cut the carrot into little solid shapes. Strip garlic and slash finely. Wash marjoram, shake dry, and pluck leaves. Heat the oil during a dish, sauté the garlic and carrot shapes over medium warmth for five minutes. At that point include mushrooms and braise for 7 minutes. Season with marjoram, salt, pepper, and caraway. Include oat cream and blend in. Flush the lemon quarter, grind the strip, and crush out the juice. Season ragout with lemon get-up-and-go and squeeze.

Bring plenty of salted water to the bubble. Clean, wash, and separation broccoli into florets and cook in water for five minutes. Orchestrate the mushroom ragout with broccoli on plates and serve everything sprinkled with pepper.

Turkey Skinny Satay Skewers

Ingredients::

- two teaspoons minced garlic

one tablespoons fresh nutty unfold (change in accordance in conjunction with your preferences)
two tablespoons earthy colored sugar, stuffed

Salt to season
one cup light-weight coconut milk
one teaspoon turmeric
three tablespoons powdery nutty unfold
600 g | 1/2lbs turkey bosom filets, cubed
Additional water if necessary
Contemporary coriander leaves
Twelve picket sticks
Oil splash

Directions:

Unit of time to splash sticks. Parts of turkey string onto sticks at that point place throughout a secure spot.

Combine all the Ingredients: throughout a serious, shallow dish and race till mingling. Supplement sticks and marinade to a lot of profound preference for around an hour or nightlong.

Drain the turkey sticks till they are attending to cook, holding the marinade. Splash the oil shower on a non-stick dish/skillet and fry over medium heat in 2 parcels till the bottom is cooked. Flip over and cook for more and more five minutes or till the turkey has steamed entirely. On the other hand, prepare throughout a pre-warmed stove at medium-high heat beneath the barbecue/sear settings till heated, turning once around ten minutes.

Switch the saved marinade to barely pot or pan and over high heat convey to a bubble. Reduce heat to normal, and stew for 5 minutes whereas intermixture or till the sauce is sweet-scented and thick. (Include extra water per table space simply if the sauce looks to be overly thick)

Serve sticks with leaves of coriander, steamed rice or vegetables, and sprinkle with satay sauce.

Courgette dish

Ingredients::

two tablespoons oil
Four cloves garlic, finely slashed
1.5 pounds Arborio rice
6 tomatoes, slashed
two teaspoons slashed rosemary
5 courgettes, finely diced
One ¼ cups peas, new or coagulated
twelve cups hot vegetable stock
one cup slashed
Salt to style
Freshly ground pepper

Headings:

Place an enormous substantial flat-bottom instrumentation over medium heat. Embody oil. At the aim once the oil is warm, embody onion and sauté till clear.

Stir inside the tomatoes and cook till delicate. Next combine inside the rice and rosemary. Blend well.

Add a large portion of the stock and cook till dry. Combine abundant of the time.

Add staying stock and cook for 3-4 minutes.

Add courgette and peas and cook till rice is delicate. Add salt and pepper to style.

Stir inside the basil. Let it sit for 5 minutes.

Chile Con Carne

Ingredients::

one tsp hot bean stew powder
one tsp paprika
One monumental onion
two tbsp tomato purée
One red pepper
one tsp ground cumin
one tbsp oil
One hamburger stock 3D sq.
Two garlic cloves
one tsp sugar (you will likewise embody barely little of dim chocolate)
410g will red excretory organ beans

400g will cleaved tomatoes
500g minced meat
½ tsp dried marjoram
Plain bubbled long-grain rice, to serve
Cream, to serve

Directions:

Have your vegetables arranged? Cleave into tiny bones one major onion, around five millimeter long. The foremost ideal approach to accomplish therefore is to half the onion down the middle, strip it, and later on cut it the nice distance into a state of thick matchsticks systematically, not dynamical all of them to the premise finish since they are entirely unbroken along. Spherical into dice over the match sticks.

Slice a red pepper inside the 0.5 the nice distance, cut base, wash the seeds, at that point hack it. At that point strip and cut two cloves of garlic.

Begin coming up with. Spot your dish over medium heat onto the hob. Apply one tbsp of oil and keep it up for one or two minutes before warm (on the off likelihood that you simply utilize an electrical hob somewhat more).

Place the onion and cook for around five minutes, mixing moderately systematically, or till your onion is thick, squidgy, and fairly clear.

Tip the one tsp of hot bean stew powder otherwise you'll be able to likewise embody one tbsp of delicate bean stew powder, garlic, red pepper,1 tsp of paprika then one tsp of cumin ground.

Supply it a fast twirl, at that point leave for more and more five minutes to cook, intermixture often.

Brown five hundred gather hamburger throughout a minced structure. Switch the fireside up barely, add your meat to the pot, and split it with the spatula or blade. At the aim once you introduce the mince, the mix can sizzle a small indefinite quantity.

Keep mixing and nudging for 5 minutes at any rate, before all mince factor is regarding up, dainty protuberances and no pink elements are left. Keep your heat sufficiently hot to sear the meat and switch earthy colored, as against merely stewing.

Produce a sauce. Disintegrate one form of the hamburger hold into 300ml of hot stock. Pour it inside the mix being minced into the cooking pan.

Add slashed tomatoes to a four hundred g bowl. Prime with 1/2 tsp of dried marjoram, one tsp of sugar, and later on embody an honest pepper and salt shake. Sprinkle with somewhere inside vary of 2 tbsp of tomato purée and later on combine well the sauce.

Simmer finely around it. Carry the total to the bubble, mix well, and place a variety on the pan. Move the warmth down till it spills finely, at that point quit for right around twenty minutes.

Often be careful for the cooking pan to mix it, to make sure that the sauce does not stick on very cheap of the instrumentation or dried out. Assumptive typically this can be} often the case, apply 2 or 3 tablespoons of water, and guarantee that the warmth is sufficiently tiny. The saucy, minced mix ought to look soaking, thick, and delicious once finely stewing.

Drain and later on flush throughout a filter a 410 g jar of your excretory organ beans, at that point mix them into the stew pot. Bubble yet again, and pocket finely for more and more ten minutes while not the very best, you will embody barely water a lot of inside the event that it's dry.

Style a small indefinite quantity little of the number and bean stew. Perhaps, it'd need

unquestionably a lot of flavored than you suspected.
Currently expel unfold, clean up the fireside and allow the bean stew to stay till serving for about10 minutes. Typically. This can be} often important in light-weight of the actual fact that it needs the mixing of the flavors.
Serve with simple bubbled vast grain rice and a couple of soured cream.

Brown Basmati Rice pilaff

Ingredients::
½ tablespoon feeder oleomargarine
½ cup mushrooms, slashed
½ cup earthy coloured basmati rice
2-3 tablespoons water
1/8 teaspoon dried thyme
Ground pepper to style
½ tablespoon oil
¼ cup scallion, cleaved
one cup vegetable stock
¼ teaspoon salt
¼ cup cleaved, cooked walnuts
Headings:
Place a pan over medium-low heat. Embody unfold and oil.
Once it liquefies, embody mushrooms and cook till somewhat delicate.
Stir inside the scallion and earthy colored rice. Cook for three minutes. Combine regularly.
Stir inside the stock, water, salt, and thyme.
Once it starts to bubble, lower heat and unfold with a prime. Stew till rice is steamed. Embody a lot of water or stock whenever needed. Stir inside the walnuts and pepper.
Serve.

Thai Red Curry:

Ingredients::
One ½ cups ironed meagerly cut kale
Pinch of salt, a lot of to style
two tablespoons Thai red curry glue
one tablespoon soy
One ¼ cups long-grain earthy colored shrub rice
One very little white onion, cleaved
one tablespoon ground ginger
One red ringer pepper
one tablespoon vegetable oil or oil
½ cup of water
One ½ teaspoons of coconut sugar or turbinado sugar
Two cloves garlic
Two of teaspoons juice
Three carrots, stripped and cut
One chime pepper
One will (14 ounces) normal coconut milk
Directions:
Take a significant pot of water and place it to bubble to line up the rice. Addition the flushed rice and begin to bubble for unit of time to stay aloof from overabundance, decreasing heat once needed. Expel from heat, channel the rice, and set the rice back to the pot. Unfold and let the rice rest till you are ready to serve for ten minutes or a lot of. Season the rice to style with salt shortly before serving, and lighten it with a fork.
To render the curry, kindle AN expansive cooking pan over the medium fireplace with the profound sides. When warm, embody your oil. At that point embody the onion and a sprinkle of salt and cook, mixing routinely for around five minutes till your onion has mollified and turns clear. Embody the garlic and ginger, and cook for around 25-30 seconds whereas persistently intermixture till sweet-scented.
Add the carrots and your chime peppers. Cook, mixing systematically till these chime peppers are fork-delicate, three to 5 minutes a lot of. At that point embody your curry glue, and cook for around two minutes, intermixture each currently and once more.

Add the water, kale, coconut milk, and sugar, and rush to mix. Get the mix over medium fireplace to a stew. Decrease fireplace variable to remain a light stew and cook till the carrots, peppers, and kale have relaxed specifically as you'd like, mixing sporadically for around 5-10 minutes.

Take away your pot from fireplace and season with rice vinegar and tamari. Embody salt to taste. On the off likelihood that your curry needs a small indefinite quantity little of a lot of vitality, embody 1⁄2 teaspoon a lot of tamari, or embody 1⁄2 teaspoon a larger quantity of your rice vinegar for larger corrosiveness. Separation each curry and rice into bowls and sweetening them, inside the event that you simply like, with cut cilantro and a sprinkle of your red pepper drops. Operate AN afterthought with sriracha or bean stew aioli sauce, inside the event that you simply like zesty curries.

If you'd prefer to incorporate bean curd, 1st heat it and embody it with coconut milk in synchronize four. Inside the event that you simply apply crude bean curd, it will take up such a large quantity of the fat, therefore heating it'd improve the flavor extensively, in any case.

Moroccan Chicken Casserole

Preparation time: 20 minutes

Cooking time: 50 minutes

Servings: 4

Ingredients:

4 chicken breasts, cubed

250g tinned chickpeas (garbanzo beans) drained 4 medjool dates, halved

6 dried apricots, halved

1 red onion, sliced 1 carrot, chopped 1 teaspoon ground cumin

1 teaspoon ground cinnamon 1 teaspoon ground turmeric 1 bird's-eye chili, chopped 600mls chicken stock

25g corn flour 60mls water 2 teaspoons fresh coriander

Directions:

Place the chicken, chickpeas (garbanzo beans), onion, carrot, chili, cumin, turmeric, cinnamon and stock (broth) into a large saucepan. Bring it to the boil, reduce the heat and simmer for 25 minutes. Add in the dates and apricots and simmer for 10 minutes. In a cup, mix the corn flour together with the water until it becomes a smooth paste. Pour the mixture into the saucepan and stir until it thickens. Add in the coriander (cilantro) and mix well. Serve with buckwheat or couscous.

Nutrition:

Calories: 401 Net carbs: 3.6g Fat: 4.8g Fiber: 1.7g Protein: 29.2g

Prawn and Coconut Curry

Preparation time: 10 minutes

Cooking time: 5 minutes

Servings: 4

Ingredients:

400g tinned chopped tomatoes

400g large prawns (shrimps), shelled and raw

25g fresh coriander (cilantro) chopped

3 red onions, finely chopped 3 cloves of garlic, crushed

2 bird's eye chilies

½ teaspoon ground coriander (cilantro)

½ teaspoon turmeric

400mls (14fl Oz) coconut milk 1 teaspoons olive oil

Juice of 1 lime

Directions:

Place the onions, garlic, tomatoes, chilies, lime juice, turmeric, ground coriander (cilantro), chilies and half of the fresh coriander (cilantro) into a blender and blitz until you have a smooth curry paste. Heat the olive oil in a frying pan, add the paste and cook for 2 minutes. Stir in the coconut milk and warm it thoroughly. Add the prawns (shrimps) to the paste and cook them until they have turned pink and are completely cooked. Stir in the fresh coriander (cilantro). Serve with rice.

Nutrition:

Calories: 322 Net carbs: 98.9g Fat: 11.8g Fiber: 8g Protein: 15.6g

Chicken and Bean Casserole

Preparation time: 15 minutes

Cooking time: 55 minutes

Servings: 4

Ingredients:

400g chopped tomatoes

400g tinned cannellini beans or haricot beans

8 chicken thighs, skin removed

2 carrots, peeled and finely chopped 2 red onions, chopped

4 sticks of celery

4 large mushrooms

2 red peppers (bell peppers), de-seeded and chopped 1 clove of garlic

2 teaspoons soy sauce 1 olive oil

1.75 liters chicken stock (broth)

Directions:

Heat the olive oil in a saucepan, add the garlic and onions and cook for 5 minutes. Add in the chicken and cook for 5 minutes then add the carrots, cannellini beans, celery, red peppers (bell peppers) and mushrooms. Pour in the stock (broth) soy sauce and tomatoes. Bring it to the boil, reduce the heat and simmer for 45 minutes. Serve with rice or new potatoes.

Nutrition:

Calories: 509 Net carbs: 12.5g Fat: 6.5g Fiber: 1.1g Protein: 27.4g

Mussels in Red Wine Sauce

Preparation time: 5 minutes

Cooking time: 5 minutes

Servings: 2

Ingredients:

800g mussels

2 x 400g tins of chopped tomatoes 25g butter

1 fresh chives, chopped 1 fresh parsley, chopped

1 bird's-eye chili, finely chopped 4 cloves of garlic, crushed 400mls red wine

Juice of 1 lemon

Directions:

Wash the mussels, remove their beards and set them aside. Heat the butter in a large saucepan and add in the red wine. Reduce the heat and add the parsley, chives, chili and garlic whilst stirring. Add in the tomatoes, lemon juice and mussels. Cover the saucepan and cook for 2-3.Remove the saucepan from the heat and take out any mussels which haven't opened and discard them. Serve and eat immediately.

Nutrition:

Calories: 364 Net carbs: 3.3g Fat: 4.9g Fiber: 0.7g Protein: 8.2g

Roast Balsamic Vegetables

Preparation time: 10 minutes

Cooking time: 45 minutes

Servings: 4

Ingredients:

4 tomatoes, chopped 2 red onions, chopped 3 sweet potatoes, peeled and chopped

100g red chicory (or if unavailable, use yellow)

100g kale, finely chopped

300g potatoes, peeled and chopped 5 stalks of celery, chopped

1 bird's-eye chili, de-seeded and finely chopped 2g fresh parsley, chopped

2gs fresh coriander (cilantro) chopped 3 teaspoons olive oil

2 teaspoons balsamic vinegar 1 teaspoon mustard Sea salt Freshly ground black pepper

Directions:

Place the olive oil, balsamic, mustard, parsley and coriander (cilantro) into a bowl and mix well. Toss all the remaining ingredients into the dressing and season with salt and pepper. Transfer the vegetables to an ovenproof dish and cook in the oven at 200C/400F for 45 minutes.

Nutrition:

Calories: 310 Net carbs: 1.1g Fiber: 0.2g Protein: 0.2g

Tomato and Goat's Pizza

Preparation time: 15 minutes

Cooking time: 20 minutes

Servings: 2

Ingredients: 225g buckwheat flour

2 teaspoons dried yeast Pinch of salt 150mls slightly water 1 teaspoon olive oil For the Topping:

75g feta cheese, crumbled 75g peseta (or tomato paste)

1 tomato, sliced 1 red onion, finely chopped 25g rocket (arugula) leaves, chopped

Directions:

In a bowl, combine all the ingredients for the pizza dough then allow it to stand for at least an hour until it has doubled in size. Roll the dough out to a size to suit you. Spoon the passata onto the base and add the rest of the toppings. Bake in the oven at 200C/400F for 15-20 minutes or until browned at the edges and crispy and serve.

Nutrition:

Calories: 585 Net carbs: 77g Fat: 8.1g Fiber: 7.6g Protein: 22.9g

Tender Spiced Lamb

Preparation time: 20 minutes

Cooking time: 4 hours 20 minutes

Servings: 8

Ingredients:

1.35kg lamb shoulder 3 red onions, sliced

3 cloves of garlic, crushed

1 bird's eye chili, finely chopped 1 teaspoon turmeric

1 teaspoon ground cumin

½ teaspoon ground coriander (cilantro)

¼ teaspoon ground cinnamon 2 tablespoons olive oil

Directions:

In a bowl, combine the chili, garlic and spices with olive oil. Coat the lamb with the spice mixture and marinate it for an hour, or overnight if you can. Heat the remaining oil in a pan, add the lamb and brown it for 3-4 minutes on all sides to seal it. Place the lamb in an ovenproof dish. Add in the red onions and cover the dish with foil. Transfer to the oven and roast at 170C/325F for 4 hours. The lamb should be extremely tender and falling off the bone. Serve with rice or couscous, salad or vegetables.

Nutrition:

Calories: 455 Net carbs: 28g Fat: 9.8g Fiber: 11g Protein: 20g

Chili Cod Fillets

Preparation time: 10 minutes

Cooking time: 10 minutes

Servings: 4

Ingredients:

4 cod fillets each)

2 teaspoons fresh parsley, chopped

2 bird's-eye chilies (or more if you like it hot)

2 cloves of garlic, chopped

4 teaspoons olive oil

Directions:

Heat a of olive oil in a frying pan, add the fish and cook for 7-8 minutes or until thoroughly cooked, turning once halfway through. Remove and keep warm. Pour the remaining olive oil into the pan and add the chili, chopped garlic and parsley. Warm it thoroughly. Serve the fish onto plates and pour the warm chili oil over it.

Nutrition:

Calories: 246 Net carbs: 5.5g Fat: 0.5g Fiber: 0.7g Protein: 18.5g

Steak and Mushroom Noodles

Preparation time: 10 minutes
Cooking time: 20 minutes
Servings: 4
Ingredients:

100g shitake mushrooms, halved, if large 100g chestnut mushrooms, sliced
150g udon noodles
75g kale, finely chopped
75g baby leaf spinach, chopped 2 sirloin steaks
2 teaspoons miso paste
2.5cm piece fresh ginger, finely chopped
2 teaspoons olive oil 1 star anise
1 red chili, finely sliced
1 red onion, finely chopped
1 fresh coriander (cilantro) chopped 1 liter (1½ pints) warm water

Directions:

Pour the water into a saucepan and add in the miso, star anise and ginger. Bring it to the boil, reduce the heat and simmer gently. In the meantime, cook the noodles according to their instructions then drain them.

Heat the oil in a saucepan, add the steak and cook for around 2-3 minutes on each side (or 1-2 minutes, for rare meat).

Remove the meat and set aside.

Place the mushrooms, spinach, coriander (cilantro) and kale into the miso broth and cook for 5 minutes.

In the meantime, heat the remaining oil in a separate pan and fry the chili and onion for 4 minutes, until softened.

Serve the noodles into bowls and pour the soup on top.

Thinly slice the steaks and add them to the top. Serve immediately.

Nutrition:

Calories: 296 Net carbs: 24.6g Fat: 13.7g Fiber: 0.7g Protein: 32.9g

Masala Scallops

Preparation time: 10 minutes
Cooking time: 20 minutes
Servings: 4
Ingredients:

2 tablespoons olive oil 2 jalapenos, chopped 1 pound sea scallops
A pinch of salt and black pepper
¼ teaspoon cinnamon powder 1 teaspoon garam masala
1 teaspoon coriander, ground 1 teaspoon cumin, ground
2 tablespoons cilantro, chopped

Directions:

Heat up a pan with the oil over medium heat, add the jalapenos, cinnamon and the other ingredients except the scallops and cook for 10 minutes.

Add the rest of the ingredients, toss, cook for 10 minutes more, divide into bowls and serve.

Nutrition:

Calories: 251 Fat: 4g Fiber: 4g Carbs: 11g Protein: 17g

Tuna and Tomatoes

Preparation time: 5 minutes
Cooking time: 20 minutes
Servings: 4
Ingredients:

1 yellow onion, chopped 1 tablespoon olive oil
1 pound tuna fillets, boneless, skinless and cubed 1 cup tomatoes, chopped
1 red pepper, chopped
1 teaspoon sweet paprika
1 tablespoon coriander, chopped

Directions:

Heat up a pan with the oil over medium heat, add the onions and the pepper and cook for 5 minutes.

Add the fish and the other ingredients, cook everything for 15 minutes, divide between plates and serve.

Nutrition:

Calories: 215 Fat: 4g Fiber: 7g Carbs: 14g Protein: 7g

Tuna and Kale

Preparation time: 5 minutes
Cooking time: 20 minutes
Servings: 4
Ingredients:

1 pound tuna fillets, boneless, skinless and cubed A pinch of salt and black pepper
2 tablespoons olive oil 1 cup kale, torn
½ cup cherry tomatoes, cubed 1 yellow onion, chopped

Directions:

Heat up a pan with the oil over medium heat, add the onion and sauté for 5 minutes.

Add the tuna and the other ingredients, toss, cook everything for 15 minutes more, divide between plates and serve.

Nutrition:

Calories 251 Fat: 4g Fiber: 7g Carbs: 14g Protein: 7g

Lemongrass and Ginger Mackerel

Preparation time: 10 minutes
Cooking time: 25 minutes
Servings: 4
Ingredients:

4 mackerel fillets, skinless and boneless 2 tablespoons olive oil
1 tablespoon ginger, grated
2 lemongrass sticks, chopped
2 red chilies, chopped Juice of 1 lime
A handful parsley, chopped

Directions:

In a roasting pan, combine the mackerel with the oil, ginger and the other ingredients, toss and bake at 390 degrees F for 25 minutes.

Divide everything between plates and serve.

Nutrition:

Calories: 251 Fat: 3g Fiber: 4g Carbs: 14g Protein: 8g

Scallops with Almonds and Mushrooms

Preparation time: 5 minutes
Cooking time: 10 minutes
Servings: 4
Ingredients:

1 pound scallops
2 tablespoons olive oil 4 scallions, chopped
A pinch of salt and black pepper
½ cup mushrooms, sliced
2 tablespoon almonds, chopped 1 cup coconut cream

Directions:

Heat up a pan with the oil over medium heat, add the scallions and the mushrooms and sauté for 2 minutes.

Add the scallops and the other ingredients, toss, cook over medium heat for 8 minutes more, divide into bowls and serve.

Nutrition:

Calories: 322 Fat: 23.7g Fiber: 2.2g Carbs: 8.1g Protein: 21.6g

Scallops and Sweet Potatoes

Preparation time: 5 minutes
Cooking time: 22 minutes
Servings: 4
Ingredients: 1 pound scallops
½ teaspoon rosemary, dried
½ teaspoon oregano, dried 2 tablespoons avocado oil 1 yellow onion, chopped
2 sweet potatoes, peeled and cubed
½ cup chicken stock
1 tablespoon cilantro, chopped A pinch of salt and black pepper

Directions:
Heat up a pan with the oil over medium heat, add the onion and sauté for 2 minutes. Add the sweet potatoes and the stock, toss and cook for 10 minutes more. Add the scallops and the remaining ingredients, toss, cook for another 10 minutes, divide everything into bowls and serve.

Nutrition:
Calories: 211 Fat: 2g Fiber: 4.1g Carbs: 26.9g Protein: 20.7g

Salmon and Shrimp Salad

Preparation time: 5 minutes
Cooking time: 0 minutes
Servings: 4
Ingredients:
1 cup smoked salmon, boneless and flaked 1 cup shrimp, peeled, deveined and cooked
½ cup baby arugula
1 tablespoon lemon juice 2 spring onions, chopped 1 tablespoon olive oil
A pinch of sea salt and black pepper

Directions:
In a salad bowl, combine the salmon with the shrimp and the other ingredients, toss and serve.

Nutrition:
Calories: 210 Fat: 6g Fiber: 5g Carbs: 10g Protein: 12g

Shrimp, Tomato and Dates Salad

Preparation time: 10 minutes
Cooking time: 0 minutes
Servings: 4
Ingredients:
1 pound shrimp, cooked, peeled and deveined
2 cups baby spinach
2 tablespoons walnuts, chopped 1 cup cherry tomatoes, halved 1 tablespoon lemon juice
½ cup dates, chopped
2 tablespoons avocado oil

Directions:
In a salad bowl, mix the shrimp with the spinach, walnuts and the other ingredients, toss and serve.

Nutrition:
Calories: 243 Fat: 5.4g Fiber: 3.3g Carbs: 21.6g Protein: 28.3g

Salmon and Watercress Salad

Preparation time: 10 minutes
Cooking time: 0 minutes
Servings: 4
Ingredients:
1 pound smoked salmon, boneless, skinless and flaked 2 spring onions, chopped
2 tablespoons avocado oil
½ cup baby arugula 1 cup watercress
1 tablespoon lemon juice 1 cucumber, sliced
1 avocado, peeled, pitted and roughly cubed
A pinch of sea salt and black pepper

Directions:
In a salad bowl, mix the salmon with the spring onions, watercress and the other ingredients, toss and serve.

Nutrition:
Calories: 261 Fat: 15.8g Fiber: 4.4g Carbs: 8.2g Protein: 22.7g

Apples and Cabbage Mix

Preparation time: 5 minutes
Cooking time: 0 minutes
Servings: 4
Ingredients:

2 cored and cubed green apples
2 tablespoons Balsamic vinegar
½ tablespoon. Caraway seeds 2 tablespoons olive oil
Black pepper
1 shredded red cabbage head

Directions:

In a bowl, combine the cabbage with the apples and the other ingredients, toss and serve.

Nutrition:

Calories: 165 Fat: 7.4g Carbs: 26g Protein: 2.6g Sugars: 2.6g Sodium: 19mg

Thyme Mushrooms

Preparation time: 10 minutes
Cooking time: 30 minute
Servings: 4
Ingredients:

1 tablespoon chopped thyme 2 tablespoon olive oil
2 tablespoons chopped parsley 4 minced garlic cloves
Black pepper
2 lbs. halved white mushrooms

Directions:

In a baking pan, combine the mushrooms with the garlic and the other ingredients, toss, introduce in the oven and cook at 400 0F for 30 minutes.
Divide between plates and serve.

Nutrition:

Calories: 251 Fat: 9.3g Carbs: 13.2 g Protein: 6 g Sugars: 0.8 g Sodium: 37 mg

Rosemary Endives

Preparation time: 5 minutes
Cooking time: 20 minutes
Servings: 4
Ingredients:

2 tablespoons olive oil 1tablespoon dried rosemary 2 halved endives
¼ tablespoon black pepper
½ tablespoon turmeric powder

Directions:

In a baking pan, combine the endives with the oil and the other ingredients, toss gently, introduce in the oven and bake at 400 0F for 20 minutes.
Divide between plates and serve.

Nutrition:

Calories: 66 Fat: 7.1g Carbs: 1.2 g Protein: 0.3g Sugars: 1.3g Sodium: 113mg

Roasted Beets

Preparation time: 10 minutes
Cooking time: 30 minutes
Servings: 4
Ingredients:

2 minced garlic cloves
¼ teaspoon. Black pepper 4 peeled and sliced beets
¼ c. chopped walnuts 2 tablespoons olive oil
¼ c. chopped parsley

Directions:

In a baking dish, combine the beets with the oil and the other ingredients, toss to coat, introduce in the oven at 420 0F, and bake for 30 minutes.
Divide between plates and serve.

Nutrition:

Calories: 156 Fat: 11.8g Carbs: 11.5g Protein: 3.8g Sugars: 8g, Sodium: 670 mg

Minty Tomatoes and Corn

Preparation time: 5 minutes
Cooking time: 0 minutes
Servings: 4
Ingredients:

2 c. corn
1 tables poon rosemary vinegar 2 tablespoons chopped mint
1 lb. sliced tomatoes
¼ tablespoon black pepper 2 tablespoons olive oil Directions:
In a salad bowl, combine the tomatoes with the corn and the other ingredients, toss and serve.
Enjoy!

Nutrition:
Calories: 230 Fat: 7.2g Carbs: 11.6g Protein: 4g Sugars: 1g Sodium: 53 mg

Pesto Green Beans

Preparation time: 10 minutes
Cooking time: 15 minutes
Servings: 4
Ingredients:

2 tablespoons olive oil
2 tablespoon sweet paprika Juice of 1 lemon
2 tablespoons basil pesto
1 lb. trimmed and halved green beans
¼ tablespoon black pepper 1 sliced red onion

Directions:
Heat up a pan with the oil over medium-high heat, add the onion, stir and sauté for 5 minutes.
Add the beans and the rest of the ingredients, toss, cook over medium heat for 10 minutes, divide between plates and serve.

Nutrition:
Calories: 280 Fat: 10g Carbs: 13.9g Protein: 4.7g Sugars: 0.8g Sodium: 138mg

Spinach Salad with Green Asparagus and Salmon

Preparation time: 10 minutes
Cooking time: 0 minutes
Servings: 2
Ingredients:

2 hands Spinach
2 pieces Egg
120 g smoked salmon 100 g Asparagus tips
150 g Cherry tomatoes Lemon 1/2 pieces
1 teaspoon Olive oil

Directions:
Cook the eggs the way you like them.
Heat a pan with a little oil and fry the asparagus. Halve cherry tomatoes.
Place the spinach on a plate and spread the asparagus tips, cherry tomatoes and smoked salmon on top.
Scare, peel and halve the eggs. Add them to the salad.
Squeeze the lemon over the lettuce and drizzle some olive oil over it. Season the salad with a little salt and pepper.

Nutrition:
Calories: 107 Fat: 4.8g Net Carbs: 11.2g Fiber: 1.4g Protein: 5.1g

Brunoised Salad

Preparation time: 10 minutes
Cooking time: 0 minutes
Servings: 3
Ingredients:

1 piece Meat tomato
1/2 pieces Zucchini
1/2 pieces Red bell pepper
1/2 pieces yellow bell pepper 1/2 pieces Red onion
3 sprigs fresh parsley 1/4 pieces Lemon
2 tablespoons Olive oil

Directions:
Finely dice the tomatoes, zucchini, peppers and red onions to get a brunoise. Mix all the cubes in a bowl.
Chop parsley and mix in the salad.
Squeeze the lemon over the salad and add the olive oil. Season with salt and pepper.
Nutrition:
Calories: 170 Fat: 3.6g Net Carbs: 8.7g Fiber: 2g Protein: 1.5g

Buns with Chicken and Cucumber

Preparation time: 15 minutes
Cooking time: 0 minutes
Servings: 4
Ingredients:
12 slices Chicken Breast (Spread) 1 piece Cucumber
1 piece Red pepper 50g fresh basil
3 tablespoons Olive oil 3 tablespoons Pine nuts Garlic 1 clove
Directions:
Wash the cucumber and cut into thin strips, then cut the peppers into thin strips.
Put the basil, olive oil, pine nuts and garlic in a food processor. Stir to an even pesto.
Season the pesto and season with salt and pepper if necessary. Place a slice of chicken fillet on a plate, brush with 1 teaspoon of pesto and top the strips with cucumber and peppers. Carefully roll up the chicken fillet to create a nice roll. If necessary, secure the rolls with a cocktail skewer.
Nutrition:
Calories: 90 Fat: 8g Protein: 4g

Hazelnut Balls

Preparation time: 40 minutes
Cooking time: 0 minutes
Servings: 1
Ingredients:
130g Dates 140g Hazelnuts
2 tablespoon Cocoa powder 1 / 2 teaspoon Vanilla extract
1 teaspoon Honey
Directions:
Put the hazelnuts in a food processor and grind them until you get hazelnut flour (of course you can also use ready-made hazelnut flour).
Put the hazelnut flour in a bowl and set aside.
Put the dates in the food processor and grind them until you get a ball.
Add the hazelnut flour, vanilla extract, cocoa and honey and pulse until you get a nice and even mix.
Remove the mixture from the food processor and turn it into beautiful balls. Store the balls in the fridge.
Nutrition:
Calories: 722 Fat: 69.8g Net Carbs: 19.2g Fiber: 11.2g Protein: 17.1g

Stuffed Eggplants

Preparation time: 10 minutes
Cooking time: 30 minutes
Servings: 2
Ingredients:
4 pieces Eggplant
3 tablespoons Coconut oil 1 piece Onion
250g Ground beef 2 cloves Garlic
3 pieces Tomatoes
1 tablespoon Tomato paste 1 hand Capers
1 hand fresh basil
Directions:
Finely chop the onion and garlic. Cut the tomatoes into cubes and shred the basil leaves.
Bring a large pot of water to a boil, add the eggplants and let it cook for about 5 minutes.
Drain, let cool slightly and remove the pulp with a spoon (leave a rim about 1 cm thick around the skin). Cut the pulp finely and set aside.

Put the eggplants in a baking dish. Preheat the oven to 175 ° C.

Heat 3 tablespoons of coconut oil in a pan on a low flame and glaze the onion.

Add the minced meat and garlic and fry until the beef is loose.

Add the finely chopped eggplants, tomato pieces, capers, and basil and tomato paste and fry them on the pan with the lid for 10 minutes.

Season with salt and pepper.

Fill the eggplant with the beef mixture and bake in the oven for about 20 minutes.

Nutrition:

Calories: 166 Fat: 3.8g Net Carbs: 8.3g Fiber: 2.4g Protein: 0.8g

Chicken Teriyaki with Cauliflower Rice

Preparation time: 300 minutes

Cooking time: 40 minutes

Servings: 3

Ingredients:

500g Chicken breast 90ml Coconut aminos

2 tablespoons Coconut blossom sugar 1 tablespoon Olive oil

1 teaspoon Sesame oil 50g fresh ginger

2 cloves Garlic

250g Chinese cabbage 1 piece Leek

2 pieces Red peppers

1 piece Cauliflower (rice) 1 piece Onion

1 teaspoon Ghee 50g fresh coriander 1 piece Lime

Directions:

Cut the chicken into cubes. Mix coconut aminos, coconut blossom sugar, olive oil and sesame oil in a small bowl.

Finely chop the ginger and garlic and add to the marinade. Put the chicken in the marinade in the fridge overnight.

Roughly cut Chinese cabbage, leek, garlic and paprika and add to the slow cooker. Finally add the marinated chicken and let it cook for about 2 to 4 hours.

When the chicken is almost ready, you can cut the cauliflower into small florets. Then put the florets in a food processor and pulse briefly to prepare rice.

Finely chop an onion, heat a pan with a teaspoon of ghee and fry the onion.

Then add the cauliflower rice and fry briefly.

Spread the chicken and cauliflower rice on the plates and garnish with a little chopped coriander and a wedge of lime.

Nutrition:

Calories: 506 Fat: 4.4g Net Carbs: 90.8g Protein: 25.9g

Curry Chicken with Pumpkin Spaghetti

Preparation time: 5 minutes

Cooking time: 45 minutes

Servings: 5

Ingredients:

500 g Chicken breast

2 teaspoons Chili powder

1 piece Onion 1 clove Garlic

2 teaspoons Ghee

3 tablespoon Curry powder 500 ml Coconut milk (can) 200g Pineapple 200g Mango 1 piece Red pepper

1 piece Butternut squash

25 g Spring onion 25 g fresh coriander

Directions:

Cut the chicken into strips and season with pepper, salt and chili powder. Then put the chicken in the slow cooker.

Finely chop the onion and garlic and lightly fry with 2 teaspoons of ghee. Then add the curry powder.

Deglaze with the coconut milk after a minute. Add the sauce to the slow cooker along with the pineapple, mango cubes and chopped peppers and let it cook for

2 to 4 hours. Cut the pumpkin into long pieces and make spaghetti out of it with a spiralizer (that's not easy, it works better with a carrot).
Briefly fry the pumpkin spaghetti in the pan and spread the chicken curry on top. Garnish with thinly sliced spring onions and chopped coriander.

Nutrition:

Calories: 160Fat: 8.6gNet Carbs: 6.1g Fiber: 1.2gProtein: 14.8g

French Style Chicken Thighs

Preparation time: 10 minutes
Cooking time: 4 hours
Servings: 6
Ingredients:

700 g Chicken leg 1 tablespoon Olive oil 2 pieces Onion 4 pieces Carrot
2 cloves Garlic 8 stems Celery
25g fresh rosemary 25g Fresh thyme 25 g fresh parsley

Directions:

Season the chicken with olive oil, pepper and salt and rub it into the meat. Roughly cut onions, carrots, garlic and celery and add to the slow cooker. Place the chicken on top and finally sprinkle a few sprigs of rosemary, thyme and parsley on top. Let it cook for at least four hours. Serve with a delicious salad, enjoy your meal!

Nutrition:

Calories: 459 Fat: 34.8g Net Carbs: 6.2g Fiber: 1.3g Protein: 29.7g

Spicy Ribs with Roasted Pumpkin

Preparation time: 24 hours
Cooking time: 4 hours
Servings: 3
Ingredients:

400 g Spare ribs
4 tablespoons Coconut-Aminos
2 tablespoons Honey 1 tablespoon Olive oil
50g Spring onions Garlic 2 cloves
1 piece green chili peppers 1 piece Onion
1 piece Red pepper 1 piece Red pepper

For the roasted pumpkin:

Pumpkin 1 piece Coconut oil 1 tablespoon
Paprika powder 1 tablespoon

Directions:

Marinate the ribs the day before.
Cut the ribs into pieces with four ribs each. Place the coconut aminos, honey and olive oil in a mixing bowl and mix. Chop the spring onions, garlic and green peppers and add them. Spread the ribs on plastic containers and pour the marinade over them. Leave them in the fridge overnight.
Cut the onions, peppers and peppers into pieces and put them in the slow cooker. Spread the ribs, including the marinade, and let them cook for at least 4 hours.
Preheat the oven to 200 ° C for the pumpkin. Cut the pumpkin into moons and place on a baking sheet lined with parchment paper.
Spread a tablespoon of coconut oil on the baking sheet and season with paprika, pepper and salt. Roast the pumpkin in the oven for about 20 minutes and serve with the spare ribs.

Nutrition:

Calories: 65 Fat: 1.3g Protein: 12.4 g

Roast Beef with Grilled Vegetables

Preparation time: 10 minutes
Cooking time: 30 minutes
Servings: 4
Ingredients:

500g Roast beef
1 clove Garlic (pressed)
1 teaspoon fresh rosemary 400g Broccoli
200g Carrot 400g Zucchini
4 tablespoons Olive oil

Directions:

Rub the roast beef with freshly ground pepper, salt, garlic and rosemary.

Heat a grill pan over high heat and grill the roast beef for about 20 minutes or until the meat shows nice brown marks on all sides. Then wrap in aluminum foil and let it rest for a while. Cut the roast beef into thin slices before serving.

Preheat the oven to 205 ° C. Put all the vegetables in a baking dish.

Drizzle the vegetables with a little olive oil and season with curry powder and / or chili flakes. Put in the oven and bake for 30 minutes or until the vegetables are done.

Nutrition:

Calories: 56 Fat: 3.6g Protein: 5.4g

Vegan Thai Green Curry

Preparation time: 20 minutes

Cooking time: 4 hours 15 minutes

Servings: 2

Ingredients:

2 pieces green chilies 1 piece Onion 1 clove Garlic

1 teaspoon fresh ginger (grated) 25g fresh coriander

1 teaspoon Ground caraway 1 piece Lime (juice)

1 teaspoon Coconut oil 500 ml Coconut milk

1 piece Zucchini

1 piece Broccoli

1 piece Red pepper

For the cauliflower rice:

1 teaspoon Coconut oil 1 piece Cauliflower

Directions:

For cauliflower rice, cut the cauliflower into florets and place in the food processor. Pulse briefly until rice has formed. Put aside.

Cut the green peppers, onions, garlic, fresh ginger and coriander into large pieces and combine with the caraway seeds and the juice of 1 lime in a food processor or blender and mix to an even paste.

Heat a pan over medium heat with a teaspoon of coconut oil and gently fry the pasta. Deglaze with coconut milk and add to the slow cooker.

Cut the zucchini into pieces, the broccoli in florets, the peppers into cubes and put in the slow cooker. Simmer for 4 hours.

Briefly heat the cauliflower rice in 1 teaspoon of coconut oil, season with a little salt and pepper in a pan over medium heat.

Nutrition:

Calories: 380 Fat: 10g Net Carbs: 44g Fiber: 5g Protein: 30g

Tofu with Cauliflower

Preparation Time: 5 Minutes

Cooking Time: 45 Minutes

Servings: 2

Ingredients:

¼ cup red pepper, seeded

1 Thai chili, cut in two halves, seeded 2 cloves of garlic

1 tsp of olive oil 1 pinch of cumin

1 pinch of coriander Juice of a half lemon 8oz tofu

8oz cauliflower, roughly chopped 1 ½oz red onions, finely chopped 1 tsp finely chopped ginger

2 teaspoons turmeric

1oz dried tomatoes, finely chopped 1oz parsley, chopped

Directions:

Preheat oven to 400 °F. Slice the peppers and put them in an ovenproof dish with chili and garlic.

Pour some olive oil over it, add the dried herbs and put it in the oven until the peppers are soft about 20 minutes).

Let it cool down, put the peppers together with the lemon juice in a blender and work it into a soft mass.
Cut the tofu in half and divide the halves into triangles.
Place the tofu in a small casserole dish, cover with the paprika mixtureand place in the oven for about 20 minutes.
Chop the cauliflower until the pieces are smaller than a grain of rice.
Then, in a small saucepan, heat the garlic, onions, chili and ginger with olive oil until they become transparent. Add turmeric and cauliflower mix well and heat again.
Remove from heat and add parsley and tomatoes mix well. Serve with the tofu in the sauce.

Nutrition Facts:
Calories 298kcal, Fat 5 g, Carbohydrate 55 g, Protein 27.5g

Lemongrass and Ginger Mackerel

Preparation Time: 10 minutes
Cooking Time: 25 minutes
Servings: 4
Ingredients:
4 mackerel fillets, skinless and boneless 2 tbsp. olive oil
1 tbsp. ginger, grated
2 lemongrass sticks, chopped 2 red chilies, chopped
Juice of 1 lime
A handful parsley, chopped
Directions:
In a roasting pan, combine the mackerel with the oil, ginger and the other ingredients, toss and bake at 390° F for 25 minutes. Divide between plates and serve.
Nutrition Facts:
Calories 251kcal, Fat 3.7 g, Carbohydrate 14 g, Protein 30g

Serrano Ham & Rocket Arugula

Preparation Time: 5 Minutes
Cooking Time: 60 Minutes
Servings: 2
Ingredients:
6oz Serrano ham
4oz rocket arugula leaves 2 tbsp. olive oil
1 tbsp. orange juice
Directions:
Pour the oil and juice into a bowl and toss the rocket arugula in the mixture. Serve the rocket onto plates and top it off with the ham.
Nutrition Facts:
Calories 220kcal, Fat 7 g, Carbohydrate 7 g, Protein 33.5g

Buckwheat with Mushrooms and Green Onions

Preparation Time: 10 minutes
Cooking Time: 40 minutes
Servings: 2
Ingredients:
1 cup buckwheat groats
2 cups vegetable or chicken broth 3 green onions, thinly sliced
1 cup mushrooms, sliced Salt and pepper to taste 2 tsp oil
Directions:
Combine all ingredients in a pot and cook on low heat for about 35-40min until the broth is completely absorbed.
Divide in two plates and serve immediately.
Nutrition Facts:
Calories 340kcal, Fat 10 g, Carbohydrate 51 g, Protein 11g

Sweet and Sour Pan with Cashew Nuts:

Preparation Time: 30 minutes
Cooking Time: 0 minutes
Servings: 2
Ingredients:
2 tbsp. Coconut oil 2 pieces Red onion
2 pieces yellow bell pepper
12oz White cabbage 6oz Pak choi
1 ½oz Mung bean sprouts
4 Pineapple slices 1 ½oz Cashew nuts
¼ cup Apple cider vinegar
4 tbsp. Coconut blossom sugar 11/2 tbsp. Tomato paste
1 tsp Coconut-Aminos
2 tsp Arrowroot powder
¼ cup Water
Directions:
Roughly cut the vegetables. Mix the arrow root with five tbsp. of cold water into a paste. Then put all the other ingredients for the sauce in a saucepan and add the arrowroot paste for binding.
Melt the coconut oil in a pan and fry the onion. Add the bell pepper, cabbage, pak choi and bean sprouts and stir-fry until the vegetables become a little softer.
Add the pineapple and cashew nuts and stir a few more times. Pour a little sauce over the wok dish and serve.
Nutrition Facts:
Calories: 573 kcal Fat: 27.81 g Carbohydrates: 77.91 g Protein: 15.25 g

Casserole with Spinach and Eggplant

Preparation Time: 1 hour
Cooking Time: 40 minutes
Servings: 2
Ingredients:
1 medium Eggplant
2 medium Onion 3 tbsp. Olive oil
3 cups Spinach, fresh 4 pieces Tomatoes
2 Eggs
¼ cup Almond milk, unsweetened 2 tsp Lemon juice
4 tbsp. Parmesan
Directions:
Preheat the oven to 400 ° F. Cut the eggplants, onions and tomatoes into slices and sprinkle salt on the eggplant slices. Brush the eggplants and onions with olive oil and fry them in a grill pan.
Cook spinach in a large saucepan over moderate heat and drain in a sieve. Put the vegetables in layers in a greased baking dish: first the eggplant, then the spinach and then the onion and the tomato.
Repeat this again. Whisk eggs with almond milk, lemon juice, salt and pepper and pour over the vegetables.
Sprinkle parmesan over the dish and bake in the oven for about 30 to 40
minutes.
Nutrition Facts:
Calories: 446 kcal Fat: 31.82 g Carbohydrates: 30.5 g Protein: 13.95 g

Vegetarian Curry

Preparation Time: 15 minutes
Time: 1 hour
Servings: 2
Ingredients:
4 medium Carrots
2 medium Sweet potatoes 1 large Onion
3 cloves Garlic
4 tbsp. Curry powder
½ tsp caraway, ground
½ tsp Chili powder Sea salt to taste
1 pinch Cinnamon
½ cup Vegetable broth 1 can Tomato cubes
8oz Sweet peas
2 tbsp. Tapioca flour

Directions:

Roughly chop carrots, sweet potatoes onions potatoes and garlic and put them all in a pot. Mix tapioca flour with curry powder, cumin, chili powder, salt and cinnamon and sprinkle this mixture on the vegetables.

Add tomato cubes. Pour the vegetable broth over it.

Close the pot with a lid, bring to a boil and let it simmer for 60 minutes on a low heat. Stir in snap peas after 30min. Cauliflower rice is a great addition to this dish.

Nutrition Facts:

Calories: 397 kcal Fat: 6.07 g Carbohydrates: 81.55 g Protein: 9.35 g

Fried Cauliflower Rice:

Preparation Time: 55 minutes
Cooking Time: 10 minutes
Servings: 2
Ingredients:

1 medium Cauliflower 2 tbsp. Coconut oil
1 medium Red onion
4 cloves Garlic
¼ cup Vegetable broth 2-inch fresh ginger
1 tsp Chili flakes 1/2 Carrot
1/2 Red bell pepper 1/2 Lemon, juiced
2 tbsp. Pumpkin seeds 2 tbsp. fresh coriander

Directions:

Cut the cauliflower into small rice grains using a food processor.

Finely chop the onion, garlic and ginger, cut the carrot into thin strips, dice the bell pepper and finely chop the herbs. Melt 1 tbsp. of coconut oil in a pan and add half of the onion and garlic to the pan and fry briefly until translucent.

Add cauliflower rice and season with salt. Pour in the broth and stir everything until it evaporates, and the cauliflower rice is tender. Take the rice out of the pan and set it aside. Melt the rest of the coconutoil in the pan and add the remaining onions, garlic, ginger, carrots and peppers.

Fry for a few minutes until the vegetables are tender. Season them with a little salt.

Add the cauliflower rice again, heat the whole dish and add the lemon juice.

Garnish with pumpkin seeds and coriander before serving.

Nutrition Facts:

Calories: 230 kcal Fat: 17.81 g Carbohydrates: 17.25 g, Protein: 5.13 g

Buckwheat with Onions

Preparation Time: 10 minutes
Cooking Time: 40 minutes
Servings: 4
Ingredients:

3 cups of buckwheat, rinsed
4 medium red onions, chopped 1 big white onion, chopped
5 oz. extra-virgin olive oil 3 cups of water
Salt and pepper, to taste

Direction:

Soak the buckwheat in the warm water for around 10 minutes. Then add in the buckwheat to your pot. Add in the water, salt and pepper to your pot and stir well.

Close the lid and cook for about 30-35 minutes until the buckwheat is ready. In the meantime, in a skillet, heat the extra-virgin olive oil and fry the chopped onions for 15 minutes until clear and caramelized.

Add some salt and pepper and mix well. Portion the buckwheat into four bowls or mugs. Then dollop each bowl with the onions. Remember that this dish should be served warm.

Nutrition Facts:

Calories: 132; Fat: 32g; Carbohydrates: 64g; Protein: 22g

Tuna, Egg & Caper Salad

Preparation Time: 5 Minutes
Cooking Time: 20 Minutes
Servings: 2
Ingredients:
3½ oz. red chicory
5oz tinned tuna, drained 3 ½ oz. cucumbers
1oz rocket arugula
6 black olives, pitted
2 hard-boiled eggs, quartered 2 tomatoes, chopped
2 tbsp. fresh parsley, chopped
1 red onion, chopped 1 stalk of celery
1 tbsp. capers
2 tbsp. extra virgin olive oil 1 tbsp. white vinegar
1 clove garlic, crushed
Directions:
Place the tuna, cucumber, olives, tomatoes, onion, chicory, celery, and parsley and rocket arugula into a bowl.
Combine olive oil, vinegar, garlic and a pinch of salt in a vinaigrette dressing.
Pour in the vinaigrette and toss the salad in the dressing. Serve onto plates and scatter the eggs and capers on top.
Nutrition Facts:
Calories: 309 kcal, Fat: 12.23 g, Carbohydrates: 25.76 g, Protein: 26.72 g

Dahl with Kale, Red Onions and Buckwheat

Preparation Time: 5 Minutes
Cooking Time: 20 Minutes
Servings: 2
Ingredients:
1 tsp. of extra virgin olive oil 1 tsp. of mustard seeds
1 ½ oz. red onions, finely chopped
1 clove of garlic, very finely chopped 1 tsp very finely chopped ginger
1 Thai chili, very finely chopped
1 tsp. curry powder 2 tsp. turmeric
10 fl. oz. vegetable broth 1 ½ oz. red lentils
1 ⅝ oz. kale, chopped
1.70 fl. oz. coconut milk 1 ⅝ oz. buckwheat
Directions:
Heat oil in a pan at medium temperature and add mustard seeds. When they crack, add onion, garlic, ginger and chili. Heat until everything is soft.
Add the curry powder and turmeric, mix well.
Add the vegetable stock, bring to the boil.
Add the lentils and cook them for 25 to 30 minutes until they are ready. Then add the kale and coconut milk and simmer for 5 minutes.
The dahl is ready. While the lentils are cooking, prepare the buckwheat. Serve buckwheat with the dahl.
Nutrition Facts:
Calories: 273 kcal Fat: 2.41 g Carbohydrates: 24.83 g Protein: 7.67 g

Miso Caramelized Tofu

Preparation Time: 55 minutes
Cooking Time: 15 minutes
Servings: 2
Ingredients:
1 tbsp. mirin
¾ oz. miso paste 5 ¼ oz. firm tofu
1 ½ oz. celery, trimmed 1 ¼ oz. red onion
4 ¼ oz. zucchini
1 bird's eye chili
1 garlic clove, finely chopped
1 tsp. fresh ginger, finely chopped 1 ⅝ oz. kale, chopped
2 tsp. sesame seeds 1 ¼ oz. buckwheat
1 tsp. ground turmeric
2 tsp. extra virgin olive oil 1 tsp. tamari (or soy sauce)

Directions

Pre-heat your over to 400°F. Cover a tray with parchment paper the mirin and miso together. Dice the tofu and let it marinate it in the mirin-miso mixture. Chop the vegetables (except for the kale) at a diagonal angle to produce long slices.

Using a steamer, cook for the kale for 5 minutes and set aside. Disperse the tofu across the lined tray and garnish with sesame seeds. Roast for 20 minutes, or until caramelized. Rinse the buckwheat using running water and a sieve.

Add to a pan of boiling water alongside turmeric and cook the buckwheat according to the packet instructions.

Heat the oil in a skillet over high heat. Toss in the vegetables, herbs and spices then fry for 2-3 minutes. Reduce to a medium heat and fry for a further 5 minutes or until cooked but still crunchy.

Nutrition Facts:

Calories: 101 kcal Fat: 4.7 g Carbohydrates: 12.38 g Protein: 4.22 g

Sirtfood Cauliflower Couscous & Turkey Steak

Preparation Time: 45 minutes

Cooking Time: 10 minutes

Servings: 2

Ingredients:

5 ¼ oz. cauliflower, roughly chopped 1 garlic clove, finely chopped

1 ½ oz. red onion, finely chopped 1 bird's eye chili, finely chopped 1 tsp. fresh ginger, finely chopped 2 tbsp. extra virgin olive oil

2 tsp. ground turmeric

1 oz. sun dried tomatoes, finely chopped

⅜ oz. parsley

5 ¼ oz. turkey steaks 1 tsp. dried sage

½ lemon, juiced 1 tbsp. capers

Directions:

Put the cauliflower using in the food processor and blend it in 1-2 pulses until it has a breadcrumb-like consistency.

In a skillet, fry garlic, chili, ginger and red onion in 1 tsp. olive oil for 2-3 minutes.

Throw in the turmeric and cauliflower then cook for another 1-2 minutes. Remove from heat and add tomatoes and parsley. Marinate the turkey steak with sage, capers, lemon juice and olive oil for 10 minutes..

In a skillet, over medium heat, fry the turkey steak, turning occasionally. Serve with the couscous.

Nutrition Facts:

Calories: 462 kcal Fat: 39.86 g Carbohydrates: 9.94 g Protein: 16.81 g

Mushroom & Tofu Scramble

Preparation Time: 30 minutes

Cooking Time: 15 minutes

Servings: 1

Ingredients:

3 ½ oz. tofu, extra firm 1 tsp. ground turmeric

1 tsp. mild curry powder

¾ oz. kale, roughly chopped 1 tsp. extra virgin olive oil

¾ oz. red onion, thinly sliced

1 ⅝ oz. mushrooms, thinly sliced

A few parsley leaves, finely chopped

Directions:

Place 2 sheets of kitchen towel under and on-top of the tofu, then rest a considerable weight such as saucepan onto the tofu, to ensure it drains off the liquid.

Combine the curry powder, turmeric and 1-2 tsp. of water to form a paste. Using a steamer, cook kale for 3-4 minutes.

In a skillet, warm oil over a medium heat. Add the chili, mushrooms and onion, cooking for several minutes or until brown and tender.

Break the tofu in to small pieces and toss in the skillet. Coat with the spice paste and stir, ensuring everything becomes evenly coated. Cook for up to 5 minutes, or until the tofu has browned then add the kale
and fry for 2 more minutes. Garnish with parsley before serving.

Nutrition Facts:

Calories: 333 kcal Fat: 22.89 g Carbohydrates: 18.8 g Protein: 20.9 g

Prawn & Chili Pak Choi

Preparation Time: 30 minutes
Cooking Time: 15 minutes
Servings: 1

Ingredients:

2 ¼ oz. brown rice 1 pak choi
2 fl. oz. chicken stock
1 tbsp. extra virgin olive oil
1 garlic clove, finely chopped
1 ⅝ oz. red onion, finely chopped
½ bird's eye chili, finely chopped 1 tsp. freshly grated ginger
4 ¼ oz. raw king prawns 1 tbsp. soy sauce
1 tsp. five-spice
1 tbsp. freshly chopped flat-leaf parsley

Directions:

Bring a medium sized saucepan of water to the boil and cook the brown rice for 25-30 minutes, or until softened.

Tear the pak choi into pieces. Warm the chicken stock in a skillet over medium heat and toss in the pak choi, cooking until the pak choi has slightly wilted.

In another skillet, warm olive oil over high heat. Toss in the ginger, chili, red onions and garlic frying for 2-3 minutes.

Put in the prawns, five-spice and soy sauce and cook for 6-8 minutes, or until the cooked. Drain the brown rice and add to the skillet, stirring and cooking for 2-3 minutes. Add the pak choi, garnish with parsley and serve.

Nutrition Facts:

Calories 403 kcal Fat: 15.28 g Carbohydrates: 50.87 g Protein: 16.15 g

Smoky Bean And Tempeh Patties

Preparation Time: 20 minutes
Cooking Time: 30 minutes
Servings: 4

Ingredients:

1 cup cooked cannellini beans 8 oz. tempeh
'¼ cup cooked bulgur
2 cloves garlic, pressed
¼ tsp onion powder 1 tsp liquid smoke
4 tsp Worcestershire sauce 1 tsp smoked paprika
2 tbsp. organic ketchup 2 tbsp. maple syrup
2 tbsp. neutral-flavored oil 3 tbsp. tamari.
¼ cup chickpea flour Nonstick cooking spray

Directions:

Mash the beans in a large bowl: it's okay if a few small pieces of beans are left. Crumble the tempeh into small pieces on top. Add the bulgur and garlic.

In a medium bowl, whisk together the remaining ingredients, except the flour and cooking spray. Stir into the crumbled tempeh preparation. Add the flour and mix until well combined. Chill for 1 hour before shaping into patties.

Preheat the oven to 350°F. Line a baking tray with parchment paper. Scoop out 1/3 cup per patty, shaping into an approximately 3-inch circle and flattening slightly on the tray. You should get eight 3.5-inch patties in all. Lightly coat the top of the patties with cooking spray. Bake for 15 minutes, carefully flip, and lightly coat the top of the patties with cooking spray and bake for another 15 minutes until lightly browned and firm.

Leftovers can be stored in an airtight container in the refrigerator for up to 4 days.

The patties can also be frozen, tightly wrapped in foil, for up to 3 months. If you don't eat all the patties at once, reheat the leftovers on low heat in a skillet lightly greased with olive oil or cooking spray for about 5 minutes on each side until heated through.

Nutrition Facts:

Calories: 200kcal, Fat: 9g, Carbohydrate: 18g, Protein: 14g

Tomato & Goat's Cheese Pizza

Preparation Time: 5 Minutes + 2 hours
Cooking Time: 50 Minutes
Servings: 2
Ingredients:

8oz buckwheat flour 2 tsp. dried yeast Pinch of salt
5fl oz. slightly water 1 tsp. olive oil
3oz feta cheese, crumbled
3oz passata or tomato paste 1 tomato, sliced
1 medium red onion, finely chopped 1oz rocket leaves, chopped

Directions:

In a bowl, combine all the ingredients for the pizza dough then allow it to stand for at least two hours until it has doubled in size.

Roll the dough out to a size to suit you. Spoon the passata onto the base and add the rest of the toppings. Bake in the oven at 400F for 15-20 minutes or until browned at the edges and crispy and serve.

Nutrition Facts:

Calories: 417kcal Fat: 16g Carbohydrate: 50g Protein: 16g

Cashew Raita

Preparation Time: 10 minutes + 1 day
Cooking Time: 45 minutes
Servings: 12
Ingredients:
For the cashew base:

1 cup raw cashew pieces
¼ cup water, plus more to soak cashews, divided
¼ cup coconut cream
2 tbsp. fresh lemon juice
1 English cucumber, chopped

For the raita:

1 recipe cashew base
3 tbsp. fresh mint leaves 3 tbsp. fresh parsley
3 tbsp. fresh cilantro
2 cloves garlic, crushed
1 tsp organic lemon zest and juice

Direction:

To make the cashew base: Place the cashews in a medium bowl and cover with water.

Cover with plastic wrap, or a lid, and let stand at room temperature overnight (or about 8 hours) to soften. Drain the cashews and rinse. Put in a high-speed food processor with a cup of water, coconut cream, lemon juice, and salt.

To keep it soft, occasionally scrape the sides with a rubber spatula. This may take up to 10 minutes, depending on the power of the device. Put the cashew paste to container covered with a lid and let it sit for 24 hours at room temperature.

You will obtain a yogurt-like consistency.Chop the cucumber finely and let it rest a few minutes with a pinch of salt ultil it releases part of its water. Drain it, add the remaining ingredients and mix.

Adjust seasonings if necessary. Refrigerate for at least 2 hours or overnight to allow the flavors to melt. Leftovers can be stored in the fridge up to 4 days.

Nutrition Facts:

Calories: 129.1. Fat 8.2 g Carbohydrate 13.1 g Protein 3.7 g

Green Beans With Crispy Chickpeas

Preparation Time: 30 minutes
Cooking Time: 10 minutes
Servings: 4
Ingredients:
1 can chickpeas, rinsed 1 tsp. whole coriander
1 lb. green beans, trimmed
2 tbsp. olive oil, divided
Kosher salt and freshly ground black pepper
1 tsp. cumin seeds
Grilled lemons, for serving
Directions
Heat grill to medium. Gather chickpeas, coriander, cumin, and 1 tbsp. oil in a medium cast-iron skillet. Put skillet on grill and cook chickpeas, mixing occasionally, until golden brown and coriander begins to pop, 5 to 6 minutes. Season with salt and pepper.
Transfer to a bowl. Add green beans and remaining tbsp. olive oil to the skillet. Add salt and pepper. Cook, turning once, until charred and barely tender, 3 to 4 minutes.
Toss green beans with chickpea mixture and serve with grilled lemons alongside.
Nutrition Facts:
Calories: 460 Fat: 15g Carbs: 57g Protein: 16g

Sloppy Joe Scramble Stuffed Spuds

Preparation Time: 25 minutes
Cooking Time: 50 minutes
Servings: 6 potato halves
Ingredients:
1 tbsp. high heat neutral-flavored oil
1 pound extra-firm tofu, drained, pressed, and crumbled
¼ tsp fine sea salt
¼ tsp ground black pepper
¾ cup onion, finely chopped
¼ cup bell pepper (any color), finely chopped
3 cloves garlic, finely chopped
1 tbsp. ground cumin
2 tsp chili powder, or to taste 1 can (15 oz.) tomato sauce 2 tbsp. organic ketchup
1 tbsp. tamari
1 tbsp. Worcestershire sauce 1 tbsp. yellow mustard
1 4-inch dill pickle, minced
¾ cup water
3 baked potatoes, cooled 1 tbsp. olive oil
Directions:
Heat 1 tbsp. of oil in a large skillet over medium-high heat. If the skillet is not well-seasoned, add the remaining tbsp. of oil.
Add the tofu, salt, and pepper. Cook for 8 to 10 minutes, occasionally stirring until the tofu is firm and golden. Stir in the onion, bell pepper, garlic, cumin, and chili powder.
Reduce the heat to medium and cook for 3 minutes, occasionally stirring, until fragrant.
Add the tomato sauce, ketchup, tamari, Worcestershire sauce, mustard, and dill pickle. Bring to a boil, and then reduce the heat to simmer. Swish the water in the tomato sauce can to clean the sides.
Simmer for 30 minutes, occasionally stirring, adding the water from the tomato sauce can. As needed for the desired consistency. Preheat the oven to broil. Cut the baked potatoes in half lengthwise.
Scoop the insides from the potatoes, leaving about 1 inch of the skin intact.
Brush both the insides and the outsides of the potato skins with the olive oil and place them on a baking sheet.
Broil for 3 to 4 minutes until lightly browned. Remove from the oven and divide the filling evenly in the potatoes, using about ¼ cup in each.
Nutrition Facts:
Calories: 306 Fat: 21g Carbohydrate: 6g Protein: 23g

Baked Salmon Salad With Creamy Mint Dressing

Preparation Time: 20 minutes
Cooking Time: 25 minutes
Servings: 1
Ingredients:
1 salmon fillet
1 cup mixed salad leaves 1 cup lettuce leaves
Two radishes, thinly sliced
½ cucumber, sliced
2 spring onions, trimmed and chopped
½ oz. parsley, roughly sliced
For the dressing:
1 tsp low-carb mayonnaise 1 tbsp. natural yogurt
1 tbsp. rice vinegar
2 stalks mint, finely chopped
Directions:
Put the salmon fillet onto a baking tray and bake for 16--18 minutes until cooked
In a bowl, blend together the mayonnaise, yogurt, rice vinegar, mint leaves and salt and set aside 5 minutes to the flavors to mix well.
Arrange the salad leaves and lettuce onto a serving plate and top with all
the radishes, cucumber, lettuce, celery, spring onions and parsley. Drizzle the dressing.
Nutrition Facts:
Calories: 433 Fat: 9g Carbohydrate: 32g Protein: 18g

Fragrant Asian Hot Pot

Preparation Time: 15 minutes
Cooking Time: 25 minutes
Servings: 2
Ingredients:
1 tsp tomato purée 1 star anise, crushed
½ oz. parsley, finely chopped
½ oz. coriander, finely chopped Juice of 1/2 lime
2 cups chicken stock
½ carrot, cut into matchsticks
½ cup cauliflower cut into small florets 2oz beansprouts
4oz raw tiger prawns
2oz rice noodles, cooked as per packet directions 2oz cooked water chestnuts, drained
20g sushi ginger, sliced 1 tbsp. high miso paste
Directions:
Set the tomato purée, star anise, parsley stalks, coriander stalks, lime juice and chicken stock in a large pan and bring to a simmer for about 10 minutes.
Add the beansprouts, cauliflower, carrot, prawns, tofu, noodles and water
chestnuts and simmer gently until the prawns are cooked.
Remove from the heat and stir at the skillet along with miso paste. Serve sprinkled with the parsley and coriander leaves.
Nutrition Facts:
Calories: 397 Fat: 15g Carbohydrate: 33g Protein: 19g

Tofu Scramble With Mushrooms

Preparation Time: 15 minutes
Cooking Time: 10 minutes
Servings: 2
Ingredients:
3 tbsp. olive oil
½ yellow onion, diced
3 cloves garlic, finely chopped 1 tsp. soy sauce
12oz firm tofu, cubed
½ red bell pepper, diced
¾ cup mushrooms, cut 3 green onions, diced
2 tomatoes, cleaved
½ tsp. ground ginger
½ tsp. bean stew powder
¼ tsp. cayenne pepper Salt and pepper to taste

Directions:
Gently sauté onion and garlic in the olive oil for 3 to 5 minutes, until they are soft. Add the remaining ingredients, except salt and pepper. Sautee for another 6 to 8 minutes, until veggies are done and tofu absorbed the liquid. Add salt and pepper, to taste.
Nutrition Facts:
Calories: 330 Fat: 9g Carbohydrate: 36g Protein: 18g

Prawn Arrabbiata

Preparation Time: 40 minutes
Cooking Time: 60 minutes
Servings: 1
Ingredients:
5oz raw prawns
2oz Buckwheat pasta
1 tbsp. extra virgin olive oil
½ Red onion, finely chopped 1 Garlic clove, finely chopped 1oz Celery, thinly sliced
1 Bird's eye chili, thinly sliced 1 tsp Dried mixed herbs
1 tsp extra virgin olive oil 2 tbsp. White wine
½ tin chopped tomatoes 1 tbsp. Chopped parsley
Directions:
Fry the garlic, onion, celery and herbs in oil on low heat for 1--2 minutes. Turn up the heat to medium, add the wine and cook until evaporated Add the tomatoes and leave the sauce simmer for 20--30 minutes, until it will reduce and get a rich texture.
While the sauce is cooking bring some water to the boil and cook the pasta
as per the package directions. When cooked, drain it and put it aside.
Put prawns into the sauce and cook for a further 3--4 minutes, till they've turned opaque and pink, then add the parsley and the cooked pasta into the sauce, mix and serve.
Nutrition Facts:
Calories: 335 Fat: 12g Carbohydrate: 38g Protein: 19g

Turmeric Baked Salmon

Preparation Time: 15 minutes
Cooking Time: 30 minutes
Servings: 1
Ingredients:
6 oz. Salmon fillet, skinned 1 tsp. extra virgin olive oil 1 tsp. Ground turmeric
¼ lemon, juiced
For the sauce:
1 tsp. extra virgin olive oil
1 oz. Red onion, finely chopped 1 oz. Tinned green peas
1 Garlic clove, finely chopped
1-inch fresh ginger, finely chopped 1 Bird's eye chili, thinly sliced
4 oz. Celery cut into small cubes
1 tsp Mild curry powder 1 Tomato, chopped
½ cup vegetable stock
1 tbsp. parsley, chopped
Directions:
Heat the oven to 400°F. Start cooking the sauce. Heat a skillet over a moderate --low heat, then add the olive oil then the garlic, onion, ginger, chili, celery.
Stir lightly for two --3 minutes until softened but not colored, then add the curry powder and cook for a further minute. Put in tomato, green peas and stock and simmer for 10/15 minutes depending on how thick you enjoy your sauce. Meanwhile, combine turmeric, oil and lemon juice and rub the salmon. Put on a baking tray and cook for 10 minutes in the oven. Serve the salmon with the celery sauce.
Nutrition Facts:
Calories: 360 Fat: 8g Carbs: 10g Protein: 40g

Baked Potatoes With Spicy Chickpea Stew

Preparation Time: 10 minutes
Cooking Time: 60 minutes
Servings: 4
Ingredients:
4 baking potatoes, pricked around 2 tbsp. olive oil
2 red onions, finely chopped
4 tsp. garlic, crushed or grated 1-inch ginger, grated
1/2 tsp chili flakes
2 tbsp. cumin seeds 2 tbsp. turmeric Splash of water
2 tins chopped tomatoes
2 tbsp. cocoa powder, unsweetened 2 tins chickpeas – do not drain
2 yellow peppers, chopped 2 tbsp.
Directions:
Preheat the oven to 400F; and start preparing all ingredients. When the oven is ready, put in baking potatoes and cook for 50min-1 hour until they are done.
While potatoes are cooking, put olive oil and sliced red onion into a large
wide saucepan and cook lightly, using the lid, for 5 minutes until the onions are tender but not brown.
Remove the lid and add ginger, garlic, cumin and cook for a further minute on a very low heat. Then add the turmeric and a tiny dab of water and cook for a few more minutes until it becomes thicker and the consistency is ok.
Then add tomatoes, cocoa powder, peppers, chickpeas with their water and salt. Bring to the boil, and then simmer on a very low heat for 45-50 minutes until it's thick. Finally stir in the 2 tbsp. of parsley, and some pepper and salt if you desire, and also serve the stew with the potatoes.
Nutrition Facts:
Calories: 520 Fat: 8g Carbohydrate: 91g Protein: 32g

Kale And Red Onion Dhal With Buckwheat

Preparation Time: 5 minutes
Cooking Time: 35 minutes
Servings: 4
Ingredients:
1 tbsp. olive oil
1 small red onion, sliced
3 garlic cloves, crushed or grated 2-inch ginger, grated
1 bird's eye chili deseeded, chopped 2 tsp. turmeric
2 tsp. garam masala 6oz snow peas
2 cups coconut milk, unsweetened 1 cup water
1 cup carrot, thinly sliced 6oz buckwheat
Directions:
Place the olive oil into a large, deep skillet and then add the chopped onion. Cook on a very low heat, with the lid for 5 minutes until softened.
Add the ginger, garlic and chili and cook 1 minute. Add turmeric and garam masala along with a dash of water and then cook for 1 minute.
Insert the snow peas, coconut milk and 1 cup water. Mix everything
together and cook for 20 minutes on low heat with the lid. Stir occasionally and add a bit more water if the dhal begins to stick.
After 20 minutes add the carrot, stir thoroughly and cook for a further 5 minutes.
While the dhal is cooking, steam the buckwheat in salted boiling water for 15 minutes, drain it and serve it with the dhal.
Nutrition Facts:
Calories: 340 Fat: 4g Carbohydrate: 30g Protein: 4g

Kale, Edamame And Tofu Curry

Preparation Time: 30 minutes
Cooking Time: 45 minutes
Servings: 4
Ingredients:
1 tbsp. oil - 1 big onion, chopped
4 cloves garlic, peeled and grated
1 3-inch fresh ginger, peeled and grated 1 red chili, deseeded and thinly sliced 1/2 tsp. ground turmeric
1/4 tsp. cayenne pepper 1 tsp. paprika
1/2 tsp. ground cumin 1 tsp. salt
8 oz. dried red lentils
2 oz. soya edamame beans 8 oz. firm tofu, cubed
2 tomatoes, roughly chopped
Juice of 1 lime
½ cup parsley, stalks removed
Directions:
Put the oil in a pan on medium heat. When the oil is hot, add the onion and cook 5 minutes. Add ginger, garlic and chili and cook for further 2 minutes. Add turmeric, cayenne, paprika, cumin and salt. Stir and add red lentils, soya edamame beans and tomatoes. Pour in 4 cups boiling water and then bring to a simmer for about 10 minutes, then lower the heat and cook for a further 40 minutes until the curry becomes thicker and all flavors are blended together. Add lime juice and parsley, stir and serve.
Nutrition Facts:
Calories: 325 Fat: 6g Carbs: 77g Protein: 28g

Lemon Chicken With Spinach, Red Onion, And Salsa

Preparation Time: 30 minutes
Cooking Time: 35 minutes
Servings: 1
Ingredients:
4oz chicken breast, skinless, boneless 1 large tomato
1 chili, finely chopped
1oz capers
Juice of 1/2 lemon
2 tbsp. extra-virgin olive oil 2 cups spinach
20g red onion, chopped
2 tsp chopped garlic 3oz buckwheat
Directions:
Heat the oven to 400°F.To make the salsa, chop the tomato very finely and put it with its liquid in a bowl. The liquid is very important because it's very tasty.
Mix with chili, capers, onion, 1tbsp oil and some drops of lemon juice. Marinate the chicken breast with garlic, lemon juice and ½tbsp oil for 10 minutes.
Heat an ovenproof skillet until warm, add the chicken and cook for a minute on every side, until light gold, then move to the oven (put on a
baking tray if your pan is not ovenproof) for 5 minutes until cooked.
Remove from the oven, and cover with foil. Leave to rest for 5 minutes before serving. Meanwhile, sauté the spinach for 5 minutes with ½tbsp oil and 1tbsp garlic. Serve alongside chicken with salsa and spinach.
Nutrition Facts:
Calories: 342 Fat: 8g Carbs: 18g Protein: 33g

Smoked Salmon Omelet

Preparation Time: 10 minutes
Cooking Time: 15 minutes
Servings: 1
Ingredients:
2 eggs
4oz Smoked salmon, chopped 1/2 tsp. Capers
½ cup Rocket, chopped 1 tsp Parsley, chopped
1 tsp extra virgin olive oil

Directions:
Crack the eggs into a bowl and whisk well. Add the salmon, capers, rocket and parsley. Heat the olive oil in a skillet.
Add the egg mixture and, with a spatula, move the mix round the pan until it's even.
Reduce the heat and allow the omelet cook. Twist the spatula around the edges to lift them, add salmon and rocket and fold the omelet in 2.
Nutrition Facts:
Calories: 303 Fat: 22g Carbohydrate: 12g Protein: 23g

Broccoli And Pasta

Preparation Time: 20 minutes
Cooking Time: 10 minutes
Servings: 2
Ingredients:
5 oz. spaghetti
5 oz. broccoli
1 garlic clove, finely chopped 3 tbsp. extra virgin olive oil
2 Shallots sliced
¼ tsp. crushed chilies 12 sage shredded leaves
Grated parmesan (optional)
Directions:
Put broccoli in boiling water for 5 minute, then add spaghetti and cook until both pasta and broccoli are done (around 8 to 10 minutes).
In the meantime, heat the oil in a frying pan and add shallots and garlic. Cook for 5 minutes until it becomes golden.
Mix chilies and sage to the pan and gently cook for more 1 minute. Drain pasta and broccoli; mix with the shallot mixture in the pan, add some Parmesan, if desired and serve.
Nutrition Facts:
Calories: 350 Fat: 8g Carbs: 38g Protein: 6g

Artichokes and Kale with Walnuts

Preparation Time: 10 minutes
Cooking Time: 30 minutes
Servings: 2
Ingredients:
1 cup of artichoke hearts 1 tbsp. parsley, chopped
½ cup of walnuts
1 cup of kale, torn
1 cup of Cheddar cheese, crumbled
½ tbsp. balsamic vinegar 1 tbsp. olive oil
Salt and black pepper, to taste
Directions:
Preheat the oven to 250°-270°Fahrenheit and roast the walnuts in the oven for 10 minutes until lightly browned and crispy and then set aside.
Add artichoke hearts, kale, oil, salt and pepper to a pot and cook for 20-25 minutes until done.
Add cheese and balsamic vinegar and stir well. Divide the vegetables in two plates and garnish with roasted walnuts and parsley.
Nutrition Facts:
Calories: 152 kcal; Fat: 32g; Carbohydrates: 59g; Protein: 23g

Pecan Crusted Chicken Breast

Preparation Time: 20 minutes
Cooking Time: 35 minutes
Servings: 4
Ingredients:
½ cup whole wheat bread, dried 1/3 cup pecans
2 tbsp. Parmesan
Salt and ground pepper 1 egg white
4 chicken breasts slices, boneless and skinless (6 to 8 oz. each)
1 tbsp. grapeseed oil Lemon cuts, for serving
1 cup mixed greens 1tbsp olive oil

Directions:
Preheat oven to 425°F. In a food processor, blitz bread, pecans and Parmesan; season with salt and pepper until you get thin breadcrumbs.
Move to a bowl. In another bowl, beat egg white until foamy. Season chicken with salt and pepper. Coat each chicken breast slice with egg white first, then put it in the breadcrumb bowl and mix until completely covered.
In a large nonstick ovenproof skillet heat grapeseed oil over medium heat. When hot, put in chicken breasts cook until gently seared, 1 to 3 minutes.
Turn chicken over and put the skillet in the oven. Cook until chicken is
done (around 8 to 12 minutes). Serve chicken with lemon cuts and a plate of mixed greens with olive oil lemon and salt.
Nutrition Facts:
Calories: 250 Fat: 8g Carbohydrates: 27g Protein: 17g

Tuna And Tomatoes

Preparation Time: 5 minutes
Cooking Time: 20 minutes
Servings: 4
Ingredients:
1 yellow onion, chopped 1 tbsp. olive oil
1 lb. tuna fillets, skinless and cubed
1 cup tomatoes, chopped 1 red pepper, chopped
1 tsp sweet paprika
1 tbsp. coriander, chopped
Directions:
Heat up a pan with the oil over medium heat, add the onions and thepepper and cook for 5 minutes, they have to be crispy and crunchy: don't overcook.
Add tuna, tomato and paprika and quickly cook 1 minute on high heat. Add coriander and serve immediately..
Nutrition Facts:
Calories 215 kcal, Fat 4g, Carbs 14g, Protein 7g

Tuna And Kale

Preparation Time: 5 minutes
Cooking Time: 20 minutes
Servings: 4
Ingredients:
1lb tuna fillets, skinless and cubed A pinch of salt and black pepper
2 tbsp. olive oil
1 cup kale
½ cup cherry tomatoes, cubed 1 yellow onion, chopped
Directions:
Steam kale for 6 minutes, drizzle 1tbsp olive it and a pinch of salt and mix well.
Heat up a pan with the remaining oil over medium heat; add the onion and sauté for 5 minutes.
Add tuna and cherry tomatoes and cook for 5 minutes. Serve the tuna with the kale on the side.
Nutrition Facts:
Calories 251 kcal, Fat 4g, Carbohydrate 14g, Protein 7g

Salmon & Kale Omelet

Preparation Time: 10 minutes
Cooking Time: 7 minutes
Servings: 4
Ingredients:
6 eggs
2 tbsp. almond milk, unsweetened Salt and ground black pepper, to taste 2 tbsp. olive oil
4 oz. smoked salmon, cut into bite-sized chunks

2 cup fresh kale, tough ribs removed and chopped finely 4 scallions, chopped finely

Directions:

In a bowl, put eggs, almond milk, salt, and black pepper, and whisk well. Set aside.

In a non-stick skillet, heat the oil over medium heat.

Place a scoop of egg mixture, distribute it evenly by rotating the skillet and cook for about 1 minute.

Place salmon kale and scallions on top of egg mixture evenly. Reduce heat to low and cook for about 4–5 minutes, or until omelet is done completely.

Carefully, transfer the omelet onto a serving plate and serve.

Nutrition Facts:

Calories 210 kcal Fat 14.9 g Carbohydrates 5.2 g Protein 14.8 g

Moroccan Spiced Eggs

Preparation Time: 1 hour
Cooking Time: 50 minutes
Servings: 2
Ingredients:

1 tsp. olive oil
1 shallot, finely chopped
1 red bell pepper, finely chopped 1 garlic clove, finely chopped
1 zucchini, finely chopped 1 tbsp. tomato paste
½ tsp. mild curry
¼ tsp. ground cinnamon
¼ tsp. ground cumin
½ tsp. salt
1 can tomatoes
1 can chickpeas, drained 1/3oz parsley
4 medium eggs at room temperature

Directions:

Heat the oil in a pan; include the shallot and red bell pepper and fry on low heat for 5 minutes. Add garlic and zucchini and cook for 2 minutes. Add tomato paste, spices and salt and stir well.

Add tomatoes and chickpeas and bring to a medium heat. Put a lid on and simmer for 30 minutes until thicker. Remove from heat and add chopped parsley. Preheat the grill to 350F.

Put the tomato sauce up into a cooking tray and crack the eggs in the middle. Put the tray under the grill for 10 minutes and serve.

Nutrition Facts:

Calories: 316 kcal Fat: 5.22 g Carbohydrates: 13.14 g Protein: 6.97 g

Chickpea, Quinoa And Turmeric Curry Recipe

Preparation Time: 10 minutes
Cooking Time: 1 hour
Servings: 4
Ingredients:

1lb potatoes
3 garlic cloves, squashed 3 tsp ground turmeric
1 tsp ground coriander 1 tsp mild curry
1 tsp ground ginger
2 cups coconut milk, unsweetened 1 tbsp. tomato purée
1 can of tomatoes 6oz quinoa
1 can chickpeas, drained 2 cups spinach

Directions:

Put the potatoes in a pan, covered in cold water and bring to the boil, then cook for 25 minutes they are soft (always check with a stick). Drain them well, remove the skin and put them a side.

Put garlic, turmeric, coriander, bean stew, ginger, coconut milk, tomato purée and tomatoes in a skillet. Bring to the boil, season with salt and pepper; at that point include the quinoa with an additional cup water.

Put on low heat, put a lid on and let simmer for 30 minutes, stirring occasionally. Halfway

through cooking, put in the chickpeas. When there are only 5 minutes left, put in the spinach and potatoes, roughly chopped.
Split in 4 portions and serve immediately.

Nutrition Facts:

Calories: 609 kcal Fat: 12.15 g Carbohydrates: 85.27 Protein: 23.04 g

Chili Sweetcorn And Wild Garlic Fritters

Preparation Time: 5 min
Cooking Time: 10 min
Servings: 4

Ingredients:

¾ cup Self-rising flour
2 cups Tinned or frozen sweetcorn 3 Medium free-range eggs
1 Red chili, finely chopped
Fry-light extra virgin olive oil spray
¾ cup Wild garlic leaves and bulbs, finely diced 2 cups lettuce, chopped

Direction:

Mix the eggs, flour, chili, diced wild garlic and sweetcorn in a bowl, season with the pepper and the salt.
Spray a large non-stick fry pan and put it on medium heat.
Use a spoon to scoop the egg mixture into the fry pan batch by batch. The mixture will give you two large fritters per person or four small fritters.
Fry the pancakes for about four minutes on one side, and then gently turn it to the other side and fry for another 3 min until it is set and golden brown.
Serve immediately with salad.

Nutrition Facts:

Calories: 198 Fat: 7g Carbohydrates: 30g Protein: 3g

Roast Mackerel And Simple Veggies

Preparation Time: 5 min
Cooking Time: 25 min
Servings: 4

Ingredients:

2oz Pitted black olives 2 Leeks, chopped
7oz Cherry tomatoes
2 Sweet potatoes, chopped 1tbsp extra virgin olive oil 1 Lemon, juiced
11oz Mackerel fillets
¼ pint Vegetable stock

Directions:

Heat your oven to 375 degrees F. Place the chopped leeks and sweet potatoes in a roasting tray. Pour the vegetable stock over them and drizzle with the extra virgin oil.
Place the tray in the oven to roast for about 15 to 20 minutes.
Take out of the oven, add the black olives, cherry tomatoes, and mackerel fillets, and then squeeze the lemon juice all over. Return to the oven to roast other 10 minutes.
Serve immediately.

Nutrition Facts:

Calories: 374 Fat: 12g Carbohydrate: 48g Protein: 17g

Baked Root Veg With Chili

Preparation Time: 20 minutes
Cooking Time: 50 minutes
Servings: 4

Ingredients:

3 medium Potatoes
3 medium Sweet potatoes 3 small Yam
2 cups Vegetable broth 1 can Red kidney beans
1 can White kidney beans
2 cans Diced tomatoes 1 can Black beans
1 tbsp. Dried oregano 2 tbsp. Paprika
1 tsp Cumin
2 tsp Chili powder 2 stalks Celery

2 medium Carrots
1 Bell pepper
2 Red onions
3 tbsp. Olive oil
½ oz. Cilantro
2 Avocados
1 Bay leaf
1 can Sweet corn 2 Tomatoes
2 Limes, juiced
1 head Romaine

Directions:

Scrub and fork the potatoes and yams. Drizzle them with oil. Sprinkle with salt and put on a baking tray for 45 minutes or until you can pierce easily with a knife.

Heat the oil in a frying pan on medium heat and add the diced onion with the chopped bell pepper, diced carrots, and celery along with a quarter tsp of salt.

Cook until the carrot is tender then add the paprika, oregano, cumin, and chili powder.

Put in tomato, the bay leaf, and the vegetable broth. Rinse the beans and drain well before adding to the pot.

Stir well and leave to simmer for a further 30 minutes. After this time has passed, get a potato masher and mash the chili a few times to crush part of the beans and thicken the mixture.

Add the juice of one lime, and salt and pepper to taste. In a bowl, finely dice the avocado and lightly mash with salt, pepper and the juice of another lime.

In another bowl, drain and rinse the corn and toss in cilantro, finely chopped, shredded romaine lettuce a pinch of salt and a tbsp. olive oil. Serve potatoes, chili, avocado and salad so that everyone can assemble his/her masterpiece. Enjoy!

Nutrition Facts:

Calories: 493kcal; Fat: 14g; Carbohydrates: 96g Protein: 14g;

Autumn Stuffed Enchiladas

Preparation Time: 35 minutes
Cooking Time: 50 minutes
Servings: 2
Ingredients:

1 Lemon, juiced
1 cup raw Cashews
½ oz. Cilantro
1 oz. Roasted pumpkin seeds 12 Corn tortillas
2 cups Butternut squash
1 cup Salsa
1 can Black beans 2 tbsp. Olive oil
¼ tbsp. Cayenne pepper
1 tsp Chili flakes 1 tsp Cumin
3 cloves Garlic
1 Jalapeno
1 Red onion
1 cup Brussel sprouts

Directions:

Soak the cashews in boiling water and set aside.

Cut the squash in half and after scooping out the seeds; lightly rub olive oil. Sprinkle with a little salt and pepper before putting on a baking sheet face down. Cook for about forty-five minutes at 400F until it is cooked. Heat one tbsp. olive oil in a pan on medium heat and put chopped onion in, stirring until soft. Finely dice the jalapeno and garlic and finely slice the Brussel sprouts. Add these three things to the fry pan and cook until the Brussels begin to wilt through.

Strain and rinse the black beans then add them to the fry pan and mix well.

When the squash is cooked and cool enough to handle, scrape out the soft insides away from the skin and put in a big bowl along with the Brussels mixture. Mix well again with salt and pepper to taste.

Put the tortillas in the oven to soften up (don't let them get crispy)

Spoon the squash mixture into the middle of the soft tortillas. Carefully roll them up to make little open-ended wraps, and then put in on baking tray with the open ends down to stop them from unrolling.

Do this for all twelve tortillas then pour the rest of the salsa on top and spread to coat evenly.

Change the temperature of the oven to 350F and bake for 30 minutes.

While these cooks put the drained, soaked cashews into a blender with one and a half cups cold water, lemon juice, and a quarter tsp salt.

Blend until smooth, adding water if it becomes too thick. This is your sour cream.

When enchiladas are done, leave to cool while you chop cilantro.

Then drizzle the sour cream generously over the dish and top with cilantro and pumpkin seeds.

Nutrition Facts:

Calories: 333kcal; Fat: 11g Carbohydrate: 36g; Protein:14g;

Creamy Vegetable Casserole

Preparation Time: 30 minutes

Cooking Time: 60 minutes

Servings: 2

Ingredients:

2 tbsp. Fresh rosemary 1 tsp Dried basil

1tsp Dried oregano

3 cloves Garlic

¼ cup Nutritional yeast 2tbsp Olive oil

2 tbsp. Apple cider vinegar 1 cup raw cashews

2 Zucchini

1 stalk Broccoli

1 Cauliflower

10 Russet potatoes

Directions:

Pour boiled water over the cashews and leave to soak. Cut up the cauliflower into small florets and boil until soft. When the cauliflower is done, drain it and put it in a blender along with the drained cashews and one and a half cups of cold water.

Add a good half tsp of salt along with the apple cider vinegar and
nutritional yeast. Blend until creamy.

Wash and grate the zucchini, set aside. Cut the broccoli into small bite- sized pieces and set aside.

Spread the sides and bottom of a baking tray with olive oil. Cut the potatoes as thin as you can and spread them in the tray forming an even layer. Pour half of the cauliflower sauce to cover and spread evenly.

Add the grated zucchini and spread out to cover the sauce. Sprinkle the oregano and basil over the zucchini, then push the pieces of broccoli into the zucchini to keep the surface as even as possible.

Drizzle a little more cauliflower sauce around the broccoli pieces to fill in the gaps.

Do another layer to use up the rest of the potatoes, then pour the rest of the remaining cauliflower sauce over top of that.

Spread it out as evenly as possible, right to the edges to fill in all the gaps around the sides.

Sprinkle the top with a half tsp of black pepper and a generous pinch or two of salt. Finely chop the fresh rosemary and sprinkle that on top also.

Put in the oven on 400F for 45 minutes. It will be done when a knife pierces the potatoes without pulling them up and the top should be beautifully browned. Let it cool before serving.

Nutrition Facts:

Calories: 389kcal; Fat: 4g; Carbohydrate: 37g; Protein: 26g

Vegan Mac And Cheese

Preparation Time: 25 minutes
Cooking Time: 30 minutes
Servings: 2
Ingredients:
1 cup raw Cashews
½ tsp Chili flakes
½ cup Nutritional yeast Salt and pepper to taste
½ tsp mustard powder
½ tsp Onion powder
½ tsp Garlic powder 3 cloves Garlic
1 Russet potato
1 White onion 2tbsp Avocado oil 1 head Broccoli
1 ½ tsp Apple cider vinegar 2 cups Macaroni
Directions:
Peel and grate the potato. Finely dice the garlic. Heat a large saucepan and oil over medium heat. Put onion and a little salt in the pot and cook until soft.
Add potato, chili flakes, garlic, mustard, onion and garlic powders into the pot. Stir well until their flavors release, then add one cup of water and cashews. Keep stirring at a simmer until the potatoes are soft.
Pour entire mixture into a blender along with the apple cider vinegar and nutritional yeast, salt and pepper. The consistency should be that of cheese sauce that is thick yet runny. If it is too thick, add more water, if it needs more salt or garlic powder, chili flakes or vinegar, do so now according to your taste.
Boil the pasta in salted water. In another pot, boil the broccoli in bite-sized florets until tender. When both are ready, transfer everything into one pot and cover with the cheese sauce. Combine well, serve and enjoy!
Nutrition Facts:
Calories: 263kcal; Fat: 14g; carbohydrates: 36g; Protein: 4g;

Butternut Squash Alfredo

Preparation Time: 15 minutes
Cooking Time: 25 minutes
Servings: 4
Ingredients:
9oz Whole grain linguine 2 cups Vegetable broth
3 cups Butternut Squash, diced
Salt and pepper to taste 1 tsp Paprika
2 cloves Garlic
1 White onion
1 cup Green peas 1 Zucchini
2tbsp Olive oil
2 tbsp. Sage
Directions:
Heat the oil in a large fry pan with medium heat. While it heats, ensures the sage leaves are clean and dry, then them put in the oil to fry, moving around not to burn.
Pull them out and put them on a paper towel. Into the fry pan, put the peeled and diced squash along with paprika, diced onion, and black pepper.
Cook until the onion is soft then add the broth and salt to taste.
Bring to a boil before turning down to low heat and leaving the squash to cook through. In another pot, cook the linguine in water with a little salt.
When the squash is tender, put it in a blender along with all the liquid and other ingredients. Blend until creamy and taste to see if more salt, pepper or spice is needed.
Put it back in the fry pan to keep warm on low heat.
Using a grater, grate the zucchini lengthwise to make long noodles. Make as many long ones as you can to blend in with the linguine. Add them to the sauce along with the green peas and cook in the butternut squash for five minutes.

When the pasta is done, save one cup of liquid before you drain it. Add the linguine to the pasta and stir well to coat the linguine.
If the sauce is too thick, add a little of pasta water. Serve the pasta topped with the fried sage leaves and a little blacker pepper.
Nutrition Facts: Calories: 432; Fat: 14g; Carbohydrate: 36g; Protein: 34g;

Vegan Lasagna

Preparation Time: 25 minutes
Cooking Time: 60 minutes
Servings: 2
Ingredients:
4 tbsp. tapioca starch
¼ tsp salt
1 tbsp. Apple cider vinegar 4 medium lemons, juiced 1 cup raw cashews
3 cups Baby spinach
1 box Lasagna noodles 2 Zucchini
½ tsp Garlic powder 2 tsp Dried oregano 2 tsp Dried basil
Salt and pepper to taste 2 tbsp. Olive oil
½ cup Nutritional yeast
16 oz. firm tofu
3 tbsp. Tomato puree 1 tbsp. onion powder 6 cloves of garlic
1 medium white onion Salt and pepper
2 cans crushed tomatoes
1 cup red lentils, drained
Directions:
Put three cups of water in a saucepan with the lentils, then bring to a boil before reducing to a simmer for around twenty minutes. Drain the lentils and set aside. In the same saucepan, add oil and the diced onion and let it cool down. When the onion is soft, add finely diced garlic, generous pinches of salt and pepper, and one tsp of dried oregano and basil, the two cans of tomato and the tomato puree. Leave to simmer for 15 minutes, stirring every 5 minutes. Add the lentils to this then set aside. This is the marinara sauce.
Put one cup of cashews into a bowl with two cups of boiled water and set aside.
Wash and slice the zucchini into lengthwise strips that are long and relatively thin then set aside.
Break up the tofu and add to the blender along with the juice from one lemon, one tsp each of basil and oregano, the nutritional yeast, garlic powder, and a little salt. Keep pulsing until it is mostly smooth but still a little textured. Put into a bowl and set aside, this is your ricotta. Drain the soaked cashews and put them into a clean blender with the apple cider vinegar, the juice from one lemon, tapioca starch, and a little salt. Pour in one and a half cups of water and blend until smooth. Pour this into a saucepan on medium heat and stir until it becomes stretchy then set aside. This is the cheese sauce. In a large baking dish, place a few spoonsful of the marinara sauce and spread it to cover the bottom and sides of the dish. Begin to layer the lasagna noodles, the ricotta, the zucchini, and the cheese sauce. Follow this with half of the spinach, more marinara, lasagna noodles, spinach, and the cheese sauce. Keep repeating until all ingredients have been used except for a small portion of the cheese sauce. Put into a 350F oven for 45 minutes on the highest shelf. Remove after 40 minutes and spoon the remainder of the cheese sauce over the top to resemble mozzarella blobs, then return to the oven for 5 to 10 more minutes. Let rest then serve and enjoy!
Nutrition Facts:
Calories: 543kcal; Fat: 14g; Carbohydrate: 76g; Protein: 34g

Cajun Turkey Rice

Preparation Time: 10 minutes
Cooking Time: 25 minutes
Servings: 4
Ingredients:
5 quarts chicken broth
2 cups uncooked white rice 1 ½ cups celery, chopped
1 ½ cups red onion, chopped 1 tbsp. garlic, minced
8oz ground pork
8oz ground beef
2 tbsp. Cajun seasoning 1 tbsp. dried thyme
1 tbsp. dried parsley
1 tbsp. dried oregano
Directions:
Place the chicken broth, rice, celery, and 1 cup of chopped onion into a large pot. Bring to a boil over high heat. Reduce heat to medium-low, cover, and simmer until the rice is tender, 20 to 25 minutes.
Meanwhile, place the remaining ½ cup of onion into a large skillet along with the garlic, pork, and beef.
Cook and stir over medium-high heat until the meat is brown and crumbly. Pour off excess grease, and then stir the meat into the cooked rice along with the thyme, parsley, and oregano.
Stir well and serve.
Nutrition Facts:
Calories: 134 Carbs: 27g Fat: 2g Protein: 4g

Tomato & Goat's Cheese Pizza

Preparation Time: 5 Minutes
Cooking Time: 50 Minutes
Servings: 2
Ingredients:
8oz buckwheat flour
2 teaspoons dried yeast Pinch of salt
5fl oz. slightly water 1 tsp olive oil
3oz feta cheese, crumbled
3ozpassata or tomato paste 1 tomato, sliced
1 red onion, finely chopped
1oz rocket arugula leaves, chopped
Directions:
In a bowl, combine all the ingredients for the pizza dough then allow it to stand for at least an hour until it has doubled in size.
Roll the dough out to a size to suit you. Spoon the passata onto the base and add the rest of the toppings. Bake in the oven at 400F for 15-20 minutes or until browned at the edges and crispy and serve.
Nutrition Facts:
Calories 387 kcal, Fat 9.9g, Carbohydrate 52g, Protein 8.4g

CHAPTER 8:

SIDE DISHES

Sage Carrots

Preparation Time: 10 minutes
Cooking Time: 25 minutes
Servings: 2
Ingredients:
2 tsps. Sweet paprika 1 tbsp. chopped sage 2 tbsps. Olive oil
1 lb. peeled and roughly cubed carrots
¼ tsp. black pepper 1 chopped red onion
Directions:
In a baking pan, combine the carrots with the oil and the other ingredients, toss and bake at 380 0F for 30 minutes. Divide between plates and serve.
Nutrition Facts:
Calories: 200 kcal, Fat: 8.7 g, Carbs: 7.9 g, Protein: 4 g,

Pesto Green Beans

Preparation Time: 10 minutes
Cooking Time: 55 minutes
Servings: 2
Ingredients:
2 tbsps. Olive oil
2 tsps. Sweet paprika Juice of 1 lemon
2 tbsp. Basil pesto
1 lb. trimmed and halved green beans
¼ tsp. black pepper 1 sliced red onion
Directions:
Heat up a pan with the oil over medium-high heat; add the onion, stir and sauté for 5 minutes. Add the beans and the rest of the ingredients, toss, cook over medium heat for 10 minutes, divide between plates and serve.
Nutrition Facts:
Calories: 280 kcal, Fat: 10 g, Carbs: 13.9 g, Protein: 4.7 g,

Minty Tomatoes and Corn

Preparation Time: 10 minutes
Cooking Time: 65 minutes
Servings: 2
Ingredients:
2 cups corn
1 tbsp. rosemary vinegar 2 tbsp. Chopped mint
1 lb. sliced tomatoes
¼ tsp. black pepper 2 tbsp. Olive oil
Directions: In a salad bowl, combine the tomatoes with the corn and the other ingredients, toss and serve. Enjoy!
Nutrition Facts:
Calories: 230 kcal, Fat: 7.2 g, Carbs: 11.6 g, Protein: 4 g

Roasted Beets

Preparation Time: 10 minutes
Cooking Time: 40 minutes
Servings: 2
Ingredients:
2 minced garlic cloves
¼ tsp black pepper
4 peeled and sliced beets
¼ cup chopped walnuts 2 tbsp. Olive oil
¼ cup chopped parsley

Directions:
In a baking dish, combine the beets with the oil and the other ingredients, toss to coat, put in the oven at 420°F, and bake for 30 minutes. Divide between plates and serve.
Nutrition Facts:
Calories: 156 kcal, Fat: 11.8 g, Carbs: 11.5 g, Protein: 3.8 g

Kale Sauté

Preparation Time: 10 minutes
Cooking Time: 15 minutes
Servings: 2
Ingredients:
1 chopped red onion
3 tbsp. Coconut aminos 2 tbsp. Olive oil
1 lb. torn kale
1 tbsp. chopped cilantro 1 tbsp. lime juice
2 minced garlic cloves
Directions:
Heat up a pan with the olive oil over medium heat; add the onion and the garlic and sauté for 5 minutes. Add the kale and the other ingredients, toss, cook over medium heat for 10 minutes, divide between plates and serve.
Nutrition Facts:
Calories: 200 kcal, Fat: 7.1 g, Carbs: 6.4 g, Protein: 6 g

Rosemary Endives

Preparation Time: 10 minutes
Cooking Time: 20 minutes
Servings: 2
Ingredients: 2 tbsp. Olive oil
1 tsp. dried rosemary 2 halved endives
¼ tsp. black pepper
½ tsp. turmeric powder
Directions:
In a baking pan, combine the endives with the oil and the other ingredients, toss gently, introduce in the oven and bake at 400 0F for 20 minutes. Divide between plates and serve.
Nutrition Facts:
Calories: 66 kcal, Fat: 7.1 g, Carbs: 1.2 g, Protein: 0.3 g

Scallops with Almonds and Mushrooms

Preparation Time: 5 minutes
Cooking Time: 10 minutes
Servings: 4
Ingredients:
1-pound scallops 2 tbsp. olive oil
4 scallions, chopped
½ cup mushrooms, sliced 2 tbsp. almonds, chopped 1 cup coconut cream
Directions:
Heat up a pan with the oil over medium heat; add the scallions and the mushrooms and sauté for 2 minutes. Add the scallops cook over medium heat for 8 minutes more, divide into bowls and serve.
Nutrition Facts:
Calories 322 kcal, Fat 23.7g, Carbohydrate 8.1g, Protein 21.6g

Thyme Mushrooms

Preparation Time: 10 minutes
Cooking Time: 30 minutes
Servings: 2
Ingredients:
1 tbsp. chopped thyme 2 tbsp. Olive oil
2 tbsp. Chopped parsley
4 minced garlic cloves
Salt and Black pepper to taste 2 lbs. halved white mushrooms
Directions:
In a baking pan, combine the mushrooms with the garlic and the other ingredients, toss, introduce in the oven and cook at 400°F for 30 minutes. Divide between plates and serve.
Nutrition Facts:
Calories: 251kcal, Fat: 9.3 g, Carbs: 13.2 g, Protein: 6 g

Apples and Cabbage Mix

Preparation Time: 10 minutes
Cooking Time:
Servings: 4
Ingredients:
2 cored and cubed green apples 2 tbsp. Balsamic vinegar
½ tsp. caraway seeds
2 tbsp. Olive oil Black pepper
1 shredded red cabbage head
Directions:
In a bowl, combine the cabbage with the apples and the other ingredients, toss and serve.
Nutrition Facts:
Calories: 165 kcal, Fat: 7.4 g, Carbs: 26 g, Protein: 2.6 g

Carrot, Tomato, And Arugula Quinoa Pilaf

Preparation Time: 10 minutes
Cooking Time: 35 minutes
Servings: 4
Ingredients:
2 teaspoons extra virgin olive oil
½ red onion, chopped 1 cup quinoa, raw
2 cups vegetable or chicken broth 1 tsp fresh lovage, chopped
1 carrot, chopped
1 tomato, chopped 1 cup baby arugula
Directions:
Heat the olive oil in a saucepan over medium heat and add the red onion. Cook and stir until translucent, about 5 minutes.
Lower the heat, stir in quinoa, and toast, stirring constantly, for 2 minutes. Stir in the broth, black pepper, and thyme.
Raise the heat to high and bring to a boil. Cover, reduce heat to low, and simmer for 5 minutes.
Stir in the carrots, cover and simmer until all water is absorbed, about 10 more minutes.
Turn off the heat, add tomatoes, arugula and lovage and let sit for 5 minutes. Add salt and pepper to taste.
Nutrition Facts:
Calories: 165 kcal Fat: 4g Carbs: 27g Protein: 6g

Bake Kale Walnut

Preparation Time: 10 minutes
Cooking Time: 30 minutes
Servings: 4
Ingredients
1 medium red onion, finely chopped
¼ cup extra virgin olive oil 2 cups baby kale
½ cup half-and-half cream
½ cup walnuts, coarsely chopped 1/3 cup dry breadcrumbs
½ tsp ground nutmeg Salt and pepper to taste
¼ cup dry breadcrumbs
2 tbsp. extra virgin olive oil
Directions
Preheat oven to 350 degrees F. In a skillet, sauté onion in olive oil until tender. In a large bowl, combine cooked onion, kale, cream, walnuts, breadcrumbs, nutmeg and salt and pepper to taste, mixing well.
Transfer to a greased 1-1/2-qt. baking dish. Combine topping ingredients and sprinkle over the kale mixture. Bake, uncovered, for 30 minutes or until lightly browned.
Nutrition Facts:
Calories: 555 Fat: 31g Carbs: 65g Protein: 26g

Arugula With Apples And Pine Nuts

Preparation Time: 10 minutes
Cooking Time: 8 minutes
Servings: 4
Ingredients:
2 tbsp. extra virgin olive oil 2 cloves garlic, slivered
2 tbsp. pine nuts

1 apple, peeled, cored and chopped 10 oz. arugula
Salt and pepper to taste

Directions:

Heat the olive oil in a large skillet or wok over low heat. Add the garlic, pine nuts, and apple. Cook until the nuts and garlic are golden, and the apple is just starting to soften, 3 to 5 minutes. Increase the heat to medium and add the arugula. Stir and cook another 2 to 3 minutes. Season with salt and pepper to taste.

Nutrition Facts:

Calories: 121 Fat: 9g Carbs: 8g Protein: 3g

Kale Green Bean Casserole

Preparation Time: 5 minutes
Cooking Time: 40 minutes
Servings: 4
Ingredients:

1 ½ cups milk
1 cup sour cream
1 cup mushrooms, chopped 2 cups green beans, chopped 2 cups kale, chopped
¼ cup capers, drained
¼ cup walnuts, crushed

Directions:

Preheat the oven to 375 degrees F and lightly grease a casserole dish. Whisk the milk and sour cream together in a large bowl.

Add mushrooms, green beans, kale, and capers. Pour into the casserole dish and top with the crushed walnuts.

Bake uncovered in the preheated oven until bubbly and browned on top, about 40 minutes.

Nutrition Facts:

Calories: 130 Fat: 6g Carbs: 14g Protein: 2g

Rice With Lemon And Arugula

Preparation Time: 10 minutes
Cooking Time: 35 minutes
Servings: 4
Ingredients:

1 small red onion, chopped
1 cup fresh mushrooms, sliced 2 cloves garlic, minced
1 tbsp. extra-virgin olive oil
3 cups long-grain rice, steamed 10 oz. fresh arugula
3 tbsp. lemon juice
¼ tsp dill weed
Salt and pepper to taste
1/3 cup feta cheese, crumbled

Directions:

Pre-heat and oven to 350°F. In a skillet, sauté the onion, mushrooms and garlic in oil until tender. Stir in the rice, arugula, lemon juice, dill and salt and pepper to taste.

Reserve 1 tbsp. cheese and stir the rest into skillet; mix well. Transfer to an 8-in. square baking dish coated with nonstick cooking spray. Sprinkle with reserved cheese. Cover and bake for 25 minutes.

Uncover and bake for an additional 5-10 minutes or until heated through and cheese is melted.

Nutrition Facts:

Calories 290kcal, Fat 6g, Carbohydrate 55g, Protein 13g

Easy Cajun Grilled Veggies

Preparation Time: 50 minutes
Cooking Time: 5 minutes
Servings: 4
Ingredients:

¼ cup extra virgin olive oil 1 tsp Cajun seasoning
1/2 tsp cayenne pepper
1 tbsp. Worcestershire sauce
2 zucchinis cut into 1/2-inch slices

2 large red onions, sliced into ½" wedges 2 yellow squash, cut into 1/2-inch slices

Directions:

In a small bowl, mix together olive oil, Cajun seasoning, cayenne pepper, and Worcestershire sauce. Place zucchinis, onions, and yellow squash in a bowl, and cover with the olive oil mixture. Salt to taste.

Cover bowl and marinate vegetables in the refrigerator at least 30 minutes. Preheat an outdoor grill for high heat and lightly oil grate. Place marinated vegetable pieces on skewers or directly on the grill. Cook 5 minutes until done.

Nutrition Facts:

Calories: 95kcal, Fat: 7g Carbs: 8g, Protein: 2g

Purple Potatoes With Onions, Mushrooms And Capers

Preparation Time: 10 minutes
Cooking Time: 25 minutes
Servings: 4
Ingredients:

6 purple potatoes, scrubbed 3 tbsp. extra virgin olive oil 1 large red onion, chopped
8 oz. fresh mushrooms, sliced Salt and pepper to taste
¼ tsp chili pepper flakes
1 tbsp. capers, drained and chopped 1 tsp fresh tarragon, chopped

Directions:

Cut each potato into wedges by quartering the potatoes, then cutting each quarter in half. Heat 1 tbsp. of olive oil over medium heat in a large skillet and cook the onion and mushrooms until the mushrooms start to release their liquid and the onion becomes translucent, about 5 minutes. Transfer the onion and mushrooms into a bowl and set aside.

Heat 2 more tbsp. of olive oil over high heat in the same skillet and add the potato wedges into the hot oil. Sprinkle with salt and pepper, and allow to cook, stirring occasionally, until the wedges are browned on both sides, about 10 minutes.

Reduce heat to medium, sprinkle the potato wedges with red pepper flakes, and allow to cook until the potatoes are tender, about 10 more minutes. Stir in the onion and mushroom mixture, toss the vegetables together, and mix in the capers and fresh tarragon.

Nutrition Facts:

Calories: 215 Fat: 6gCarbs: 23g Protein: 3g

Vegetarian Stuffed Peppers

Preparation Time: 10 minutes
Cooking Time: 70 minutes
Servings: 6
Ingredients:

1 ½ cups brown rice, uncooked 6 large green bell peppers
3 tbsp. soy sauce
3 tbsp. dry red wine
1 tsp vegetarian Worcestershire sauce 1 ½ cups extra firm tofu
1/2 cup sweetened dried cranberries
¼ cup walnuts, chopped
½ cup Parmesan, grated Salt and pepper, to taste 2 cups tomato sauce
2 tbsp. brown sugar

Directions:

Preheat oven to 350°F. In a saucepan bring 3 cups water to a boil. Stir in rice. Reduce heat, cover and simmer for 40 minutes. Meanwhile, core and seed green peppers, leaving bottoms intact.

Place peppers in a microwavable dish with about ½" of water in the bottom. Microwave on high for 6 minutes. In a small saucepan, bring soy sauce, wine and Worcestershire sauce to a simmer. Add tofu and simmer until the liquid is absorbed.

Combine rice, tofu, cranberries, nuts, cheese, salt and pepper in a large bowl and mix well. Pack rice firmly into peppers. Return peppers to the dish you first microwaved them in and bake for 25 to 30 minutes, or until lightly browned on top.

Meanwhile, in a small saucepan over low heat, combine tomato sauce and brown sugar. Heat until hot.

Serve stuffed peppers with the tomato sauce spooned over each serving.

Nutrition Facts:

Calories: 250 Carbs: 22g Fat: 10g Protein: 17g

Roasted Red Endive With Caper Butter

Preparation Time: 10 minutes
Cooking Time: 25 minutes
Servings: 4
Ingredients:

10 red endives
2 tsp. extra virgin olive oil
2 anchovy fillets, packed in oil 1 small lemon, juiced
3 tbsp. capers, drained
5 tbsp. cold butter, cut into cubes 1 tbsp. fresh parsley, chopped Salt and pepper as needed

Directions:

Preheat the oven to 425°F. Toss endives with olive oil, salt, and pepper, and spread out on to a baking sheet cut side down.

Bake for about 20-25 minutes or until caramelized.

While they're roasting, add the anchovies to a large pan over medium heat and use a fork to mash them until broken up.

Add lemon juice and mix well, then add capers.

Lower the heat and slowly stir in the butter and parsley. Drizzle butter over roasted endives, season as necessary and garnish with more fresh parsley.

Nutrition Facts:

Calories 109 fat 8.6g protein1.5 g, carbohydrates 4.9 g, Fiber 4 g

Chickpeas With Caramelized Onion And Endive

Preparation Time: 10 minutes
Cooking Time: 25 minutes
Servings: 4
Ingredients:

2 large red endives
¼ cup extra-virgin olive oil
2 medium red onions, sliced thinly 2 tsp sugar
¼ cup Medjool dates, chopped Salt and pepper, to taste
2 cans of chickpeas

Directions:

Prepare the endives discarding the external leaves and the core. Wash them in a large bowl of cold water then cut them into large pieces and set aside.

Heat the oil over medium heat in a large skillet.

Add the onions and cook until translucent, about 5 minutes. Stir in the sugar, and continue cooking until the onions are golden brown, about 10 minutes.

Add the dates and the endive leaves.

Cook, stirring occasionally, until the leaves are tender, about 6 minutes. Season with salt and pepper to taste.

Stir in the chickpeas and let cook until the flavors have blended, for about
5 minutes.

Nutrition Facts:

Calories: 288 Fat: 6g Carbohydrate: 52g Protein: 10g

CHAPTER 9:

SAUCES AND DRESSINGS

Salsa Verde

Preparation Time: 20 minutes
Cooking Time: 10minutes
Servings: 4
Ingredients:
½ cup fresh parsley, finely chopped 3 tbsp. fresh basil, finely chopped
2 cloves garlic, crushed
¾ cup olive oil
2 tbsp. small capers
½ lemon, the juice
½ tsp ground black pepper 1 tsp sea salt
Directions:
Add all of the ingredients to a deep bowl and mix with an immersion blender until the sauce has the desired consistency.
Store the sauce in the refrigerator for up to 4-5 days or in the freezer.
Nutrition Facts:
Calories 323, Fat 37g, Carbohydrates 2g, Protein 1g

Tzatziki

Preparation Time: 30 minutes
Cooking Time: 0 minutes
Servings: 6
Ingredients:
½ cucumber
1 cup Greek yogurt 1 tbsp. olive oil
2 cloves garlic
1 tbsp. fresh mint, finely chopped Pinch of ground black pepper
1 tsp salt
Directions:
Rinse the cucumber grate it with a grater without peeling it. The green skin adds color and texture to the sauce.
Put the grated cucumber in a strainer and sprinkle salt on top. Mix well and let the liquid drain for 5-10 minutes. Wrap cucumber in a tea towel and squeeze out excess liquid.
Crush garlic and place it in a bowl. Add cucumber, oil and fresh mint.
Stir in the yogurt and add black pepper and salt to taste. Let the sauce sitin the refrigerator for at least 10 minutes for the flavors to develop.
Nutrition Facts:
Calories 81, Fat 7g, Carbohydrates 3g, Protein 1g

Guacamole

Preparation Time: 15 minutes
Cooking Time: 0 minutes
Servings: 4
Ingredients:
2 ripe avocados
1 clove garlic
3 tbsp. olive oil
½ white onion 1 tomato, diced
5 1/3 tbsp. fresh cilantro
½ lime, the juice Salt and pepper
Directions:
Peel the avocados and mash with a fork. Grate or chop the onion finely and add to the mash. Squeeze the lime and add the juice.

Add tomato, olive oil and finely chopped cilantro. Season with salt and pepper and mix well.
Let the sauce sit in the refrigerator for at least 10 minutes for the flavors to develop.
Nutrition Facts:
Calories 244, Fat 25g, Carbohydrates 5g, Protein 3g

Avocado Caesar Dressing

Preparation Time: 10 minutes
Cooking Time: 0 minutes
Servings: 4
Ingredients:
1/3 cup avocado, mashed 2 cloves garlic, minced
1 tbsp. olive oil
2 anchovy fillets or 1 tsp anchovy paste 3 tbsp. lemon juice
¼ cup Parmesan cheese, shredded
2 tbsp. almond milk, unsweetened 2 teaspoons Worcestershire sauce
½ tsp mustard 2 tbsp. water
¾ tsp sea salt
¼ tsp ground pepper
Directions:
Add all ingredients into a high-powered blender or food processor and blend until smooth.
Taste and add additional salt and pepper if needed.
Nutrition Facts:
Calories 58, Fat 5g, Carbohydrates 2g, Protein 2g

Italian Veggie Salsa

Preparation Time: 10 minutes
Cooking Time: 10 minutes
Servings: 4 Ingredients:
2 red bell peppers cut into wedges 3 zucchinis, sliced
½ cup garlic, minced
2 tbsp. olive oil
A pinch of black pepper 1 tsp Italian seasoning
Directions:
Heat up a pan with the oil over medium-high heat, add bell peppers and zucchini, toss and cook for 5 minutes.
Add garlic, black pepper and Italian seasoning, toss, cook for 5 minutes more.
Blitz in a food processor when done until completely smooth.
Nutrition Facts:
Calories 132 kcal, Fat 3g, Carbohydrate 7g, Protein 4g

Black Bean Salsa

Preparation Time: 10 minutes
Cooking Time: 0 minutes
Servings: 6
Ingredients:
1 tbsp. coconut aminos
½ tsp cumin, ground
1 cup canned black beans, drained 1 cup salsa
6 cups romaine lettuce leaves, torn
½ cup avocado, pitted and cubed
Directions:
In a bowl, combine the beans with the aminos, cumin, salsa, lettuce and avocado, toss, divide into small bowls and serve as a snack.
Nutrition Facts:
Calories 181 kcal, Fat 4g, Carbohydrate 14g, Protein 7g

Mung Sprouts Salsa

Preparation Time: 10 minutes
Cooking Time: 0 minutes
Servings: 2
Ingredients:
1 red onion, chopped
2 cups mung beans, sprouted A pinch of red chili powder

1 green chili pepper, chopped 1 tomato, chopped
1 tsp chaat masala
1 tsp lemon juice
1 tbsp. coriander, chopped

Directions:

In a salad bowl, mix onion with mung sprouts, chili pepper, tomato, chili powder, chaat masala, lemon juice, coriander and pepper, toss well, divide into small cups and serve.

Nutrition Facts:

Calories 100 kcal, Fat 2g, Carbohydrate 3g, Protein 6g

Jerusalem Artichoke Gratin

Preparation Time: 10 minutes
Cooking Time: 45 minutes
Servings: 3
Ingredients:

1lb Jerusalem artichoke 1 cup milk
3tbsp grated cheese
1 tbsp. crème Fraiche 1tsp butter
Curry, paprika powder, nutmeg, salt, pepper

Directions:

Wash and peel the Jerusalem artichokes and slice them into approx. ½ inch thick slices. Bring them to a boil with the milk in a saucepan. Then stir in the spices and crème Fraiche.

Grease a baking dish with butter and add the Jerusalem artichoke and milk mixture. Bake on the middle shelf in the oven for about half an hour at 325°F..

Sprinkle with grated cheese and bake five minutes before the end of the baking time.

Nutrition Facts:

Calories: 133 Net carbs: 9.9g Fat: 8.1g Fiber: 1.1g Protein: 4.7g

CHAPTER 10:

DINNER RECIPES

Aromatic chicken breast with kale, red onions, tomato and chilli salsa

Ingredients::

4 oz skinless, boneless pigeon breast 2 tsp ground turmeric

Juice of ¼ leemon

1 tbsp extra virgin vegetable oil 2 oz kale, chopped

¼ red onion, sliced

1 tsp chopped fresh ginger 2 oz buckwheat

For the salsa:

1 tomato

1 bird's eye chilli, finely chopped 1 tbsp capers, finely chopped

2 tbsp parsley, finely chopped Juice of ¼ lemon

Planning steps:

To make the salsa, remove the attention from the tomato and chop it very finely, taking care to stay the maximum amount of the liquid as possible. Mix with the chili, capers, parsley and juice. You'll put everything in a blender but the top result's a touch different.

Heat the oven to 420 °F. Marinate the pigeon breast in 1 teaspoon of the turmeric, the lemon juice and a touch oil. Leave for 5–10 minutes.Heat an ovenproof frypan until hot, then add the marinated chicken and cook for a moment approximately on all sides , until pale golden, then transfer to the oven (place on a baking tray if your pan isn't ovenproof) for 8–10 minutes or until cooked through. Remove from the oven, cover with foil and leave to rest for five minutes before serving. Meanwhile, cook the kale during a steamer for five minutes. Fry the red onions and therefore the ginger during a little oil, until soft but not coloured, then add the cooked kale and fry for another minute. Cook the buckwheat according to the packet instructions with the remaining tsp of turmeric. Serve alongside the chicken, vegetables and salsa.

Sirtfood bites

Ingredients:

4 oz walnuts

1 oz dark chocolate (85 per cent cocoa solids), broken into pieces; or cocoa nibs

9 oz Medjool dates, pitted 1 tbsp cocoa powder

1 tbsp ground turmeric

1 tbsp extra virgin vegetable oil the scraped seeds of 1 vanilla pod or 1 tsp vanilla 1–2 tbsp water

Directions:

Place the walnuts and chocolate during a kitchen appliance and process until you have a fine powder. Add all the opposite ingredients except the water and blend until the mixture forms a ball. You'll or might not have to feature the water depending on the consistency of the mixture – you don't want it to be too sticky. Using your hands, form the mixture into bite-sized balls and refrigerate in an airtight container for at least 1 hour before eating them. You'll roll some of the balls in some more cocoa or desiccated coconut to realize a different finish if you wish. They will keep for up to 1 week in your fridge.

Asian king prawn stir-fry with buckwheat noodles

Ingredients:

5 oz shelled raw king prawns, deveined
2 tsp tamari (you can use soy sauce if you're not avoiding gluten) 2 tsp extra virgin olive oil
2.5 oz soba (buckwheat noodles) 1 clove , finely chopped
1 bird's eye chilli, finely chopped 1 tsp finely chopped fresh ginger
¼ red onions, sliced
1.5 oz celery, trimmed and sliced 3 oz green beans, chopped
2 oz kale, roughly chopped
½ cup chicken broth
1 tbsp lovage or celery leaves

Directions:

Heat a frypan over a high heat, then cook the prawns in 1 teaspoon of the
tamari and 1 teaspoon of the oil for 2–3 minutes. Transfer the prawns to a plate. Wipe the pan out with kitchen paper, as you're getting to use it again.
Cook the noodles in boiling water for 5–8 minutes or as directed on the packet. Drain and set aside.
Meanwhile, fry the garlic, chilli and ginger, red onion, celery, beans and kale within the remaining oil over an medium–high heat for 2–3 minutes. Add the stock and convey to the boil, then simmer for a minute or two, until the vegetables are cooked but still crunchy.
Add the prawns, noodles and lovage/celery leaves to the pan, bring back to the boil then remove from the heat and serve.

Strawberry buckwheat tabouleh

Ingredients:

2 oz buckwheat
1 tbsp ground turmeric
½ avocado
½ tomato
¼ red onion
1 oz Medjool dates, pitted
1 tbsp capers
1 oz parsley
3 oz strawberries, hulled
1 tbsp extra virgin olive oil
juce of ½ lemon
1 oz rocket

Directions:

Cook the buckwheat with the turmeric consistent with the packet instructions. Drain and keep to one side to chill.
Finely chop the avocado, tomato, red onion, dates, capers and parsley and blend with the cool buckwheat. Slice the strawberries and gently mix into the salad with the oil and juice. Serve on a bed of rocket.

Chicken Skewers with Satay Sauce

Ingredients:

5 oz pigeon breast, dig chunks 1 tsp. Ground turmeric
1/2 tsp. extra virgin vegetable oil
1.5 oz Buckwheat
1 oz Kale, stalks removed and sliced 1 oz Celery, sliced
4 Walnut halves, chopped, to garnish
¼ purple onion , diced 1 clove , chopped
1 tsp. Extra virgin vegetable oil 1 tsp. favorer
1 tsp. Ground turmeric
¼ cup chicken broth
½ cup Coconut milk
1 tbsp. Walnut butter or spread 1 tbsp. Coriander, chopped

Directions:

Mix the chicken with the turmeric and vegetable oil and put aside to marinate 30 minutes to 1 hour would be best, but if you're short on time, just leave it for as long as you'll
.

Cook the buckwheat consistent with the packet instruc tions, adding the kale and celery for the last 5–7 minutes of the cooking time. Drain. Heat the grill on a high setting. For the sauce, gently fry the purple onion and garlic within the vegetable oil for 2–3 minutes until soft. Add the spices and cook for an extra minute. Add the stock and coconut milk and convey to the boil, then add the walnut butter and stir through. Reduce the warmth and simmer the sauce for 8 or 10 minutes, or till creamy and rich. As the sauce is simmering, thread the chicken on to the skewers and place under the recent grill for 10 minutes, turning them after 5 minutes. To serve, stir the coriander through the sauce and pour it over the skewers, then scatter over the chopped walnuts.

Smoked salmon omelette

Ingredients:

2 _Medium eggs

4 oz Smoked salmon, sliced 1/2 tsp. Capers

0.5 oz Rocket, chopped 1 tsp. Parsley, chopped

1 tsp. Extra virgin olive oil

Directions:

Crack the eggs into a bowl and whisk well. Add the salmon, capers, rocket and parsley.

Heat the olive oil during a non-stick frypan until hot but not smoking. Add the egg mixture and, employing a spatula or turner, move the mixture round the pan until it's even. Reduce the warmth and let the omelette cook through. Slide the spatula around the edges and roll up or fold the omelette in half to serve.

The Sirtfood Diet's Shakshuka

Ingredients:

1 tsp. extra virgin vegetable oil

½ purple onion, finely chopped 1 Garlic clove, finely chopped 1 oz Celery, finely chopped

1 Bird's eye chilli, finely chopped 1 tsp. Groud cumin

1 tsp. Ground turmeric 1 tsp. Paprika

3 Tinned chopped tomatoes

1 __oz Kale, stems removed and roughly chopped 1 tbsp. Chopped parsley

2 _Medium eggs D

Irections:

Heat alittle , deep-sided frypan over a medium–low heat. Add the oil and fry the onion, garlic, celery, chilli and spices for 1–2 minutes.

Add the tomatoes, then leave the sauce to simmer gently for 20 minutes, stirring occasionally.

Add the kale and cook for an extra 5 minutes. If you are feeling the sauce is getting too thick, simply add a touch water. When your sauce features a nice rich consistency, stir within the parsley.

Make two little wells within the sauce and crack each egg into them. Reduce the heat to its lowest setting and canopy the pan with a lid or foil. Leave the eggs to cook for 10–12 minutes, at which point the whites should be firm while the yolks are still runny. Cook for a further 3–4 minutes if you favor the yolks to be firm. Serve immediately – ideally straight from the pan.

Prawn Arrabbiata

Ingredients:

Raw or cooked prawns (Ideally king prawns)

2 oz Buckwheat pasta

1 tbsp. extra virgin olive oil

½ Red onion, finely chopped 1 Garlic clove, finely chopped 1 oz Celery, finely chopped

1 germander speedwell chilli, finely chopped

1 tsp. dried mixed herbs

1 tsp. extra virgin olive oil

2 tbsp. White wine (optional) 3 Tinned chopped tomatoes 1 tbsp. chopped parsley

Directions:

Fry the onion, garlic, celery and chilli and dried herbs within the oil over an medium–low heat for 1–2 minutes. Turn the warmth up to medium, add the wine and cook for 1 minute. Add the tomatoes and leave the sauce to simmer over a medium–low heat for 20–30 minutes, until ithas a nice rich consistency. If you feel the sauce is getting too thick simply add a little water.

While the sauce is cooking bring a pan of water to the boil and cook the pasta consistent with the packet instructions. When cooked to your liking, drain, toss with the vegetable oil and confine the pan until needed.

If you're using raw prawns add them to the sauce and cook for a further 3–4 minutes, until they have turned pink and opaque, add the parsley and serve. If you are using cooked prawns add them with the parsley, bring the sauce to the boil and serve.

Add the cooked pasta to the sauce, mix thoroughly but gently and serve.

Turmeric baked salmon

Ingredients:

Skinned Salmon

1 tsp. extra virgin vegetable oil 1 tsp. Ground turmeric

1/4 Juice of a lemon

1 tsp. extra virgin vegetable oil

¼ purple onion, finely chopped 2 oz Tinned green lentils

1 clove, finely chopped

1 Bire's eye chilli, finely chopped 5 oz Celery, dig 2cm lengths

1 tsp. Mild flavorer

1 Tomato, dig 8 wedges

½ cup Chicken or vegetable stock 1 tbsp. Chopped parsley

Directions:

Heat the oven to 390 °F.

Start with the spicy celery. Heat a frypan over a medium–low heat, add the vegetable oil, then the onion, garlic, ginger, chilli and celery. Fry gently for 2–3 minutes or until softened but not coloured, then add the flavorer and cook for an extra minute.

Add the tomatoes then the stock and lentils and simmer gently for 10 minutes. You'll want to extend or decrease the cooking time depending on how crunchy you wish your celery.

Meanwhile, mix the turmeric, oil and juice and rub over the salmon. Place on a baking tray and cook for 8–10 minutes.

To finish, stir the parsley through the celery and serve with the salmon.

Turmeric chicken & kale salad (honey lime dressing)

Ingredients

For the chicken:

1 teaspoon ghee or 1 tbsp copra oil

½ medium brown onion, diced

9 oz. chicken mince or diced up chicken thighs 1 large clove, finely diced

1 tsp turmeric powder 1 tsp lime zest

juice of ½ lime

½ tsp salt + pepper For the salad:

6 broccolini stalks or 2 cups of broccoli florets 2 tbsp pumpkin seeds (pepitas)

3 large kale leaves, stems removed and chopped - ½ avocado, sliceed

Handful of fresh coriander leaves, chopped

Handful of fresh parsley leaves, chopped

For the dressing

3 tbsp lime juice

1 small clove, finely diced or grated

3 tbsp extra-virgin olive oil 1 tsp raw honey

½ tsp wholegrain or Dijon mustard

½ tsp sea salt and pepper

Directions:
Heat the ghee or copra oil during a small frypan over mediumhigh heat.
Add the onion and sauté on medium heat for 4-5 minutes, until golden. Add the chicken mince and garlic and stir for 2-3 minutes over medium-high heat, breaking it apart. Add the turmeric, lime zest, lime juice, salt and pepper and cook, stirring frequently, for a further 3-4 minutes. Set the cooked mince aside.
While the chicken is cooking, bring alittle saucepan of water to boil. Add the broccolini and cook for two minutes. Rinse under cold water and dig 3-4 pieces each.
Add the pumpkin seeds to the frypan from the chicken and toast over medium heat for two minutes, stirring frequently to stop burning. Season with a little salt. Set aside. Raw pumpkin seeds are also fine to use.
Place chopped kale during a salad bowl and pour over the dressing. Using your hands, toss and massage the kale with the dressing. This will soften the kale, quite like what citrus juice does to fish or beef carpaccio – it 'cooks' it slightly.
Finally toss through the cooked chicken, broccolini, fresh herbs, pumpkin seeds and avocado slices.

Buckwheat noodles with chicken kale & miso dressing

Ingredients
For the noodles:
2-3 handfuls of kale leaves
5 oz buckwheat noodles (100% buckwheat, no wheat) 3-4 shiitake mushrooms, sliced
1 tsp copra oil or ghee
1 brown onion, finely diced
1 _medium free-range pigeon breast , sliced or diced 1 long red chilli, thinly sliced
2 large garlic cloves, finely diced
2-3 tbsp Tamari sauce (gluten-free soy sauce)
For the miso dressing:
1½ tablespoon fresh organic miso 1 tbsp Tamari sauce
1 tbsp extra-virgin vegetable oil 1 tbsp lemon or juice
1 tsp sesame oil (optional)
Directions:
Bring an medium saucepan of water to boil. Add the kale and cook for 1 minute, until slightly wilted. Remove and set aside but reserve the water and convey it back to the boil. Add the soba noodles and cook consistent with the package instructions (usually about 5 minutes). Rinse under cold water and put aside.
Within the meantime, pan fry the shiitake mushrooms during a little ghee or coconut oil (about a teaspoon) for 2-3 minutes, until lightly browned on all sides. Sprinkle with sea salt and put aside.
Within the same frypan , heat more copra oil or ghee over medium-high heat. Sauté onion and chilli for 2-3 minutes and then add the chicken pieces. Cook 5 minutes over medium heat, stirring a couple of times, then add the garlic, tamari sauce and a touch splash of water. Cook for a further 2-3 minutes, stirring frequently until chicken is cooked through.
Finally, add the kale and soba noodles and toss through the chicken to warm up.
Mix the miso dressing and drizzle over the noodles right at the end of cooking, this manner you'll keep all those beneficial probiotics in the miso alive and active.

Baked salmon salad (creamy mint dressing)

Ingredients:
1 salmon fillet (4 oz)
1.5 oz mixed salad leaves
1.5 oz young spinach leaves

2 radishes, trimmed and thinly sliced 2 oz cucumber, dig chunks
2 spring onions, trimmed and sliced
1 small handful parsley, roughly chopped
For the dressing:
1 tsp low-fat mayonnaise 1 tbsp natural yogurt
1 tbsp rice vinegar
2 leaves mint, finely chopped
Salt and freshly ground black pepper

Directions:

Preheat the oven to 390 °F.

Place the salmon fillet on a baking tray and bake for 16–18 minutes until just cooked through. Remove from the oven and set aside. The salmon is equally nice hot or cold in the salad. If your salmon has skin, simply cook skin side down and remove the salmon from the skin employing a turner after cooking. It should slide off easily when cooked.

during a small bowl, mix together the mayonnaise, yogurt, rice wine vinegar, mint leaves and salt and pepper together and leave to face for a minimum of 5 minutes to permit the flavors to develop.

Arrange the salad leaves and spinach on a serving plate and top with the radishes, cucumber, spring onions and parsley. Flake the cooked salmon onto the salad and drizzle the dressing over.

Choco chip granola

Ingredients:

7 oz jumbo oats
2 oz pecans, roughly chopped 3 tbsp light vegetable oil
1 oz butter
1 _tbsp dark sugar
2 _tbsp rice malt syrup
2 oz good-quality (70%) bittersweet chocolate chips

Direction:

Preheat the oven to 320 °F. Line an outsized baking tray with a silicone sheet or baking parchment.

Mix the oats and pecans together during a large bowl. During a small nonstick pan, gently heat the olive oil, butter, sugar and rice malt syrup until the butter has melted and therefore the sugar and syrup have dissolved. Don't allow to boil. Pour the syrup over the oats and stir thoroughly until the oats are fully covered.

Distribute the granola over the baking tray, spreading right into the corners. Leave clumps of mixture with spacing instead of an even spread. Bake within the oven for 20 minutes until just tinged golden brown at the edges. Remove from the oven and leave to chill on the tray completely.

When cool, hack any bigger lumps on the tray together with your fingers and then mix within the chocolate chips. Scoop or pour the granola into an airtight tub or jar. The granola will keep for a minimum of 2 weeks.

Lamb butternut squash and date tagine

Ingredients:

2 tbsp vegetable oil
1 purple onion, sliced 1 tsp ginger, grated
3 garlic cloves, grated or crushed
1 tsp chilli flakes (or to taste) 2 tsp cumin seeds
1 _cinnamon stick
2 _tsp ground turmeric
2 _lb lamb neck fillet, dig small chunks
½ teaspoon salt
3 _oz medjool dates, pitted and chopped
3 tin chopped tomatoes, plus half a can of water 1 lb butternut squash, chopped into 1cm cubes 1 lb tin chickpeas, drained

2 tbsp fresh coriander (plus extra for garnish)
Buckwheat, couscous, flatbreads or rice to serve

Directions:

Preheat your oven to 280 °F.

Drizzle about 2 tbsp of vegetable oil into an outsized ovenproof saucepan or cast iron casserole dish. Add the sliced onion and cook on a mild heeat, with the lid on, for about 5 minutes, until the onions are softened but not brown.

Add the grated garlic and ginger, chilli, cumin, cinnamon and turmeric. Stir well and cook for 1 more minute with the lid off. Add a splash of water if it gets too dry.

Next add in the lamb chunks. Stir well to coat the meat in the onions and spices then add the salt, chopped dates and tomatoes, plus about 1 cup of water.

Bring the tagine to the boil then put the lid on and put in your preheated oven for 1 hour and 15 minutes.

Thirty minutes before the end of the cooking time, add within the chopped butternut squash and drained chickpeas. Stir everything together, put the lid back on and return to the oven for the ultimate 30 minutes of cooking.

When the tagine is prepared, remove from the oven and stir through the chopped coriander. Serve with buckwheat, couscous, flatbreads or basmati rice.

Baked potatoes with spicy chickpea stew

Ingredients:

4-6 baking potatoes, pricked everywhere 2 tbsp olive oil
2 red onions, finely chopped
4 cloves garlic, grated or crushed 1 tsp ginger, grated
½ tsp chilli flakes 2 tbsp cumin seeds 2 tbsp turmeric Splash of water
3 chopped tomatoes
2 tbsp unsweetened chocolate (or cacao)
1 lb tins chickpeas (or kidney beans if you prefer) including the chickpea water DON'T DRAIN!!
2 yellow peppers chopped into bitesize pieces
2 tbsp parsley plus extra for garnish
Salt and pepper to taste (optional) Side salad (optional)

Directions:

Preheat the oven to 390 °F, meanwhile you'll prepare all of your ingredients.

When the oven is hot enough put your baking potatoes within the oven and cook for 1 hour or until they are done how you wish them.

Once the potatoes are within the oven, place the vegetable oil and chopped red onion during a large wide saucepan and cook gently, with the lid on for 5 minutes, until the onions are soft but not brown.

Remove the lid and add the garlic, ginger, cumin and chilli. Cook for a further minute on a coffee heat, then add the turmeric and a really small splash of water and cook for an additional minute, taking care to not let the pan get too dry.

Next, add within the tomatoes, cocoa powder (or cacao), chickpeas (including the chickpea water) and yellow pepper. Bring back the boil, then simmer on a coffee heat for 45 minutes until the sauce is thick and unctuous (but don't let it burn!). The stew should be done at roughly the same time because the potatoes.

Finally, stir within the 2 tablespoons of parsley, and a few salt and pepper if you would like, and serve the stew on top of the baked potatoes, perhaps with an easy side salad.

Chargrilled beef

Ingredients:

1 potato, peeled, and dig small dice 1 tbsp extra virgin olive oil

1 tbsp parsley, finely chopped

½ red onion, sliced into rings 2 oz kale, sliced

1 clove, finely chopped

4 oz 1½"-thick beef fillet steak or 1"-thick beefsteak 3 tbsp red wine

½ cup beef broth 1 tsp tomato purée

1 tsp cornflour, dissolved in 1 tbsp water

Directions:

Heat the oven to 430 °F.

Place the potatoes during a saucepan of boiling water, bring back to the boil and cook for 4–5 minutes, then drain. Place during a roasting tin with 1 teaspoon of the oil and roast in the hot oven for 35–45 minutes. Turn the potatoes every 10 minutes to make sure even cooking. When cooked, remove from the oven, sprinkle with the chopped parsley and mix well.

Fry the onion in 1 teaspoon of the oil over medium heat for 5–7 minutes, until soft and nicely caramelized. Keep warm. Steam the kale for 2–3 minutes then drain. Fry the garlic gently in ½ teaspoon of oil for 1 minute, till soft but not colored. Add the kale and fry for a further 1–2 minutes, until tender. Keep warm.

Heat an ovenproof frypan over high heat until smoking. Coat the meat in ½ a teaspoon of the oil and fry within the hot pan over an medium–high heat consistent with how you wish your meat done.If you like your meat medium, it might be better to sear the meat then transfer the pan to an oven set at 430°F and finish the cooking that the way for the prescribed times.

Remove the meat from the pan and set aside to rest. Add the wine to the hot pan to mention any meat residue — Bubble to scale back the wine by half, until syrupy and with a concentrated flavor. Add the stock and tomato purée to the steak pan and convey to the boil, then add the cornflour paste to thicken your sauce, adding it a little at a time until you've got your desired consistency. Stir in any of the juices from the rested steak and serve with the roasted potatoes, kale, onion rings and wine sauce.

Kale, edamame and tofu curry

Ingredients:

1 tbsp rapeseed oil

1 large onion, chopped

4 cloves garlic, peeled and grated

1 large finger fresh ginger, peeled and grated

1 red chilli, deseeded and thinly sliced

1/2 tsp ground turmeric 1/4 tsp cayenne pepper 1 tsp paprika

1/2 tsp ground cumin 1 tsp salt

9 oz dried red lentils 4 cups boiling water

2 oz frozen soyaedamame beans

6 oz firm tofu, chopped into cubes 2 tomatoes, roughly chopped Juice of 1 lime

6 oz kale leaves, stalks removed, and torn

Directions:

Put the oil during a heavy-bottomed pan over a low-medium heat. Add the onion and cook for five minutes before adding the garlic, ginger, and chilli and cooking for an extra 2 minutes. Add the turmeric, cayenne, paprika, cumin and salt. Stir through

before adding the red lentils and stirring again. Pour in the boiling water and convey to a hearty simmer for 10 minutes, then reduce the heat and cook for an extra 20-30 minutes until the curry features a thick '•porridge' consistency.

Add the soya beans, tofu and tomatoes and cook for a further 5 minutes. Add the juice and kale leaves and cook until the kale is just tender.

Veal Cabbage Rolls – Smarter with Capers, Garlic and Caraway Seeds

Ingredients:

1 kg white cabbage (1 white cabbage)
Salt
2 onions
1 clove of garlic
3 tbsp oil
700 g veal mince (request from the butcher)
40 g escapades (glass; depleted weight)
2 eggs
Pepper
1 tsp favorer
1 tbsp paprika powder (sweet)
400 ml veal stock
125 ml soy cream

Directions:

Wash the cabbage and evacuate the external leaves. Cut out the tail during a wedge. Spot a huge pot of salted water and heat it to the aim of boiling.

Within the interim, expel 16 leaves from the cabbage during a gentle progression, increase the bubbling water and cook for 3-4 minutes

Lift out, flush under running virus water and channel. Spot on a kitchen towel, spread with a subsequent towel and pat dry

Cut out the hard, center leaf ribs.

Peel and finely cleave onions and garlic. Warmth 1 tablespoon of oil. Braise the onions and garlic until translucent.

Let cool during a bowl. Include minced meat, tricks, eggs, salt, and pepper and blend everything into a meat player.

Put 2 cabbage leaves together and put 1 serving of mince on each leaf. Move up firmly and fasten it with kitchen string.

Heat the rest of the oil during a pan and earthy colored the 8 cabbage abounds in it from all sides.

Add the caraway and paprika powder. Empty veal stock into the pot and heat to the aim of boiling. Cover and braise the cabbage turns over medium warmth for 35–40 minutes, turn within the center. Mix the soy cream into the sauce and let it bubble for an extra 5 minutes. Season with salt and pepper. Put the cabbage roulades on a plate and present with earthy colored rice or pureed potatoes.

Prawns Sweet and Spicy Glaze with China-Cole-Slav

Ingredients:

250 g Chinese cabbage (0.25 Chinese cabbage)
Salt
50 g little carrots (1 little carrot)
1 little red onion
½ lime
75 ml coconut milk (9% fat)
2 tsp sugar
1 tsp vinegar
Pepper
2 stems coriander
3 tbsp pure sweetener
1 dried stew pepper
2 tbsp Thai fish sauce
1 clove of garlic
3 spring onions
400 g shrimps (with shell, 8 shrimps)
2 tbsp oil

Arrangement Steps

Clean the cabbage and evacuate the tail. Cut the cabbage into fine strips over the rib. Sprinkle with somewhat salt, blend vivaciously and let steep for half-hour.

Within the interim, strip the carrot, dig fine strips. Strip the red onion and furthermore dig strips. Crush the lime.

Mix coconut milk with sugar, vinegar, 1 tbsp juice, and slightly pepper. Channel the cabbage and blend it in with the carrot and onion strips with the coconut milk.

Wash the coriander leaves, shake dry, pluck the leaves, cleave and blend within the plate of mixed greens. Let it steep for an extra half-hour.

Boil the natural sweetener, stew pepper, fish sauce, and three tablespoons of water during a touch pot and cook while mixing until the sugar has totally weakened. Allow chill to off.

Peel and smash garlic. Wash and clean the spring onions and cut them into pieces around 2 cm long.

Break the shrimp out of the shells, however, leave the rear ends on the shrimp.

Cut open the rear, evacuate the dark digestion tracts. Wash shrimp and pat dry.

Heat oil within the wok and to the aim of smoke. Include the shrimp and garlic and fry quickly. Season with pepper.

Add 3-4 tablespoons of the bean stew fish sauce and cook while mixing until the sauce adheres to the shrimp; that takes around 2 minutes.

Add the onion pieces and fry for an extra 45 seconds. Season the coleslaw once more. Put the shrimp on a plate and present it with the serving of mixed greens.

Vegetarian Lasagna - Smarter with Seitan and Spinach

Ingredients:

225 g spinach leaves (solidified)
300 g seitan
2nd little carrots
2 sticks celery
1 onion
1 clove of garlic
2 tbsp oil
Salt
Pepper
850 g canned tomatoes
200 ml exemplary vegetable stock
1 tsp fennel seeds
30 g parmesan (1 piece)
Nutmeg
225 g ricotta
16 entire grain lasagna sheets
Butter for the form
150 g mozzarella

Arrangement Steps

Let the spinach defrost. Hack the seitan finely or put it through the center cut of the meat processor.

Wash and strip carrots. Wash, clean, expel, and finely dice the celery. Strip and cleave the onion and garlic.

Heat the oil during a pan and braise the carrots, celery, onions, and garlic for 3 minutes over medium warmth. Include from that point forward and braise for 3 minutes while mixing. Season with salt and pepper.

Put the canned tomatoes and stock within the pan and spread and cook over medium warmth for 20 minutes, mixing every so often. Pulverize the fennel seeds, include, and season the sauce with salt and pepper.

Meanwhile, finely grind the Parmesan. Concentrate on some nutmeg. Crush the spinach enthusiastically, generally slash, and blend during a bowl with the ricotta, parmesan, salt, pepper, and nutmeg.

Lightly oil a preparing dish (approx. 30 x 20 cm). Spread rock bottom of the shape with slightly sauce and smooth it out. Spot 4 sheets of lasagna on the brink of every other, if essential slice to estimate. Add 1/3 of the spinach blend and smooth. Spread 1/4 of the sauce on top. Layer 4 lasagna sheets, 1/3 spinach, and 1/4 sauce once more, rehash the procedure.

Place the keep going lasagna sheets on top and spread the
remainder of the sauce over them.

Drain the mozzarella and attack enormous pieces. Spread on the lasagna. Heat veggie-lover lasagna during a preheated stove at 180 ° C (fan broiler: 160 ° C, gas: levels 2–3) on the center rack for 35–40 minutes. Let the veggie lover lasagna rest for around 5 minutes before serving.

Asparagus and Ham Omelet with Potatoes and Parsley

Ingredients:

200 g new potatoes
Salt
150 g white asparagus
1 onion
50 g bresaola (Italian meat ham)
2 stems parsley
3 eggs
1 tbsp rapeseed oil
Pepper

Directions:

Wash the potatoes well. Cook in bubbling salted water for approx. 20 minutes, channel and let cool. While the potatoes are cooking, strip the asparagus, remove the lower woody closures. Cook asparagus in salted water for around quarter-hour, scoop of the water, channel well and let cool. Strip the onion and hack finely.

Cut the asparagus and potatoes into little pieces.

Cut the bresaola into strips.

Wash parsley, shake dry, pluck leaves, and slash. Beat the eggs during a bowl and race with the hacked parsley.

Heat the oil during a covered skillet and sauté the onion solid shapes until medium-high warmth until translucent.

Add potatoes and keep it up simmering for 2 minutes.

Add asparagus and fry for 1 moment.

Add the bresaola and season everything with salt and pepper.

Put the eggs within the skillet and spread and stew for 5–6 minutes over low warmth. Drop out of the skillet and serve directly.

Poached Eggs on Spinach with sauce

Ingredients:

1 clove of garlic
3 tsp. oil
1 tsp. sugar
200 ml wine
Salt
Pepper
1 shallot
250 g youthful spinach leaves
Nutmeg
2 tbsp vinegar
4 eggs
2 cuts entire grain toast

Directions:

Peel and finely slash the garlic and braise in 1 teaspoon of oil. Sprinkle sugar, include wine, and convey to the bubble. Lessen to 1/3 over medium warmth. Salt, pepper and keep warm. Peel the shallot and shakers finely. Wash the spinach well and let it channel. Warmth the rest of the oil during a skillet, sauté the shallot during a smooth warmth. Include the spinach and let it a breakdown in 3-4 minutes. Include slightly nutmeg, salt, and pepper.

Boil 1 liter of water with the vinegar. Painstakingly beat the eggs during a bowl with the goal that the yolks stay flawless.

Stir the bubbling vinegar water energetically with a whisk.

Now let the eggs slide in (by the pivot of the water they separate right away).

Boil the water once more. At that point expel the pot from the hob and let the eggs cook (poach) for 3-4 minutes.

Scoop the eggs with a froth trowel and permit them to channel. Put the spinach on a plate and put the eggs thereon. Shower with the sauce and serve. Toast the bread within the toaster and present with it.

Pasta with Minced Lamb Balls and Eggplant, Tomatoes and Sultanas

Ingredients:

250 gleans minced sheep
2 tbsp low-fat quark
1 egg
2 tbsp breadcrumbs
Salt
Pepper
1 tsp. cinnamon
200 g little eggplant (1 little eggplant)
1 onion
1 clove of garlic
2 tbsp oil
150 g orecchiette pasta
2 tbsp sultanas
400 g pizza tomatoes (can)
1 straight leaf
125 ml great vegetable stock

Directions:

Mix minced sheep, quark, egg, and breadcrumbs during a bowl. Season with salt, pepper, and cinnamon.

Using wet hands, transform the slash into balls the size of a cherry. Chill quickly.

Clean, wash, dry the eggplant, and dig 5 mm blocks. Strip onion and garlic and hack finely.

Heat 1 tablespoon of oil during a skillet and fry the meatballs in it until brilliant earthy colored. Expel and put during a secure spot.

Wipe out the dish and afterward heat up the rest of the oil. Include the eggplant shapes, onion, and garlic and braise for 4-5 minutes, mixing. Meanwhile, cook the pasta nibble verification during tons of bubbling salted water as per the bundle guidelines.

Add the sultanas, tomatoes, and sound leave to the skillet. Pour within the stock and convey it to the bubble.

Cover and cook for 4 minutes over medium warmth. At that point put the meatballs within the dish and cook secured for an extra 5

Salad

Ingredients:

600 g huge waxy potatoes
Salt
100 g red onion (2 red onions)
3 tbsp fruit crush vinegar
150 ml exemplary vegetable stock
½ tsp. agave syrup
1½ tbsp rapeseed oil
500 g cucumber (1 cucumber)
Pepper
3 stems dill

Arrangement Steps

Wash potatoes and cook in bubbling water for around 20 minutes. Channel, extinguish, strip while hot and let cool.

Cut the potatoes into cuts and salt. Strip the onions and finely dice them.

Boil the onion 3D shapes with vinegar, stock, and agave syrup. Pour the bubbling stock over the potatoes.

Add oil and blend everything. Let represent half-hour, mixing tenderly more regularly.

Clean, wash, and hack the cucumber into exceptionally fine cuts. Blend within the serving of mixed greens, season with salt and pepper, and let the plate of mixed greens steep for an extra 10 minutes.

Within the interim, wash the dill, shake it dry, pluck the banners, cut them finely, blend them within the potato plate of mixed greens, and serve.

Vegetable Spaghetti

Ingredients:

200 g red chime pepper (1 red ringer pepper)
200 g yellow chime pepper (1 yellow ringer pepper)
150 g carrots (2 carrots)
300 g broccoli
12 yellow cherry tomatoes
½ pack parsley
20 g tawny (8 leaves)
3 spring onions
300 g entire grain spaghetti
Salt
½ lemon
4 tbsp oil
Pepper

Arrangement Steps

Quarter the peppers, center them, wash and spot them on a heating sheet, skin side up. Broil under the recent flame broil until the skin turns dark and rankles.

Cover and let cool during a bowl secured for 10 minutes (steam). At that point skin and dig fine strips.

Peel the carrots and cut them into flimsy cuts. Clean broccoli, dig little florets and wash. Wash and split tomatoes.

Wash parsley, shake dry and pluck the leaves, clean and wash roan, generally hack both. Clean, wash and cut the spring onions into meager cuts.

Cook the spaghetti nibble evidence during tons of salted water as indicated by the bundle directions. Include broccoli and carrots 4 minutes before the finish of the cooking time. Squeeze lemon. Channel the pasta and blend during a bowl with the readied Ingredients:, 1 teaspoon lemon squeeze, and oil.

Spaghetti with Salmon in Lemon Sauce

Ingredients:

150 g salmon filet (without skin)
100 g leek (1 flimsy stick)
100 g little carrots (2 little carrots)
½ natural lemon
2 stems parsley
150 g entire grain spaghetti
Salt
2 tbsp oil
Pepper
100 ml of fish stock
150 ml of soy cream

Planning Steps

Wash salmon, pat dry, and dig 2 cm 3D squares.

Clean the leek, wash it, and cut it into dainty rings. Strip the carrots and cut them into flimsy strips.

Within the interim, wash the lemon half hot and rub dry. Strip the lemon strip meagerly and dig fine strips. Crush juice. Wash parsley, shake dry, pluck leaves and cleave finely.

Cook the pasta chomp verification in saltwater as indicated by the bundle guidelines.

Heat oil during a dish. Season the salmon with pepper and fry everywhere within the recent oil for 3-4 minutes.

Remove the salmon, braise the leek rings, and carrot strips within the dish over medium warmth for 3-4 minutes.

Remove the salmon, braise the leek rings, and carrot strips within the dish over medium warmth for 3-4 minutes.

If fundamental, salt the salmon, set it back within the container, and warmth quickly. Blend within the parsley. Drain the pasta during a strainer and blend tenderly with the sauce. Season with salt and pepper and serve the spaghetti with salmon directly.

Kale and red onion dahl with Buckwheat

Ingredients::

one tablespoon olive oil
One very little very little onion sliced
Two cm ginger grated
One eye chilli deseeded and finely cleaved (more on the off likelihood that you just that you just things hot!)
two teaspoons turmeric
Two teaspoons garam masala
One hundred sixty g very little lentils
four hundred cc cc milk
two hundred cc cc
A hundred g kale or spinach would be a unprecedented unprecedented
One hundred sixty g buckwheat or brown rice

Instructions:

Place the olive oil in a very vast, deep saucepan and embody the cut onion. Cook on a low heat, with the lid on for 5.
Add the garlic, ginger and chilli and cook for one more minute.
Add the turmeric, garam masala and a splash of water and cook for one a lot of a lot of.
Add the red lentils, coconut milk, and 200ml water (do this simply by half filling embody coconut milk can with water and tipping it into the saucepan).
Combine everything together altogether and embody for twenty 5 associate degree a twenty heat with the cover cover. Stir once throughout a jiffy and embody water if the dhal starts to stick.
After twenty minutes add the kale, stir thoroughly and replace the cover, embody for a further five 5 7. About fifteen ready, place embody buckwheat in a medium pot and add plenty of effervescent water. Bring the water back dahl the boil and cook for ten minutes

Miso-marinated Baked Cod with Stir-Fried Greens and benny

Ingredients::

Three 1/2 teaspoons (20g) miso
One tablespoon mirin
One tablespoon further virgin olive oil
One x 7-ounce (200g) skinless cod filet
1/8 cup (20g) red onion, sliced
3/8 cup (40g) celery, sliced
Two three three, finely cleaved
One Thai chili, finely cleaved
one teaspoon finely chopped fresh ginger
3/8 cup (60g) inexperienced beans
3/4 cup (50g) kale, roughly cleaved
One teaspoon benny benny
Two tablespoons (5g) parsley, roughly chopped
one tablespoon tamari (or soy sauce, if but avoiding gluten)
1/4 cup (40g) buckwheat
One teaspoon ground turmeric

Guidelines:

Mix the miso, mirin, and one teaspoon of the oil. Rub all associate degree the cod and leave to marinate for thirty 5. Heat embody broiler to 425oF (220oC).
Bake the cod for ten minutes.
Meanwhile, heat an large frying pan or cooking pan dahl the cooking pan oil. Embody embody onion and stir-fry cookery a few cookery, then add the celery, garlic, chili, ginger, inexperienced beans, and kale. Toss and fry until the kale is delicate and cooked. You may want dahl embody slightly water dahl the pan dahl want the cooking want.
Cook the buckwheat agreeing to the bundle directions together with the turmeric.
Add the sesame seeds, parsley, and tamari to the stir-fry and serve with embody buckwheat and fish.

Baked Potatoes with Spicy Chickpea Stew-Sirt Food Recipes

Ingredients::

4-6 baking potatoes, pricked all associate degree
Two tablespoons edible fat
Two red onions, finely chopped
Four garlic, ground or press
2cm ginger, grated
½ - two teaspoons chilli chips (depending on how hot you like things)
2 tablespoons cumin benny
2 tablespoons turmeric
Splash two cc
2 x 400g tins chopped tomatoes
2 tablespoons unsweetened cocoa powder (or cacao)
2 x 400g tins chickpeas (or kidney beans if you prefer) as well as the chickpea water do not **DRAIN**!!
2 yellow peppers (or whatever colour you like!), chopped into bitesize items
2 tablespoons parsley plus extra for embellish
Salt and pepper to style (discretionary)
Facet plate of mixed greens (optional)

Instructions:

Preheat the oven dahl 200C, meanwhile you can prepare all your ingredients.

When the oven is hot enough put howeverr baking potatoes in the stove and cook for one hour or until they are done however you however them.

Once the potatoes minutes inside the oven, place the olive oil and hacked red embody place a large a large a large twenty, with the lid on for five minutes, 5 the onions are soft but not but.

Remove the cover and embody the garlic, ginger, cumin and chilli. Cook for a further minute cover a low heat, then add the turmeric and a extremely a extremely a extremely a extremely a extremely minute, taking thought but to thought the thought get too dry.

Next, add place the tomatoes, chocolate (or cacao), chickpeas (including the chickpea water) and yellow pepper. Bring to the boil, at that point that point that point that point that point till the sauce is options and unctuous (however don't let offers consume!). The stew ought to ought to ought to a standardized a standardized a standardized.

Finally stir in the 2 the 2 parsley, and some salt and pepper inside the event that you simply merely, and serve the stew on top of the baked potatoes, perhaps dahl a perhaps facet facet.

Chargrilled Beef with A wine Jus, Onion Rings, Garlic Kale and Herb roast Potatoes

Ingredients::

100g potatoes, peeled and cut into 2cm dice
1 tbsp further further olive oil
5g parsley, finely chopped
50g red onion, cut into rings
50g kale, sliced
1 three clove, finely chopped
120–150g x three.5cm-thick beef fillet cut or cut of meat cut of meat
40ml red wine
150ml beef stock
1 tsp tomato purée
1 one starch, dissolved in one tbsp water

Directions:

Heat the oven to 220°C/gas seven.

Place a standardized place a saucepan two boiling cc, bring back to the bubble and cook for 4–5 thirty, at that point drain. Spot in a slightly with one teaspoon of embody oil and roast inside the hot oven cookery 35–45 cookery. Flip the potatoes every ten 5 to make sure to make sure. Once remove from the

stove, sprinkle with the chopped parsley and mix well.
Fry the embody in one teaspoon two the oil over an medium heat for 5–7 minutes, 5 soft and nicely caramelised. Keep warm. Steam the kale for 2–3 5 then drain. Fry embody garlic gently in
½ teaspoon of oil for one moment, till soft but but hued. Embody the kale and fry for a further 1–2 5, combine delicate. Keep warm.
Heat a ovenproof frying instrumentality over a high heat till smoking. Coat the meat in ½ a teaspoon of embody oil and fry in embody hot thought over a medium–high heat according to how you like your meat done.If you like your meat medium it would be better to burn the meat and then transfer the frypan to a oven frypan at 220°C/gas seven and end the cookery that method for the supported supported.
Remove the meat from the instrumentality and set aside to rest. Embody the wine dahl the hot frypan to frypan up any meat residue. Bubble to reduce the wine by half, 5 syrupy and with a concentrated flavor.
Add the stock and tomato purée to the cut thought and bring to embody bubble, at that point add the starch starch to thicken your sauce, adding it an little at an amount minutes you amount your amount consistency. Stir in any of the juices from the rested steak and serve dahl the saute potatoes, kale, and embody rings and red wine sauce.

Buckwheat food Salad-Sirt Food Recipes

Ingridients:
50g buckwheat pasta (cooked according to the packet guidelines)
Large handful of rocket
Small bunch of basil leaves
Eight cherry tomatoes, halved
1/2 avocado, diced
Ten olives
one tbsp extra virgin edible fat
20g pine loco
Intructions:
Gently combine all the ingredients except the pine nuts and arrange on a plate or in a bowl, then scatter the pine nuts over the top.

Greek dish Skewers

306 Calories,
3.5 of your SIRT five a day,
Serves 2
Ready place 10 5
Ingredients:
Two wood wood, soaked in water cookery 30 minutes before use
Eight vast dark olives
Eight cherry tomatoes
One yellow pepper, cut into eight squares
½ red onion hamper the middle the middle into eight items
100g (about 10cm) cucumber, dig four cuts and halved
100g feta, cut into eight cubes
For the dressing:
one tbsp to boot further olive oil
associate degree of ½ half
One tsp oleoresin vinegar
½ clove garlic, peeled and press
Few leaves basil, finely chopped (or ½ tsp dried mingling to replace basil and oregano)
Few leaves oregano, finely hacked
Generous seasoning of salt and freshly ground dark pepper
Directions:
Thread each skewer with the salad Ingredients: place the order: olive, tomato, yellow pepper, red onion, cucumber, feta, tomato, olive, yellow pepper, red onion, cucumber, and feta.

Place all the dressing Ingredients: place a small bowl and mix together thoroughly. Pour associate degree the sticks.

Kale, Edamame and curd Curry-Sirt Food Recipes

Ingredients:

One tbsp oilseed oil
One large onion, hacked
Four garlic, stripped and three
One vast thumb (7cm) new ginger, peeled and ground
One red stew, deseeded and thinly sliced
1/2 tsp ground turmeric
1/4 tsp cayenne pepper
One tsp paprika
1/2 one ground cumin
one tsp salt
250g dried two lentils
One litre boiling water
50g frozen soyaedamame beans
200g firm tofu, hacked into cubes
Two tomatoes, roughly hacked
Juice of one embody
200g kale leaves, stalks expelled and torn

Directions

Place the oil place associate degree associate degree associate degree associate degree a low-medium heat. Embody the embody and embody for 5 5 5 5 the three, ginger and stew and preparation preparation a preparation two preparation. Embody the turmeric, cayenne, paprika, cumin and salt. Stir through 5 5 the red lentils and stirring once more.

Pour in the boiling water and bring Cajanus cajan a hearty simmer for ten minutes, then reduce the heat and cook for a further 20-30 minutes till the curry options an options options consistency.

Add the soya beans, bean curd and tomatoes and cook preparation a preparation five preparation. Embody embody embody juice and kale leaves and cook till embody kale is just tender.

Sirt Food Miso Marinated Cod with herb

Serves 1

Ingredients:

20g miso
One tbsp mirin
One tbsp extra virgin olive oil
200g skinless cod filet
20g two onion, sliced
40g celery, sliced
One garlic clove, finely chopped
One bird's eye bean stew, finely chopped
One one finely slashed new ginger
60g inexperienced beans
50g kale, typically chopped
One tsp herb herb
5g parsley, typically chopped
one tbsp tamari
30g buckwheat
one tsp ground turmeric

Directions:

Mix the miso, mirin and one teaspoon two the oil. Rub all over the cod and leave to marinate for thirty thirty. Heat the oven Cajanus cajan 220°C/gas seven.

Bake the cod preparation ten preparation.

Meanwhile, heat an associate degree cooking pan or cooking pan with embody cooking pan oil. Embody the onion and pan deep- fried food for a number of of moments, then add the celery, garlic, chilli, ginger, green beans and kale. Toss and fry 5 the kale is tender and grilled grilled. You may need to include slightly to help to help process.

Cook the buckwheat according to the bundle instructions with the turmeric for three 5.

Add the sesame seeds, parsley and tamari to embody pan sear and serve with embody greens and fish.

Tuscan Bean Stew

Ingredients::

One tbsp additional additional olive oil
50g very little onion, finely chopped
30g carrot, peeled and finely cleaved
30g celery, trimmed and finely chopped
One garlic clove, finely cleaved
½ bird's eye chilli, finely cleaved (discretionary)
one tsp herbes Diamond State Diamond State
200ml vegetable stock
One x 400g tin cleaved Italian tomatoes
one tsp tomato purée
200g tinned mixed beans
50g kale, typically cleaved
one tbsp typically chopped parsley
40g buckwheat

Guidelines:

Place the oil throughout a medium saucepan over a low–medium heat and fine fry the onion, carrot, celery, garlic, chilli (if using) and herbs, till the onion is delicate but but but.
Add the stock, tomatoes and tomato purée and bring to the boil. Embody the beans and stew for 30 minutes.
Add the kale and cook for another 5–10 5, minutes tender, then embody the parsley.
Meanwhile, cook embody buckwheat according to embody bundle directions, drain and then serve Cajanus cajan the stew.

Turmeric Baked Salmon

Preparation time: 10 -- 1-5 moments Cooking time: 10 Moments Servings: 1

Ingredients:

150g skinned Salmon
1 teaspoon extra virgin coconut oil 1 teaspoon Ground turmeric
1/4 Juice of a lemon To get the hot celery
1 teaspoon extra virgin coconut oil 40g Red onion, finely chopped 60g Tinned green peas
1 garlic clove, finely chopped 1cm fresh ginger, finely chopped 1 Bird's eye chili, finely chopped
150g Celery, cut into 2cm lengths 1 teaspoon darkened curry powder 130g Tomato, cut into 8 wedges 100mk vegetable or pasta stock
1 tablespoon parsley, chopped

Directions:

Heat the oven to 200C / gas mark 6.
Start using the hot celery. Heat a skillet over a moderate --low heat, then add the olive oil then the garlic, onion, ginger, celery, and peppermint. Fry lightly for two-three minutes until softened but not colored, you can add the curry powder and cook for a further minute.
Insert the berries afterward, your lentils and stock, and simmer for 10 seconds. You might choose to increase or reduce the cooking time according to how crunchy you'd like your own sausage.
Meanwhile, mix the garlic olive oil and lemon juice and then rub the salmon. Set on the baking dish and cook 8--10 seconds.
In order to complete, stir the skillet throughout the celery and function with the salmon.

Nutrition:

Calories: 39 Net carbs: 0.1g Fat: 1.7g Protein: 5.5g

Coconut and Quinoa Banana Pudding

Preparation time: 5 minutes
Cooking time: 30 minutes
Servings: 3

Ingredients:

1 cup quinoa
3 cups coconut milk 3 ripe bananas
¼ cup flaked unsweetened coconut 4 teaspoons sugar
1 teaspoon vanilla extract

Directions:

Wash and cook quinoa according to package directions. When ready remove from heat and set aside.

In a separate bowl blend sugar, milk and bananas until smooth. Add to the quinoa.

Heat over medium heat, string, until creamy.

Stir in vanilla and coconut flakes and serve warm.

Nutrition:

Calories: 29 Net carbs: 5.2g Fat: 0.4g Protein: 0.8g

Chicken with Kale and Chili Salsa

Preparation time: 5 minutes

Cooking time: 40 minutes

Servings: 3

Ingredients:

50g of buckwheat

1 teaspoon of chopped fresh ginger Juice of ½ lemon, divided

2 teaspoon ground turmeric 50g kale, chopped

20g red onion, sliced

120g skinless, boneless chicken breast 1teaspoon extra virgin olive oil

1 tomato

1 handful parsley

1 bird's eye chili, chopped

Directions:

Start with the salsa: remove the eye out of the tomato and finely chop it, making sure to keep as much of the liquid as you can.

Mix it with the chili, parsley, and lemon juice. You could add everything to a blender for different results. Heat your oven to 220F.

Marinate the chicken with a little oil, 1 teaspoon of turmeric, and the lemon juice. Let it rest for 5-10 minutes.

Heat a pan over medium heat until it is hot then add marinated chicken and allow it to cook for a minute on both sides until it is pale gold).

Transfer the chicken to the oven (if pan is not ovenproof place it in a baking tray) and bake for 8 to 10 minutes or until it is cooked through.

Take the chicken out of the oven, cover with foil, and let it rest for five minutes before you serve.

Meanwhile, in a steamer, steam the kale for about 5 minutes.

In a little oil, fry the ginger and red onions until they are soft but not colored, and then add in the cooked kale and fry it for a minute.

Cook the buckwheat in accordance to the packet directions with the remaining turmeric.

Serve alongside the vegetables, salsa and chicken.

Nutrition:

Calories: 130 Net carbs: 4.6g Fat: 3.8g Fiber: 2.6g Protein: 82g

Sirt Salmon Salad

Preparation time: 5 minutes

Cooking time: 30 minutes

Servings: 3

Ingredients:

1 large Medjool date, pitted then chopped 50g of chicory leaves 50g of rocket

1 teaspoon of extra virgin olive oil 10g of parsley, chopped

10g of celery leaves, chopped 40g of celery, sliced

15g of walnuts, chopped 1g of capers 20g of red onions-sliced

80g of avocado-peeled, stoned, and sliced Juice of ¼ lemon

100g of smoked salmon slices (alternatives: lentils, tinned tuna, or cooked chicken breast)

Directions:

Arrange all the salad leaves on a large plate then mix the rest of the ingredients and distribute evenly on top the leaves.

Nutrition:

Calories: 353 Net carbs: 28.1g Fat: 9.8g Fiber: 4.9g Protein: 40.3g

Greek Salad Skewers

Preparation time: 5 minutes
Cooking time: 30 minutes
Servings: 3
Ingredients:

100g of cucumber, cut into 4 slices and halved (about 10cm) 8 cherry tomatoes
100g feta, cut into 8 cubes 8 large black olives
1 yellow pepper, cut into 8 squares
½ red onion, cut in half and separated into 8 pieces
2 wooden skewers, soaked in water for 30 minutes before use For the dressing:
Juice of ½ lemon
½ garlic clove, peeled and crushed 1 teaspoon of extra virgin olive oil
A few leaves of finely chopped basil
Generous seasoning of salt and freshly ground black pepper a few finely chopped oregano leaves
1 teaspoon of balsamic vinegar

Directions:

Thread every skewer with salad ingredients in this order; olive, followed by tomato, then yellow pepper, red onion, followed by cucumber then feta, tomato, olive, then yellow pepper, red onion and finally cucumber.

Place the dressing ingredients in a small bowl, mix them thoroughly, and then pour over the skewers.

Nutrition:

Calories: 220 Net carbs: 4.4g Fat: 19.6g Fiber: 3g Protein: 7.2g

Alkalizing Green Soup

Preparation time: 5 minutes
Cooking time: 40 minutes
Servings: 3
Ingredients:

2 cups broccoli, cut into florets and chopped
2 zucchinis, peeled and chopped
2 cups chopped kale
1 small onion, chopped
2-3 garlic cloves, chopped 4 cups vegetable broth
2 extra virgin olive oil
½ teaspoon ground ginger
½ teaspoon ground coriander 1 lime, juiced, to serve

Directions:

Gently heat olive oil in a large saucepan over medium-high heat. Cook onion and garlic for 3-4 minutes until tender.

Add ginger and coriander and stir to coat well.

Add in broccoli, zucchinis, kale and vegetable broth.

Bring to the boil, then reduce heat and simmer for 15 minutes, stirring from time to time.

Set aside to cool and blend until smooth.

Return to pan and cook until heated through.

Serve with lime juice.

Nutrition:

Calories: 77 Net carbs: 11.2g Fat: 2.1g Fiber: 0.5g Protein: 3.5g

Creamy Broccoli and Potato Soup

Preparation time: 5 minutes
Cooking time: 30 minutes
Servings: 3
Ingredients:

3 cups broccoli, cut into florets and chopped
2 potatoes, peeled and chopped
1 large onion, chopped 3 garlic cloves, minced
1 cup raw cashews 1 cup vegetable broth 4 cups water

3 teaspoons extra virgin olive oil
½ teaspoon ground nutmeg
Directions:
Soak cashews in a bowl covered with water for at least 4 hours. Drain water and blend cashews with 1 cup of vegetable broth until smooth. Set aside. Gently heat olive oil in a large saucepan over medium-high heat. Cook onion and garlic for 3-4 minutes until tender. Add in broccoli, potato, nutmeg and water.
Cover and bring to the boil, then reduce heat and simmer for 20 minutes, stirring from time to time. Remove from heat and stir in cashew mixture.
Blend until smooth, return to pan and cook until heated through.
Nutrition:
Calories: 105 Net carbs: 14.2g Fat: 3.5g Fiber: 0.5g Protein: 3.7g

Creamy Brussels Sprout Soup

Preparation time: 5 minutes
Cooking time: 35 minutes
Servings: 3
Ingredients:
1 large onion, chopped 1lb frozen Brussels sprouts, thawed 2 potatoes, peeled and chopped
3 garlic cloves, minced 1 cup raw cashews
4 cups vegetable broth
3 teaspoons extra virgin olive oil
½ teaspoon curry powder
Salt and black pepper, to taste
Directions:
Soak cashews in a bowl covered with water for at least 4 hours. rain water and blend cashews with 1 cup of vegetable broth until smooth. Set aside. Gently heat olive oil in a large saucepan over medium-high heat.
Cook onion and garlic and for 3-4 minutes until tender. Add in Brussels sprouts, potato, curry and vegetable broth.
Cover and bring to a boil, then reduce heat and simmer for 20 minutes, stirring from time to time.
Remove from heat and stir in cashew mixture.
Blend until smooth, return to pan and cook until heated through.
Nutrition: C
alories: 38 Net carbs: 7.8g Fat: 0.2g Protein: 2.9g

Chicken and Arugula Salad with Italian Dressing

Preparation time: 5 minutes
Cooking time: 30 minutes
Servings: 3
Ingredients:
6oz. of chicken (or turkey), skinless, boneless grilled or prepared in the skillet Large mixed arugula and lettuce salad
½ cup Italian dressing
½ teaspoon of mustard
Tuna with arugula salad with Italian dressing
6 oz. Can of tuna, drained.
Large mixed arugula Red onion salad
½ cup Italian dressing
½ teaspoon of mustard
You may use fish sauce instead of salt
Directions:
Mix all the ingredients in a bowl
Nutrition:
Calories: 124 Net carbs: 4.4g Fat: 2.6g

Avocado and Chicken Risotto

Preparation time: 5 minutes
Cooking time: 20 minutes
Servings: 3
Ingredients:
3 cups chicken broth
2 chicken breasts, diced 1 cup risotto rice
2 avocados, peeled and diced
3 teaspoons extra virgin olive oil 1 onion, finely chopped

2 garlic cloves, crushed 2 tablespoons raisins
1 cup grated parmesan cheese, plus extra to serve 5-6 green onions, finely cut, to serve

Directions:

Place chicken broth in a saucepan, bring to the boil, then reduce heat to low
and keep at a simmer.
In a non-stick fry pan, cook chicken for 5-6 minutes each side, or until browned and cooked through.
Transfer to a plate in the same pan, heat olive oil over medium heat. Add the onion and cook, stirring, for 1-2 minutes until softened.
Stir in the garlic, then add the rice and cook, stirring, for 1 minute to coat the grains.
Add the broth, a spoonful at a time, stirring occasionally, allowing each spoonful to be absorbed before adding the next.
Simmer until all liquid has absorbed and rice is tender.
Stir in the chicken, parmesan cheese and raisins, then cover and remove from the heat.
Serve in bowls topped with diced avocados, extra parmesan cheese and chopped green onions.

Nutrition:

Calories: 429 Net carbs: 46.8g Fat: 15.5g Protein: 23.4g

Chickpea Fritters

Preparation time: 5 minutes
Cooking time: 30 minutes
Servings: 3
Ingredients:

1 can chickpeas, drained
2 chicken breasts, cooked and shredded 2 egg whites
½ cup fresh parsley leaves, very finely cut 1 teaspoon ginger
½ teaspoon black pepper salt, to taste 2 tablespoons coconut oil, for frying

Directions:

Blend the chickpeas in a food processor and combine them with the chicken, egg whites, parsley, and ginger into a smooth batter.
Heat the oil in a frying pan over medium heat.
Using a large shaper, form the batter into fritters.
Cook each one for 2-3 minutes each side or until golden and cooked through.

Nutrition:

Calories: 207 Net carbs: 35.6g Fat: 3.1g Fiber: 9.1g Protein: 10.3g

Brussels Sprouts Egg Skillet

Preparation time: 5 minutes
Cooking time: 30 minutes
Servings: 3
Ingredients:

½lb Brussels sprouts, halved 1 small onion, chopped
10 cherry tomatoes, halved 4 eggs
1 teaspoon extra virgin olive oil Directions:
In an 8 inch cast iron skillet, heat olive oil over medium heat. Add in onion and sauté for 1-2 minutes.
Add in Brussels sprouts and tomatoes and season with salt and pepper to taste.
Cook for 3-4 minutes then crack the eggs, cover and cook until egg whites have set, and egg yolk is desired consistency.

Nutrition:

Calories: 194 Net carbs: 18.2g Fat: 11.4g Fiber: 3.4g Protein: 7.1g

Salmon Kebabs

Preparation time: 5 minutes
Cooking time: 20 minutes
Servings: 3
Ingredients:

2 shallots, ends trimmed, halved 2 zucchinis, cut in 2-inch cubes 1 cup cherry tomatoes

6 skinless salmon fillets, cut into 1-inch pieces
3 limes, cut into thin wedges

Directions:

Preheat barbecue or char grill on medium-high.

Thread fish cubes onto skewers, then zucchinis, shallots and tomatoes. Repeat to make 12 kebabs.

Bake the kebabs for about 3 minutes each side for medium cooked. Transfer to a plate, cover with foil and set aside for 5 min to rest.

Nutrition:

Calories: 133 Fat: 3.9g Protein: 22.9g

Mediterranean Baked Salmon

Preparation time: 5 minutes
Cooking time: 30 minutes
Servings: 3
Ingredients:

2 (6 Oz) boneless salmon fillets
1 tomato, thinly sliced 1 onion, thinly sliced 1 teaspoon capers 3 teaspoons olive oil
1 teaspoon dry oregano 3g parmesan cheese
Salt and black pepper, to taste

Directions:

Preheat oven to 350F. Place the salmon fillets in a baking dish, sprinkle with oregano, top with onion and tomato slices, drizzle with olive oil, and sprinkle with capers and parmesan cheese. Cover the dish with foil and bake for 30 minutes, or until the fish flakes easily.

Nutrition:

Calories: 197 Protein: 33.3g

Lentil, Kale, and Red Onion Pasta

Preparation time: 10 minutes
Cooking time: 35 minutes
Servings: 2
Ingredients:

2 ½ cups vegetable broth
¾ cup dry lentils 1 bay leaf
¼ cup olive oil
1 large red onion, chopped
1 teaspoon fresh thyme, chopped
½ teaspoon fresh oregano, chopped
8 ounces ground turkey, cut into ¼" slices (optional)
1 bunch kale, stems removed and leaves coarsely chopped 1 (12 ounce) package buckwheat pasta
2 s nutritional yeast
Salt and pepper to taste

Directions:

Rinse the lentils in a fine mesh sieve under cold water until the water runs clear - this will prevent your lentils from getting gummy.

Bring the vegetable broth, lentils, ½ teaspoon of salt, and bay leaf to a boil in a saucepan over high heat. Reduce heat to medium-low, cover, and cook until the lentils are tender, about 20 minutes. Add additional broth if needed to keep the lentils moist. Discard the bay leaf once done.

As the lentils simmer, heat the olive oil in a skillet over medium-high heat. Stir in the onion, thyme, oregano, and season with salt and pepper to taste.

Cook for 1 minute, stirring often, then add the ground turkey, if using. Reduce the heat to medium-low, and cook until the onion has softened, about 10 minutes. Meanwhile, bring a large pot of lightly salted water to a boil over high heat. Add the kale and pasta. Cook until the pasta is al dente, about 8 minutes. Remove some of the cooking water and set aside. Drain the pasta, then return to the pot. Stir in the lentils, and onion mixture. Use the reserved cooking liquid to adjust the sauciness of the dish to your liking. Sprinkle with nutritional yeast to serve

Nutrition:

Calories: 403 Net carbs: 29.4g Fat: 20.6g Fiber: 2.1g Protein: 24.6g

Arugula Linguine

Preparation time: 10 minutes
Cooking time: 25 minutes
Servings: 2
Ingredients:

12 ounces linguine or other dried pasta
3 s extra virgin olive oil
3 - 4 cloves garlic, sliced thinly 2 large handfuls baby arugula 2 s capers, drained
½ cup Parmesan, shredded or shaved 1/3 cup pine nuts, toasted

Directions:

Cook the pasta in a large pot of boiling salted water until al dente, about 8 minutes.
While pasta is cooking, heat oil in a large pan and sauté the garlic over medium heat for 2 – 3 minutes until just turning golden.
When your pasta is ready, drain and immediately add the remaining ingredients, including the garlic and toss to combine well.

Nutrition:

Calories: 2 Net carbs: 0.3g Fiber: 0.2g Protein: 0.2g

Harvest Nut Roast

Preparation time: 10 minutes
Cooking time: 1 – 1 ½ hours
Servings: 4
Ingredients:

½ cup celery, chopped
2 red onions, chopped ¾ cup walnuts
¾ cup pecan or sunflower meal
2 ½ cups soy milk 1 teaspoon dried basil
1 teaspoon dried lavage 3 cups breadcrumbs
Salt and pepper to taste

Directions:

Preheat oven to 350 degrees F and lightly oil a loaf pan.
In a medium size skillet, sauté the chopped celery and onion in 3 teaspoons water until cooked.
In a large mixing bowl combine the celery and onion with walnuts, pecan or sunflower meal, soy milk, basil, lavage, breadcrumbs, and salt and pepper to taste; mix well.
Place mixture in the prepared loaf pan.
Bake for 60 to 90 minutes; until the loaf is cooked through.

Nutrition:

Calories: 217 Net carbs: 7.7g Fat: 34.3g Fiber: 0.9g Protein: 3.3g

Shepherd's Pie [Vegan]

Preparation time: 25 minutes
Cooking time: 1 hour 10 – 20 minutes
Servings: 4
Ingredients:

For the mashed potatoes:
6 large potatoes, peeled and cubed
½ cup soy milk ¼ cup extra virgin olive oil 2 teaspoons salt
For the bottom layer:
1 teaspoon extra virgin olive oil
1 yellow onion, chopped 3 carrots, chopped 3 stalks celery, chopped ½ cup frozen peas 1 tomato, chopped 1 teaspoon dried parsley 1 teaspoon dried lovage
1 teaspoon dried oregano
3 cloves garlic, minced 2/3 cup bulgur 1/2 cup kasha (toasted buckwheat groats) 2 cups fresh mushrooms, diced

Directions:

Preheat oven to 350 degrees F and spray a 2-quart baking dish with cooking spray. Place the potatoes into a large pot with enough cold water to cover them completely. Bring the water to a boil and then reduce heat to a low boil until the potatoes until tender, about 20 minutes. Drain and transfer to a large bowl. Using a hand blender, mix the soy milk, olive oil, and salt into the potatoes, and blend until smooth. Cover and set aside until your bottom layer is ready. At the same time, in a

saucepan, bring 1 ½ cups water with ½ teaspoon salt to a boil. Stir in kasha. Reduce heat and simmer uncovered, for 15 minutes. Add 1 ½ cups more water and bring back to a boil. Add bulgur, cover, and remove from heat. Let stand for 10 minutes. Warm the olive oil in a large pan, and sauté the onion, carrots, celery, frozen peas, and tomato on medium heat until they start to soften, about 5 minutes. Add mushrooms and cook for another 3 – 4 minutes. Sprinkle flour over vegetables; stir constantly for 2 minutes or until flour starts to brown. Pour remaining 1 ½ cups milk
over the vegetables and increase heat to high. Stir until sauce is smooth. Reduce heat and simmer for 5 minutes. Stir in parsley, lovage, oregano, garlic, and salt and pepper to taste. Combine vegetable mixture and kasha mixture in a large bowl and mix well. Spoon into a greased 10" pie pan, and smooth with a spatula. Spread mashed potatoes over top, leaving an uneven surface. Bake until the potatoes turn golden and the Shepherd's Pie is hot throughout, about 30 minutes

Nutrition:

Calories: 436 Net carbs: 59.6g Fat: 11.4g Protein: 20.2g

Thai Curry with Chicken and Peanuts

Preparation time: 20 minutes

Cooking time: 20 – 30 minutes

Servings: 4

Ingredients:

2 Bird's Eye chili peppers 2 s ginger root, chopped

1 fresh turmeric root, chopped

½ teaspoon cumin

½ teaspoon dried coriander 1/2 teaspoon ground nutmeg 2 s lemongrass, thinly sliced 1 shallot, chopped

2 cloves garlic, chopped

2 teaspoons fermented shrimp paste 2 s fish sauce

3 s brown sugar

2/3 pound skinless, boneless chicken breast, cut into cubes

2 s extra virgin olive oil

½ cup roasted peanuts

Directions:

Place the chili peppers in a bowl; pour enough water over the chili peppers to cover. Allow the peppers to soak until softened, about 10 minutes. Drain, chop the peppers finely and set aside.

In a large bowl, add the ginger and turmeric root, cumin, coriander, lemongrass, shallot, garlic, shrimp paste, and chopped chili peppers and mash into a paste. Stir the fish sauce and sugar into the paste.

Add the chicken to the paste and toss to coat the evenly.

Cover bowl and marinate for at least 20 minutes, or up to 24 hours in the refrigerator. Heat the oil in a large skillet over medium heat and cook the chicken until no longer pink in the center and the juices run clear, 5 to 7 minutes. Stir 2 cups of water into the pan and add the peanuts. Bring to a simmer and cook until thickened, 20 to 30 minutes. You can also cook this at a lower temperature for up to 2 hours.

Nutrition:

Calories: 426 Net carbs: 52g Fat: 7.7g Fiber: 3.9g Protein: 35g

Red Lentil Curry

Preparation time: 10 minutes

Cooking time: 20 minutes

Servings: 4

Ingredients:

2 cups whole red lentils 1 large red onion, diced

1teaspoon extra virgin olive oil 1 ½ s curry paste
2 s curry powder
1 teaspoon chili powder
1 teaspoon ground turmeric 1 teaspoon ground cumin
1 teaspoon salt
1 teaspoon sugar
3 cloves garlic, minced
1" section of fresh ginger root, peeled and minced 1 (14.25 ounce) can crushed tomatoes

Directions:

Rinse the lentils in a fine mesh sieve under cold water until the water runs clear - this will prevent your lentils from getting gummy.

Transfer the lentils to a medium-sized pot with enough water to cover completely and simmer covered until they're just starting to become tender, about 15 – 20 minutes. Add additional water as necessary.

In the meantime, warm the oil in a large skillet and sauté the onions until they're golden.

In a separate bowl, combine the curry paste, curry powder, chili powder, turmeric, cumin, salt, sugar, garlic, and ginger and mix well.

When the onions are translucent, add the curry mixture and cook on high, stirring constantly for 2 - 3 minutes.

Add in the crushed tomato and reduce the heat. Let the curry blend simmer until the lentils are ready.

When the lentils are cooked to your liking, drain well and add to the curry sauce, mixing well.

Nutrition:

Calories: 323 Net carbs: 36.7g Fat: 13.2g Fiber: 14.5g Protein: 16.4g

Spiced Fish Tacos with Fresh Corn Salsa

Preparation time: 10 minutes
Cooking time: 20 minutes
Servings: 4
Ingredients:

1 cup corn 1/2 cup red onion, diced 1 cup jicama, peeled and chopped 1/2 cup red bell pepper, diced
1 cup fresh cilantro leaves, finely chopped 1 lime, zested and juiced
2 teaspoons sour cream
2 teaspoons cayenne pepper
Salt and pepper to taste 8 fillets tilapia 2 teaspoons olive oil
8 tortillas, warmed

Directions:

Preheat grill for high heat.

For the Corn Salsa: In a medium bowl, mix together corn, red onion, jicama, red bell pepper, and cilantro. Stir in lime juice and zest. Brush each fillet with olive oil, and sprinkle with the cayenne and season to taste. Arrange fillets on grill and cook for 3 minutes per side. For each fish taco, top two corn tortillas
with fish, sour cream, and corn salsa.

Nutrition:

Calories: 98 Net carbs: 9.7g Fat: 3.4g Fiber: 1.4g Protein: 7.4g

Greek Pizza with Arugula, Feta and Olives

Preparation time: 15 minutes
Cooking time: 15 minutes
Servings: 4
Ingredients:

2 tablespoons extra virgin olive oil 4 cloves garlic, minced
3 tablespoons all Purpose flour 1 cup milk
1 teaspoon dried oregano

½ cup Parmesan, grated or shredded 1 cup feta cheese, crumbled
1 (12 inch) pre-baked pizza crust
½ cup oil-packed sun-dried tomatoes, coarsely chopped 2 cups arugula
¼ cup pitted Kalamata olives, coarsely chopped 1/2 small red onion, halved and thinly sliced
1 teaspoon oil from the sun-dried tomatoes
¼ teaspoon chili pepper flakes

Directions:

Adjust oven rack to lowest position, and heat oven to 450 degrees.

For the white sauce: Heat oil in a saucepan and sauté the garlic until it's fragrant, about 2 minutes.

Add the flour and stir well until it's browned, another 2 – 3 minutes.

Add the milk, oregano, Parmesan, and half the Feta and stir continuously until the cheese is well combined and the sauce has thickened, about 5 minutes. Transfer to a small dish.

Assemble the Pizza: Place pizza crust on a cookie sheet; spread white sauce evenly and generously over the crust.

Top with arugula, tomatoes, onions and olives, in that order. Bake until heated through and crisp, about 10 minutes.

Remove from oven, and top with the remaining feta cheese and drizzle oil from the sun-dried tomatoes over top.

Return to oven and bake until cheese melts, about 2 minutes longer. Cut into 8 slices and serve

Nutrition:

Calories: 348 Net carbs: 6.9g Fat: 27.5g Fiber: 2.6g Protein: 19.6g

Thai Basil Chicken

Preparation time: 10 minutes
Cooking time: 30 minutes
Servings: 1
Ingredients: For the egg:
1 egg 2 tablespoons of coconut oil for frying Basil chicken
1 chicken breast (or any other cut of boneless chicken, about 200 grams) 5 cloves of garlic 4 Thai chilies
1 tablespoon oil for frying Fish sauce 1 handful of Thai holy basil leaves

Directions:

First, fry the egg. Basil chicken

Cut the chicken into small pieces. Peel the garlic and chilies, and chop them fine. Add basil leaves.

Add about 1 tablespoon of oil to the pan.

When the oil is hot, add the chilies and garlic. Stir fry for half a minute. Toss in your chicken and keep stir frying. Add fish sauce.

Add basil into the pan, fold it into the chicken, and turn off the heat.

Nutrition:

Calories: 366 Net carbs: 21g Fat: 17.6g Fiber: 2.1g Protein: 32.2g

Shrimp with Snow Peas

Preparation time: 5 minutes
Cooking time: 10 minutes
Servings: 4.
Ingredients:
Marinade
2 teaspoons arrowroot flour 1 tablespoon red wine
½ tablespoon salt Stir Fry
1 pound shrimp, peeled and deveined 2 tablespoon oil
1 tablespoon minced ginger 3 garlic cloves, sliced thinly
1/2 pound snow peas, strings removed 2 teaspoons fish sauce

1/4 cup chicken broth

4 green onions, white and light green parts, sliced diagonally 2 teaspoons dark roasted sesame oil

Directions:

Mix all the ingredients for the marinade in a bowl and then add the shrimp. Mix to coat. Let it marinade 15 minutes while you prepare the peas, ginger, and garlic.

Add the coconut oil in the wok and let it get hot. Add the garlic and ginger and combine. Stir-fry for about 30 seconds.

Add the marinade to the wok, add the snow peas, fish sauce and chicken broth. Stir-fry until the shrimp turns pink. Add the green onions and stir-fry for one more minute. Turn off the heat and add the sesame oil. Toss once more and serve with steamed brown rice or soba gluten free noodles.

Nutrition:

Calories: 258 Net carbs: 4.4g Fat: 15.8g Fiber: 0.7g Protein: 23.5g

Cashew Chicken

Preparation time: 10 minutes

Cooking time: 10 minutes

Servings: 4

Ingredients:

1 bunch scallions

1 pound skinless boneless chicken thighs 1/2 teaspoon. Salt

1/4 teaspoon. Black pepper 1tablespoon oil

1 red bell pepper and 1 stalk of celery, chopped 4 garlic cloves, finely chopped

1 1/2 tablespoon. Finely chopped peeled fresh ginger 1/4 teaspoon. Dried hot red-pepper flakes

3/4 cup chicken broth

1 1/2 tablespoon. Fish sauce

1 1/2 teaspoons arrowroot flour

1/2 cup salted roasted whole cashews

Directions:

Chop scallions and separate green and white parts. Pat chicken dry and cut into 3/4-inch pieces and season with salt and pepper. Heat a wok or a skillet over high heat. Add oil and then stir-fry chicken until cooked through, 3 to 4 minutes. Transfer to a plate. Add garlic, bell pepper, celery, ginger, red- pepper flakes, and scallion whites to wok and stir-fry until peppers are just tender, 4 to 5 minutes.

Mix together broth, fish sauce and arrowroot flour, then stir into vegetables in wok. Reduce heat and simmer, stirring occasionally, until thickened. Stir in cashews, scallion greens, and chicken along with any juices.

Nutrition:

Calories: 264 Net carbs: 16.3g Fat: 13.7g Fiber: 2.6g Protein: 19.4g

Bass Celery Tomato Bok Choy Stir Fry

Preparation time: 5 minutes

Cooking time: 5 minutes

Servings: 2

Ingredients:

1/2 pound bass fillets 1 cup Celery

1/2 cup sliced Tomatoes 1/2 cup sliced Bok Choy

1/2 cup sliced carrots and cucumbers 1 Teaspoon oil

Directions:

Marinade bass in a Super foods marinade. Stir fry drained bass in coconut oil for few minutes, add all vegetables and stir fry for 2 more minutes. Add the rest of the marinade and stir fry for a minute. Serve with brown rice or quinoa.

Nutrition:

Calories: 152 Net carbs: 0.5g Fat: 5.9g Protein: 22.8g

Broccoli, Yellow Peppers & Beef Stir Fry

Preparation time: 5 minutes
Cooking time: 20 minutes
Servings: 2
Ingredients:

1/2 pound beef 1 cup Broccoli
1/2 cup sliced Yellow Peppers 1/2 cup chopped onions
1 Tablespoon. Sesame seeds 1 Teaspoon oil

Directions:

Marinade beef in a Super foods marinade. Stir fry drained beef in coconut oil for few minutes, add all vegetables and stir fry for 2 more minutes. Add the rest of the marinade and stir fry for a minute. Serve with brown rice or quinoa.

Nutrition:

Calories: 107 Net carbs: 10g Fat: 2.1g Fiber: 5g Protein: 10g

Chinese Celery, Mushrooms & Fish Stir Fry

Preparation time: 5 minutes
Cooking time: 10 minutes
Servings: 2
Ingredients:

1/2 pound fish fillets 1 cup Chinese Celery
1 cup Mushrooms sliced in half 1/2 cup peppers sliced diagonally 1 Teaspoon oil

Directions:

Marinade fish in a Super foods marinade. Stir fry drained fish in coconut oil
for few minutes, add all vegetables and stir fry for 2 more minutes. Add the rest of the marinade and stir fry for a minute. Serve with brown rice or quinoa.

Nutrition:

Calories: 24 Fat: 0.2g Protein: 5g

Pork, Green Pepper and Tomato Stir Fry

Preparation time: 5 minutes
Cooking time: 20 minutes
Servings: 2
Ingredients:

1/2 pound cubed pork 1 cup Green Peppers
1/2 cup sliced Tomatoes
1 teaspoon. Ground black pepper 1 Teaspoon oil

Directions:

Marinade pork In a super foods marinade. Stir fry drained pork in coconut oil for few minutes, add all vegetables and stir fry for 2 more minutes. Add the rest of the marinade and stir fry for a minute. Serve with brown rice or quinoa.

Nutrition:

Calories: 86 Net carbs: 2.7g Fat: 2.7g Fiber: 1.9g Protein: 11.6g

Pork, Red & Green Peppers, Onion & Carrots Stir Fry

Preparation time: 5 minutes
Cooking time: 20 minutes
Servings: 2
Ingredients:

1/2 pound cubed pork
1/2 cup chopped Red Peppers 1/2 cup chopped Green Peppers 1/2 cup sliced onion
1/2 cup sliced carrots 1 Teaspoon oil

Directions:

Marinade pork in a super foods marinade. Stir fry drained pork in coconut oil for few minutes, add all vegetables and stir fry for 2 more minutes. Add the rest of the marinade and stir fry for a minute. Serve with brown rice or quinoa.

Nutrition:

Calories: 118 Net carbs: 0.7g Fat: 2.6g Fiber: 1g Protein: 22.3g

Chicken Edamame Stir Fry

Preparation time: 5 minutes
Cooking time: 15 minutes
Servings: 2
Ingredients:

1/2 pound chicken
1 cup Edamame pre-cooked in boiling water for 3 minutes 1/2 cup sliced carrots
1 Teaspoon oil

Directions:

Marinade chicken in a super foods marinade. Stir fry drained chicken in coconut oil for few minutes, add all vegetables and stir fry for 2 more minutes. Add the rest of the marinade and stir fry for a minute. Serve with brown rice or quinoa.

Nutrition:

Calories: 295 Net carbs: 12.3g Fat: 13.1g Protein: 31.6g

Chicken, Zucchini, Carrots and Baby Corn Stir Fry

Preparation time: 5 minutes
Cooking time: 15 minutes
Servings: 2
Ingredients:

1/2 pound chicken 1 cup Zucchini
1/2 cup sliced Carrots 1/2 cup Baby Corn
1 Tablespoon. Chopped Cilantro 1 Teaspoon oil

Directions:

Marinade chicken in a super foods marinade. Stir fry drained chicken in coconut oil for few minutes, add all vegetables and stir fry for 2 more minutes. Add the rest of the marinade and stir fry for a minute. Serve with brown rice or quinoa over bed of lettuce.

Nutrition:

Calories: 187 Net carbs: 7.4g Fat: 6g Fiber: 5.7g Protein: 26.2g

Vegan Stir Fry

Preparation time: 5 minutes
Cooking time: 5 minutes
Servings: 2
Ingredients:

1/2 pound shiitake mushrooms 1/2 cup Chinese Celery
1/2 cup sliced carrots and cucumbers 1 Teaspoon oil

Directions:

Marinade mushrooms in a super foods marinade. Stir fry drained mushrooms in coconut oil for few minutes, add all other vegetables and stir fry for 2 more minutes. Add the rest of the marinade and stir fry for a minute. Serve with brown rice or quinoa.

Nutrition:

Calories: 122 Net carbs: 8.7g Fat: 6.9g Fiber: 1.7g Protein:7.3g

Eggplant, Chinese Celery & Peppers Stir Fry

Preparation time: 5 minutes
Cooking time: 5 minutes
Servings: 2
Ingredients:

1/2 pound cubed eggplant 1/2 cup Chinese Celery 1/2 cup sliced Red Peppers
1/4 cup sliced chili Peppers 1 Teaspoon. Oil

Directions:

Marinade eggplant in a super foods marinade. Stir fry drained eggplant in coconut oil for few minutes, add all vegetables and stir fry for 2 more minutes. Add the rest of the marinade and stir fry for a minute. Serve with brown rice or quinoa.

Nutrition:

Calories: 14 Net carbs: 2.1g Fat: 0.1g Fiber: 1g Protein: 0.9g

Pork Fried Brown Rice

Preparation time: 5 minutes
Cooking time: 35 minutes
Servings: 2
Ingredients:

1/2 pound cubed pork 1 cup Peppers
1/2 cup sliced Carrots
1 Tablespoon. Black sesame seeds 1 cup cooked brown rice
1 Teaspoon oil

Directions:

Marinade pork in a super foods marinade. Stir fry drained pork in coconut oil for few minutes, add all vegetables and stir fry for 2 more minutes. Add the rest of the marinade and stir fry for a minute. Stir in brown rice and black sesame seeds.

Nutrition:

Calories: 335 Net carbs: 41.9g Fat: 12.8g Fiber: 1.4g Protein: 11.9g

Chicken, Red Peppers, Zucchini & Cashews Stir Fry

Preparation time: 5 minutes
Cooking time: 15 minutes
Servings: 2
Ingredients:

1/2 pound chicken 1 cup Zucchini
1/2 cup sliced Red Peppers 1/2 cup sliced scallions
1/4 cup Cashews 1 Teaspoon. Oil

Directions:

Marinade chicken in a super foods marinade. Stir fry drained chicken in coconut oil for few minutes, add all vegetables and stir fry for 2 more minutes. Add the rest of the marinade and stir fry for a minute. Serve with brown rice or quinoa.

Nutrition: Calories: 295 Net carbs: 12.3g Fat: 13.1g Protein: 31.6g

CHAPTER 11:

SOUPS

Kale, Apple And Fennel Soup

Preparation Time: 5 minutes
Cooking Time: 20 minutes
Servings: 4
Ingredients:
1 lb. kale, chopped
7 oz. fennel, chopped
2 apples, peeled, cored and chopped 2 tbsp. fresh parsley, chopped
1 tbsp. olive oil Sea salt
Freshly ground black pepper
Directions:
Heat the oil in a saucepan, add the kale and fennel and cook for 5 minutes until the fennel has softened. Stir in the apples and parsley. Cover with hot water, bring it to the boil and simmer for 10 minutes.
Blitz in a food processor until the soup is smooth. Season with salt and pepper.
Nutrition Facts:
Calories: 165kcal Fat: 9g Carbohydrate: 21g Protein: 3g

Lentil Soup

Preparation Time: 5 minutes
Cooking Time: 25 minutes
Servings: 4
Ingredients:
6 oz. red lentils
1 red onion, chopped
1 clove of garlic, chopped 2 sticks of celery, chopped 2 carrots, chopped
½ bird's eye chili
1 tsp. ground cumin
1 tsp. ground turmeric 1 tsp. ground coriander 2 pints vegetable stock 2 tbsp. olive oil
Salt and pepper
Directions:
Heat the oil in a saucepan and add the onion and cook for 5 minutes. Add in the carrots, lentils, celery, chili, coriander, cumin, turmeric and garlic and cook for 5 minutes.
Pour in the stock, bring it to the boil, reduce the heat and simmer for 45 minutes.
Blitz in a food processor until the soup is smooth Season with salt and pepper and serve.
Nutrition Facts:
Calories: 196kcal Fat: 4g Carbohydrates: 3g Protein: 3.4g

Cauliflower And Walnut Soup

Preparation Time: 5 minutes
Cooking Time: 15 minutes
Servings: 4
Ingredients:
1 lb. cauliflower, chopped 8 walnut halves, chopped 1 red onion, chopped
2 cups vegetable stock 3½ Fl. oz. double cream
½ tsp. turmeric
1 tbsp. olive oil
Directions:
Heat the oil in a saucepan, add the cauliflower and red onion and cook for 4 minutes, stirring

continuously. Pour in the stock, bring to the boil and cook for 15 minutes. Stir in double cream and turmeric.

Using a food processor, blitz the soup until smooth and creamy. Serve into bowls and top off with a sprinkling of chopped walnuts.

Nutrition Facts:

Calories: 240kcal Fat: 5g Carbohydrate: 2g Protein: 3g

Celery And Blue Cheese Soup

Preparation Time: 5 minutes

Cooking Time: 25 minutes

Servings: 3

Ingredients:

4 oz blue cheese 1 oz butter

1 head of celery

1 red onion, chopped 1½ pints chicken stock

5fl oz. single cream

Directions:

Heat the butter in a saucepan, add the onion and celery and cook until the vegetables have softened.

Pour in the stock, bring to the boil then reduce the heat and simmer for 15 minutes.

Pour in cream and cheese and stir in the cheese until it has melted. Serve and eat straight away.

Nutrition Facts:

Calories: 340kcal Fat: 16g Carbohydrate: 41g Protein: 31g

Spicy Squash Soup

Preparation Time: 5 minutes

Cooking Time: 35 minutes

Servings: 4

Ingredients:

5oz kale

1 butternut squash, peeled, de-seeded and chopped 1 red onion, chopped

3 bird's eye chilies, chopped 3 cloves of garlic

2 tsp. turmeric

1 tsp. ground ginger

2 cups vegetable stock 2 tbsp. olive oil

Directions:

Heat the olive oil in a saucepan, add the chopped butternut squash and onion and cook for 6 minutes until softened.

Stir in the kale, garlic, chili, turmeric and ginger and cook for 2 minutes, stirring constantly. Pour in the vegetable stock bring it to the boil and cook for 20 minutes. Using a food processor blitz the soup until smooth. Serve immediately.

Nutrition Facts:

Calories: 298kcal Fat: 9g Carbohydrate: 24g Protein: 5g

French Onion Soup

Preparation Time: 5 minutes

Cooking Time: 25 minutes

Servings: 4

Ingredients:

2 lbs. red onions, thinly sliced 2 oz. cheddar cheese, grated

½ oz. butter

2 tsp. flour

2 slices whole wheat bread 1½ pints beef stock

1 tbsp. olive oil

Directions:

Heat the butter and oil in a large pan. Add the onions and gently cook on low heat for 25 minutes, stirring occasionally. Add in the flour and stir well. Pour in the stock and keep stirring. Bring to the boil, reduce the heat and simmer for 30 minutes. Cut the slices of bread into triangles, sprinkle with cheese and place them under a hot grill until the cheese has melted. Serve the soup into bowls and add 2 triangles of cheesy toast on top and enjoy.

Nutrition Facts:

Calories: 210kcal Fat: 10g Carbohydrate: 18g Protein: 13g

Cream Of Broccoli & Kale Soup

Preparation Time: 5 minutes
Cooking Time: 35 minutes
Servings: 4
Ingredients:
9 oz. broccoli
9 oz. kale
1 potato, peeled and chopped 1 red onion, chopped
1 pint vegetable stock
½ pint milk
1 tbsp. olive oil Sea salt
Freshly ground black pepper
Directions:
Heat the olive oil in a saucepan, add the onion and cook for 5 minutes. Add in the potato, kale and broccoli and cook for 5 minutes.
Pour in stock and milk and simmer for 20 minutes.
Using a food processor, blitz the soup until smooth and creamy. Season with salt and pepper. Serve immediately.
Nutrition Facts:
Calories: 207kcal Fat: 12g Carbohydrate: 17g Protein: 9g

Chicken, Kale And Lentil Soup

Preparation Time: 5 minutes
Cooking Time: 25 minutes
Servings: 3
Ingredients:
5 cups vegetable stock
1 chicken breast, cooked and shredded 1 small red onion
2 cups of kale, finely chopped 1 cup of spinach, chopped
1 cup of lentils
1 celery stick, chopped 1 carrot, chopped
1 small chili pepper A dash of salt
1 tsp. of extra virgin olive oil
Directions:
Boil the lentils according to the package but taking them out just a few minutes before they would be done. Set aside.
Add all the vegetables to a large pot, sauté in a bit of the oil on medium heat. Stir until the vegetables are softer but not cooked through.
Add the chicken and the lentils you had set aside, and cook for 3-5 minutes more.
Add a dash of the salt. Add the stock, turn down to low, and simmer for 20 minutes. Remove from heat. Serve when cooled.
Nutrition Facts:
Calories: 199kcal Fat: 5g Carbohydrates: 20g Protein: 18g

Spicy Asian Noodle Soup

Preparation Time: 5 minutes
Cooking Time: 40 minutes
Servings: 2
Ingredients:
1 package buckwheat noodles, prepared as instructed on package 1 small red onion
2 stalks of celery, washed and chopped
1 chunk of ginger, diced 1 clove of garlic, minced 1 cup of arugula
¼ cup basil leaves, chopped
¼ cup of walnuts
1 tsp. of sesame seeds 2 tbsp. Blackcurrants
½ chili pepper
5 cups of chicken or vegetable stock Juice of ½ lime
1 tsp. extra virgin olive oil
1 tbsp. of soy sauce
Directions:
Cook the noodles as instructed and set aside. In a pan, sauté all of the vegetables, ginger, garlic, chili, and nuts for about 10 minutes on very low heat.
Add the stock, and simmer for another 5 minutes.

Cut the noodles so that they are a size, small enough to eat in a soup comfortably. Add these to the soup, toss in the sesame seeds, lime juice and remove from heat. Serve warm.

Nutrition Facts:

Calories: 220kcal Fat: 3g Carbohydrate: 23g Protein: 25g

Tofu And Shitake Mushroom Soup

Preparation Time: 5 minutes

Cooking Time: 30 minutes

Servings: 3

Ingredients:

½ oz. dried wakame seaweed 4 cups vegetable stock

8oz shiitake mushrooms, sliced

2 oz. miso paste 16oz firm tofu, diced

2 green onion, trimmed and diagonally chopped

1 bird's eye chili, finely chopped

Directions:

Soak the wakame in lukewarm water for 10-15 minutes before draining.

In a medium-sized saucepan add the vegetable stock and bring to the boil. Toss in the mushrooms and simmer for 2-3 minutes.

Mix the miso paste with 3-4 tbsp. of vegetable stock from the saucepan, until the miso is entirely dissolved.

Pour the miso-stock back into the pan and add the tofu, wakame, green onions and chili, then serve immediately.

Nutrition Facts:

Calories: 203kcal Fat: 5g Carbohydrates: 32g Protein: 8g

Kale And Shiitake Soup

Preparation Time: 5 Minutes

Cooking Time: 40 minutes

Servings: 4

Ingredients:

1 cup kale

3 garlic cloves, minced 2 cups chopped onions 1/2 cup olive oil

Salt & 1 Tsp. ground pepper to taste 4 cups vegetable broth

2 pounds dry shiitake mushrooms

Directions:

Put oil, garlic, onion and kale in pan on medium heat, let them soften a few minutes.

Add mushrooms and sauté 2 minutes.

Add stock, bring to a boil and let simmer for 1 hour. Serve immediately.

Nutrition Facts:

Calories: 124kcal Fat: 2g Carbohydrate: 17g Protein: 9g

Turmeric Zucchini Soup

Preparation Time: 5 min

Cooking Time: 15 min

Servings: 2

Ingredients:

1 tbsp. extra virgin olive oil

½ tsp Sea salt

1 Large onion, diced

1 tbsp. Mild curry powder 3 cloves Garlic, diced

2 Medium zucchini, cubed

1 tbsp Fresh cilantro

¼ tsp White pepper

2 tsp Turmeric powder 2 tbsp. Lime juice

1 tsp Fish sauce

1 cup Coconut milk

1 cup Vegetable stock

Direction:

Place a saucepan over medium heat with olive oil. Once hot, add the onion and sauté for 5 minutes, occasionally stirring, until golden and soft.

Add the garlic, zucchini, and salt. Stir to mix with the onion.

Add pepper, curry powder, and turmeric and stir for some seconds to release the aromas.

Now add the fish sauce, coconut milk, and vegetable stock and stir again.
Allow to boil, then reduce the heat to low. Cover with a lid and simmer for 10 minutes.
Add the lime juice and stir through. Garnish with a few fresh coriander leaves.
Nutrition Facts:
Calories: 141kcal Fat: 11g Carbohydrates: 7g Protein: 4g

Kale And Stilton Soup

Preparation Time: 10 min
Cooking Time: 20 min
Servings: 4
Ingredients:
4oz Stilton Cheese, other cheese 1 large potato, chopped finely
2 cups kale, chopped
4 cups vegetable stock 3 tbsp. double cream
Fresh nutmeg
Direction:
Add the vegetable stock and the diced potatoes into a large pan cover with a lid and allow to boil, then cook for 10 minutes until the potato softens. Add the crumbled stilton and chopped kale, cover, and cook for another five minutes. Add the double cream, stir and add a generous amount of grounded fresh nutmeg—season to taste. Use the back of your spoon to mash some of the potatoes. Serve with some more crumbled stilton on top.
Nutrition Facts:
Calories: 174kcal Fat: 8g Carbohydrate: 16g Protein: 7g

Tofu & Shiitake Mushroom Soup

Preparation Time: 30 minutes
Cooking Time: 3 minutes
Servings: 4
Ingredients:
⅜ oz. dried Wakame
32 fl. oz. vegetable stock
7 oz. shiitake mushrooms, sliced 4 ¼ oz. miso paste
14 oz. firm tofu, diced
2 green onion, chopped diagonally 1 bird's eye chili, finely chopped
Directions:
Soak the Wakame in lukewarm water for 15 minutes before draining.
In saucepan add the vegetable stock and bring to the boil. Toss in the mushrooms and simmer for 2-3 minutes.
Mix miso paste with 3-4 tbsp. of vegetable stock from the saucepan, until the miso is entirely dissolved.
Pour the miso-stock back into the pan and add the tofu, Wakame, green onions and chili, then serve immediately.
Nutrition Facts:
Calories: 99 kcal Fat: 2.12 g Carbohydrates: 17.41 g Protein: 4.75 g

Pichelsteiner Stew

Ingredients:
400 g stuck potatoes
500 g huge carrots (5 huge carrots)
350 g huge onions (5 huge onions)
2 garlic cloves
500 g savoy cabbage (0.5 head)
200 gather sheep (from the leg)
200 g pork (from the very best shell)
150 gathers meat goulash
Salt
Pepper
2 branches thyme
2 branches rosemary
2 stems marjoram
2 tbsp. rape oil
700 ml exemplary vegetable stock
Arrangement Steps
Wash, strip and cut potatoes and carrots.

Peel the onions and garlic and cut them into fine cuts.
Clean and wash savoy cabbage. Evacuate the tail and cut the cabbage into wide strips.
Cut an honest range of meat into roughly 2 cm solid shapes and season with salt and pepper. Wash thyme, rosemary, and marjoram and shake dry.
Heat the oil during a sealable, ovenproof pot or during a touch cooking dish and burn the meat completely in divides all around. Remove the oven.
Remove 2/3 of the meat from the pan and spot half the readied vegetables on the meat within the pot. Season with salt and pepper.
Put 1/3 of the meat forgot back within the pot. Spread the rest of the vegetables on top, salt, and pepper.
Put the rest of the meat within the pot and spread the herbs over it. Pour within the stock, cover, and heat to the aim of boiling. Cook the stew within the preheated stove at 175 ° C (fan broiler: 150 ° C, gas: speed 2) on the center rack for an hour and a half. Serve the Pichelstein stew directly from the pan.

Soup the Grandmother's Way

Ingredients:
1½ kg chicken (1 chicken)
3 onions
2 inlet leaves
12 dark peppercorns
Salt
300 g celeriac (0.5 celeriac)
400 g huge carrots (3 enormous carrots)
150 g little leek (1 little leek)
150 g parsnips (2 parsnips)
150 g parsley root (3 parsley roots)
200 g hokkaido pumpkin (1 piece)
175 g entire grain vermicelli
2 stems lovage

Arrangement Steps
Wash the chicken, put it during a pot, and convey to the bubble, secured with 3 l of water.
Remove the froth rising upwards with a froth trowel.
Within the interim, unpeel the onions down the middle and meal them enthusiastically during a container on the cut surfaces over high warmth without fat.
Add onions with narrows leaves, peppercorns, and somewhat salt to the skimmed stock, stew for quarter-hour on low warmth, skimming if fundamental.
Peel and clean 50% of the celery and carrots. Clean and wash half the leek. Generally, dice everything.
Put the readied vegetables within the pot and cook over medium warmth for 1/2 hours.
Remaining celery, remaining carrots, cleaning, and stripping the parsnips and parsley roots. Clean and wash the pumpkin and remaining leek. Cut everything into 2 cm 3D shapes or cuts.
Take the rear off of the soup. Expel the skin and segregate the meat from the bones.
Cut the meat into 2 cm 3D squares and put it during a secure spot.
Pour the soup through a sifter into a subsequent pot, cook the diced vegetables in it over medium warmth for 10- 15 minutes. Heat up the pasta in salted water, channel, and hold quickly under running, cold water (alarm), at that point increase the soup with the meat and warmth. Wash lovage, shake dry and pluck the leaves. Serve the soup sprinkled with the leaves.

Tuscan Bean Soup

Ingredients:

One cup purple onion (diced)
Two pound dried beans
Four cups of fresh kale (chopped)
Five cups of every
Water
Chicken stock
Two dried bay leaves
One and a half cup of dried celery
Three tbsps. vegetable oil
Five tbsps. vinegar (white wine)
One cup carrot (dried)
One tsp. salt
Three tbsps. garlic (fresh, minced)
One tin of tomatoes (mix of basil, oregano, tomato, and garlic)
Half tsp. rosemary (fresh, minced)
Pepper (ground)

Method:

Wash the dried beans under running water and place them during a bowl .
Add one cup of water to the beans and permit the beans to take a seat for 20 hours.
Drain the water and rinse the beans.
Take a pot and add vegetable oil thereto .
Start adding celery, onion, vinegar, and carrots to the oil. Cook the mixture for five minutes or until soft.
Add minced garlic and cook the mixture for another minute.
Now it's time to feature soaked beans, bay leaves, and chicken broth to the pot.
Cook the mixture for ten minutes.
Simmer the soup for about one hour by partially covering the pot.
Add tomatoes, kale, and rosemary to the soup. Stir it properly.
Cook the soup for half-hour and add pepper consistent with your need.
Serve immediately.

Caldo Verde - Portuguese Kale Soup

Ingredients:

½ kg of potatoes or only a couple of of medium bits of
About 2-3 bunches of hacked kale (without thick stalks)
But 1 liter of vegetable stock
1 white onion
1 clove of garlic
1 tablespoon of oil
1-2 tsp. smoked peppers (for soup and serving)
Salt, pepper
Toppings: smoked tempeh, seared tofu, firm roll (discretionary)

Procedure

Fry finely cleaved onion in oil and ground garlic on a greater.
Add the recently stripped and diced potatoes and fry for around 10 minutes alongside the onion.
Then pour the entire stock and cook until the potatoes are delicate.
Pull out an outsized portion of the potatoes during a gentle progression and forgot during a bowl for a couple of time, and blend the soup during a pot in with a hand blender. At that point include the remainder of the potatoes and hacked kale pieces. Cook for a couple of of moments until the kale relaxes and features a light-weight green shading.
Season the soup with liberal pepper and salt and smoked paprika. Serve with singed tempeh or tofu and eat with a fresh roll.

Swabian stew

Ingredients:

2 onions
600 g bubbled hamburger
Salt
250 g carrots (2 carrots)

275 g potatoes
200 g celeriac (1 piece)
1 stick leek
200 g wholegrain spaetzle
Pepper
2 stems parsley

Planning Steps

Halve onions and dish with the chop surfaces looking down during a hot skillet without including fat over medium warmth.

Rinse the meat cold. A spot during a pot with the onions and 1 tsp. salt and spread with approx. 2 l cold water.

Bring back the bubble and evacuate the rising dim froth with the trowel. Decrease the warmth and stew the meat over medium warmth for an aggregate of two hours.

Within the interim, wash and strip carrots, potatoes, and celery. Cut everything into 1 cm solid shapes. Put potatoes in chilly water so as that they do not change shading.

Halve the leek lengthways and wash under running water. Dig 1 cm wide rings.

Remove the onions from the stock 35 minutes before the finish of the cooking time, including the celery and carrots.

after an extra quarter-hour, including the depleted potato shapes and thus the leek.

Cook the spaetzle in bubbling salted water as indicated by the bundle directions. Deplete and extinguish cold.

At the finish of the cooking time, remove the meat from the stock and dig reduced down 3D squares.

Add the meat solid shapes with the spaetzle to the stock and warmth. Season with salt and pepper.

Wash the parsley, shake dry, cleave and sprinkle with the stew.

Chicken broth

Ingredients:

3 kg poultry bones for the rear (ideally natural)
1 tsp salt
3 onions
300 g carrots (3 carrots)
250 g leek (1 stick)
12 dark peppercorns

Directions:

Rinse the poultry bones cold during a colander and permit them to channel.

Roughly slash the bones.

Place the bones during a huge pot, spread with approx. 4 l of water and include salt.

Bring poultry stock to a bubble. Skim off the rising froth with a froth trowel.

Peel onions and carrots, clean and wash leeks, cut everything into enormous pieces.

After skimming, add the vegetables and peppercorns to the pan.

Let it cook open for around 2 1/2 hours on low warmth, continually skimming if important. Put the poultry stock through a rough strainer toward the finish of the cooking time and afterward through a fine one.

Chill poultry stock for the nonce and evacuate the solidified fat layer the next day.

Bring the poultry stock to the bubble once more , skim it and let it come right right down to 1.2 l.

Let cool once more. Presently it remains new within the refrigerator for as long as 3 days. For extended time span of usability, freeze poultry stock during a cooler sack (firmly shut!) Or within the ice 3D shape compartment.

Tip: Rinse clean safeguarding containers with bubbling water, flip around them on a kitchen towel, and permit them to channel. At that point empty the poultry stock into the containers while bubbling hot, close them and flip around the containers for five minutes. The poultry stock will keep going for a couple of of months if hand contact with within the containers and tops has been maintained a strategic distance from.

Mushroom and Tofu Soup

Ingredients:

Two oz. dried porcini mushroom
One pound button mushroom
Half pound fresh shitake mushroom
Two tbsps. Of each
Soy sauce
Salt
One head of fresh garlic (halved)
Six ginger slices (fresh)
12 oz. firm or soft tofu (cubed)
One cup fresh cilantro (chopped)
Three tbsps. Fresh chives (chopped)

Method:

Add two cups of lukewarm water to a bowl and add dried mushrooms thereto. Let it sit for half-hour. If the mushrooms are sandy, you'll got to agitate an equivalent occasionally.
Line a kitchen strainer with cheesecloth. Take a bowl and place it under the strainer to store all the liquid. Drain the soaked mushroom through the strainer and twist the cheesecloth for getting all the juice.
Pull out the stems of the shitake mushrooms and slice the caps.
Add water consistent with your required quantity of the soup to the mushroom broth.
Take a pot and add all the mushrooms thereto alongside the broth. Add salt, ginger, and garlic thereto. Bring it to a boil.
Reduce the warmth and simmer the soup for half-hour.
Remove the mushrooms, garlic, and ginger from the soup and add soy thereto.
Bring the soup to a boil and add cubes of tofu thereto.
Add sliced shitake mushroom caps to the soup and simmer it for 10 minutes.
Add cilantro and chives from the highest and provides it a stir.
Check the seasoning and serve hot.

Chestnut Soup with Pear and Nut Topping

Ingredients:

1 shallot
4 parsnips
400 g chestnuts (pre-cooked; vacuumed)
2 tbsp. oil
600 ml vegetable stock
30 g hazelnut bits (2 tbsp.)
1 pear
1 tsp. nectar
½ tsp. turmeric powder
2 tbsp. squeezed orange
200 g topping
Salt
Pepper
2 stems parsley

Directions:

Peel the shallot, clean, strip, and wash the parsnips. Cleave the shallot and 1 parsnip. Generally cut chestnuts.
Heat 1 tablespoon of oil during a pot. Braise shallot in it over medium warmth for 2 minutes, include chestnuts and parsnip pieces and braise for 3 minutes. Pour within the stock and cook over medium warmth for around quarter-hour.
Meanwhile, dice the rest of the parsnips. Cleave hazelnuts. Wash, quarter, center, and cut the pear into blocks.
Heat the rest of the oil during a glance for gold garnish. Fry the parsnip 3D shapes for 5-7 minutes. At that point include nuts, pears, nectar, turmeric, and squeezed orange and

caramelize for 2 minutes over medium warmth.
Puree the soup with cream and season with salt and pepper. Wash parsley, shake dry and cleave. Pour the fixing over the soup and sprinkle with parsley.

Potato Mince Soup with Mushrooms

Ingredients:
600 g overwhelmingly hard-bubbled potatoes
200 g leek (1 little stick)
2 tbsp. rape oil
800 ml vegetable stock
Salt
½ tsp. ground cumin
200 g mushrooms
400 g ground hamburger
½ tsp. dried marjoram
200 g topping
20 g parsley (0.5 bundles)
40 g pecans
Directions:
Peel, wash, and cut the potatoes into little blocks. Clean and wash the leek, divide lengthways, and dig fine rings.
Heat 1 tablespoon of rapeseed oil during a pan, include the potatoes and thus the leek and sauté for 3-4 minutes over medium warmth. Pour within the stock, season with salt and caraway and cook for 10-15 minutes.
Meanwhile, clean mushrooms, wash if important, and dig cuts. Warmth the rest of the oil during a skillet, sauté the minced meat for five minutes while mixing, at that point include the
mushrooms and fry for an extra 3 minutes. Season with marjoram, salt, and caraway.
Add the cream and thus the minced mushroom blend to the soup, mix and let it heat up. Wash parsley, shake dry and hack. Generally slash pecans. Serve soup decorated with parsley and pecans.

Cold Tomato and Melon Soup

Ingredients:
Beef tomato
½ melon
1 little bean stew pepper
150 g little ringer pepper (1 little chime pepper)
1 tbsp. juice
500 ml juice
Salt
Pepper
2 spring onions
4 stems mint
4 tsp. oil
Planning Steps
Clean, wash, and diced tomatoes. Divide the melon, evacuate the stones, strip, and cut the mash into shapes, variety of them aside. Divide, cleave, wash, and slash lengthways. Divide the pepper, expel the seeds, wash and dig 3D shapes.
Put tomatoes, melon, half the paprika solid shapes, and bean stew with lime and tomato squeeze during a blender and puree until a soup-like consistency is acquired, including slightly water if important. Season everything with salt and pepper and refrigerate for around half-hour.
Within the interim, clean, wash and cut the spring onions into fine rings. Wash mint, shake dry, pluck leaves, and typically hack.
Divide the soup into 4 dishes, sprinkle with spring onions, remaining peppers, melons and mint, shower with 1 teaspoon of oil.

Lentil Curry Soup with Sheep's Cheese

Fixing

80 g red focal points
600 ml vegetable stock
1 tsp. flavorer
100 g celery (2 stems)
Salt
Pepper
150 g sheep cheddar (45% fat in dry issue)
2 tsp. oil
2 cuts entire grain bread

Arrangement Steps

Bring the lentils and stock to the bubble during a pan. Include the flavorer and spread and cook for 10 minutes over low warmth.

Within the interim, wash celery, channel, clean, and, if vital, unwind. Put the celery green during a secure spot.

Cut the celery into around 5 mm slight cuts, increase the lentils and spread and cook for a further 3-4 minutes.

Season the curry soup with salt and pepper. Disintegrate sheep cheddar. Sprinkle with celery, organize with cheddar and oil, and present with the bread.

Carrots - Cream Soup

Ingredients:

100 g carrots (1 carrot)
20 g parsley root (1 piece)
100 g potatoes (1 potato)
220 ml exemplary vegetable stock
6 stems arugula
Salt
Pepper
Nutmeg
1 tsp. chipped almonds

Directions:

Wash the carrot and parsley root, strip and dig cuts around 1 cm thick. Strip, wash, and shakers the potato.

Bring the vegetable stock to a bubble during a pot. Include the readied vegetables, bring back the bubble, and spread and cook over low warmth for quarter-hour.

Within the interim, wash the rocket, shake it dry, expel the unpleasant stalks, and cleave.

Puree the soup during a blender or with a hand blender. Salt, pepper and include slightly nutmeg.

Fill the soup into a bowl or a profound plate, sprinkle with rocket, and chopped almonds.

Asparagus Soup with Carrots

Ingredients:

400 g asparagus
1 shallot
100 g floury potatoes
1 tbsp. spread
100 ml vegetable stock
50 g crème fraiche cheddar
Salt
Pepper
125 g shrimps (8 shrimps; without head and shell)
½ lime
1 carrot
1 stem coriander
1 tbsp. rape oil

Directions:

Peel asparagus, stop woody finishes if fundamental. Spot bowls and segments during a pot, spread with 600 ml of water and stew for approx. 10 minutes on low warmth. Include asparagus sticks, delicately salt, cook within the blend for around 20 minutes with a light-weight nibble. Expel the sticks from the blend and permit them to chill marginally. Mix through a strainer.

Peel and dice the shallot, strip, wash and cut the potatoes into pieces. Sauté quickly with the shallot during a hot pan in

margarine. Mix within the flour and deglaze with 500 ml asparagus. Cook for around quarter-hour, mixing sometimes. Within the interim, cut the asparagus lances into 3 cm pieces, increase the soup, include crème fraiche, and puree the soup.
Rinse the shrimp, pat dry, and spread on a level plate.
Squeeze the lime and sprinkle the juice over the prawns.
Clean, wash, and strip the carrot. First dig slight cuts, at that point into fine pencils.
Wash the coriander, shake dry, pluck the leaves, and put during a secure spot.
Heat the rapeseed oil during a container and sauté the carrots for 4–5 minutes.
Add shrimp and sauté for 1–2 minutes, blending much of the time. Remove the oven.
Topping the soup with carrots, shrimps, and coriander leaves and serve.

Mediterranean Vegetable Broth

Ingredients:
100 g carrots (2 carrots)
250 g fennel bulb (2 fennel bulbs)
75 g celery (4 stems)
80 g tomatoes (6 tomatoes)
50 g red onions (3 red onions)
2 garlic cloves
2 tbsp. oil
3 stems basil
8th dark peppercorns
1 squeeze saffron strings
3 narrows leaves

Directions:
Wash and clean the carrots, fennel, and celery, expel the celery if important, and slash it generally. Wash the tomatoes and cut them into little pieces.
Halve onions unpeeled. Strip cloves of garlic and squash them with the rear of a blade.
Heat oil during an enormous pan. Braise the fennel, carrots,
celery, tomatoes, onions, and garlic over low warmth, blending as often as possible, for 8-10 minutes.
Add 4 liters of water and heat to the aim of boiling.
Skim off any froth which can happen with a trowel.
Rinse the basil, shake it dry and add it to the pot with peppercorns, saffron, and sound leaves. Spread and cook over medium warmth for around hour.
Put the fluid through a fine strainer during a subsequent post. Come right down to around 1200 ml over high warmth. Either use it immediately or keep it refrigerated; the stock remains there for as long as 3 days.
To freeze: empty the cooled stock into a cooler pack utilizing a pipe, close firmly, and freeze. The time span of usability: around a half year.
To save: Put the stock in bubbling water in 3 glasses (400 ml content) washed with bubbling water, close quickly and flip around for five minutes, at that point stand upstanding and keep cool. The time span of usability: around 3 months.

Kale and Toasted Walnut Soup.

Ingredients
two tsp extra virgin olive oil
30g red onion, sliced
30g celery, sliced
One garlic clove, sliced
one tsp dried thyme
75g preserved or preserved white beans, such as cannellini or haricot
500ml vegetable stock
50g kale, usually chopped
Four pecan halves, chopped

Method

throughout a medium saucepan, heat one teaspoon of the olive oil over a low–medium heat and fry the red onion, celery and garlic for 2–3 minutes. At the aim once they have 5, add the thyme, beans and stock and bring to embrace bubble.

Simmer for twenty five thirty over low heat, then add the kale and cook for a further ten 5. When all the vegetables square measure square measure sauteed, combine. You might have to add barely barely barely is too thick. On the off likelihood that it looks flavorsome watery before you combine it, basically increase the heat and leave it cajan pea bubble 5 it's thicker.

whereas the soup is cooking, heat your stove to 160°C/gas three and toast your walnuts for 10–15 5 so as that they are pleasantly browned – watch them carefully as they will without doubt without doubt without doubt without doubt to consumed.

Serve your soup showered with the remaining teaspoon two oil oil with oil pecans.

CHAPTER 12:

SALADS

Greek Salad Skewers

Preparation Time: 10 minutes
Cooking Time: 0 minutes
Servings: 2
Ingredients:
8 big black olives 8 cherry tomatoes
1 yellow pepper, cut into 8 squares
½ red onion, split into 8 wedges 1 cucumber, cut into 8 pieces
4 oz. feta, cut into 8 cubes
1 tbsp. extra-virgin olive oil Juice of 1/2 lemon
1 tsp balsamic vinegar
1/2 teaspoons garlic, crushed Ground Black pepper
Salt
Directions:
Put the salad ingredients on the skewers following this order: cherry tomato, yellow pepper, red onion, cucumber, feta, black olive.
Repeat for each skewer and put on a serving plate.
As dressing, put in a small bowl: olive oil, a pinch of salt and pepper, lemon juice, balsamic vinegar and crushed garlic. Whisk well and drizzle on the skewers.
Nutrition Facts:
Calories: 236kcal Fat: 21g Carbohydrate: 14g Protein: 7g

Sesame Chicken Salad

Preparation Time: 12 minutes
Cooking Time: 0 minutes
Servings: 2
Ingredients:
1 tbsp. sesame seeds 1 cucumber, chopped
4 oz. baby spinach, roughly sliced
2 oz. pak choi, really finely chopped 1/2 red onion, very finely chopped
6 oz. cooked chicken, shredded
For the dressing:
1 tbsp. extra-virgin olive oil 1 tsp sesame oil
Juice of 1 lime
1 tsp clear honey 2 tsp soy sauce
Directions:
Toast the sesame seeds in a dry skillet for two minutes till lightly browned and aromatic. Transfer to a plate to cool. In a bowl mix together the olive oil, sesame oil, lime juice, honey and soy sauce to create the dressing.
Put the cucumber, peeled, halved lengthways, deseeded using a teaspoon and chopped in a large bowl. Add spinach, pak choi, red onion and mix. Pour on the dressing and mix.
Divide the salad between 2 plates and top with the shredded chicken. Distribute on the sesame seeds just before serving.
Nutrition Facts:
Calories: 391 Fat: 15g Carbohydrate: 20g Protein: 39g

Coronation Chicken Salad

Preparation Time: 15 minutes
Cooking Time: 0 minutes
Servings: 1
Ingredients:
3 oz. Natural yoghurt Juice of 1/4 of a lemon
1 tsp Coriander, chopped
1 tsp Ground turmeric
1/2 tsp. moderate curry powder 4 oz. Cooked chicken breast
6 Walnut halves, finely chopped 2 Medjool dates, thinly sliced 20 grams Red onion, diced
1 Bird's eye chili 1 oz. Rocket
Direction:
Cut the chicken breast to bite-sized pieces
In a serving plate put the rocket as a base, then sprinkle the chicken, walnuts, dates, onion.
Mix yoghurt, lemon juice, spices and coriander together in a small bowl and drizzle it over the salad.
Nutrition Facts:
Calories: 364 Fat: 12g Carbohydrate: 45g Protein: 15g

Sirt Fruit Salad

Preparation Time: 10 minutes
Cooking Time: 0 minutes
Servings: 1
Ingredients:
1/2 cup freshly produced green tea 1 tsp honey
1 orange, halved
1 apple, cored and roughly chopped 10 red seedless grapes
10 blueberries
Directions:
Stir the honey into half a cup of green tea and let it chill. When chilled, add the juice of half orange.
Slice the other half and put in a bowl with the chopped apple, blueberries and grapes.
Pour over the tea and let rest in the fridge for 30 minutes before serving.
Nutrition Facts:
Calories: 110 Fat: 0g Carbohydrate: 17g Protein: 2g.

Fresh Salad With Orange Dressing

Preparation Time: 10 minutes
Cooking Time: 0 minutes
Servings: 2
Ingredients:
½ cup lettuce
1 medium yellow bell pepper 1 medium Red pepper
4 oz. Carrot, grated 10 Almonds
Ingredients dressing:
4 tbsp. Olive oil
½ cup Orange juice
1 tbsp. Apple cider vinegar Salt and pepper to taste
Direction:
Clean the peppers and cut them into long thin strips. Tear off the lettuce leaves and cut them into smaller pieces.
Mix the salad with the peppers and the carrots in a bowl. Roughly chop the almonds and sprinkle over the salad.
Mix all the ingredients for the dressing in a bowl. Pour the dressing over the salad just before serving.
Nutrition Facts:
Calories: 150 Fat: 10g Carbohydrate: 11g Protein: 2g

Tomato And Avocado Salad

Preparation Time: 10 minutes
Cooking Time: 0 minutes
Servings: 1
Ingredients:
1 large Tomato
4 oz. Cherry tomatoes
1/2 medium Red onion

1 ripe Avocado 1tsp fresh oregano
1tbsp. extra virgin olive oil
1 tsp White wine vinegar 1 pinch Celtic sea salt

Direction:

Cut the tomato into thick slices. Cut half of the cherry tomatoes into slices and the other half in half. Cut the red onion into super thin half rings. (if you have it, use a mandolin for this)

Cut the avocado into 6 parts. Spread the tomatoes on a plate, place the avocado on top. Sprinkle red onion and oregano and drizzle olive oil, vinegar and a pinch of salt on the salad.

Nutrition Facts:

Calories: 165 Fat: 14g Carbohydrate: 7g Protein: 5g

Arugula With Fruits And Nuts

Preparation Time: 10 minutes
Cooking Time: 3 minutes
Servings: 1
Ingredients:

½ cup Arugula 1 Peach
1 /2 medium Red onion
¼ cup Blueberries 5 Pecans
dressing: 1/2 medium Peach 1 tbsp. Olive oil
2 tbsp. White wine vinegar 1 sprig fresh basil

Directions:

Halve the peach and remove the seed.

Heat a grill pan and grill it briefly on both sides. Cut the red onion into thin half rings. Roughly chop the pecans.

Heat a pan and roast the pecans in it until they are fragrant.

Place the arugula on a plate and spread peaches, red onions, blueberries and roasted pecans over it.

Put all the ingredients for the dressing in a food processor and mix to an even dressing. Drizzle the dressing over the salad.

Nutrition Facts:

Calories: 160 Fat: 7g Carbohydrate: 25g Protein: 3g

Spinach Salad With Asparagus And Salmon

Preparation Time: 20 minutes
Cooking Time: 8 minutes
Servings: 1
Ingredients:

2 cups Spinach
2 Eggs
4 oz. smoked salmon 1 cup Asparagus tips 4 oz. Cherry tomatoes Lemon 1/2 pieces
1 tsp Olive oil

Directions:

Boil the eggs until they are done (6 minutes for soft boiled, 8 minutes for hard boiled). Heat a pan with a little oil and fry the asparagus tips . Halve cherry tomatoes.

Place the spinach on a plate and spread the asparagus tips, cherry tomatoes and smoked salmon on top.

Peel and halve the eggs. Add them to the salad. Squeeze the lemon and drizzle some olive oil over it.

Season the salad with a little salt and pepper.

Nutrition Facts:

Calories: 552 Fat: 40g Carbohydrate: 6g Protein: 39g

Brunoise Salad

Preparation Time: 10 minutes
Cooking Time: 0 minutes
Servings: 1
Ingredients:

1 large tomato
1 medium zucchini
1/2 medium red bell pepper

1/2 medium yellow bell pepper 1/2 medium red onion
3 springs fresh parsley
1 /2 Lemon
2 tbsp. Olive oil

Directions:

Finely dice tomatoes, zucchini, peppers and red onions to get a brunoise. Mix all the cubes in a bowl. Chop parsley and mix in the salad. Squeeze the lemon over the salad and add the olive oil. Season with salt and pepper.

Nutrition Facts:

Calories: 84 Carbs: 3g Fat: 4g Protein: 0g

Broccoli Salad

Preparation Time: 20 minutes
Cooking Time: 5 minutes
Servings: 1
Ingredients:

1 head of Broccoli
1 /2 medium Red onion
2 Carrots, grated
¼ cup Red grapes
2 1/2 tbsp. Coconut yogurt
1 tbsp. Water
1 tsp Mustard
1 pinch Salt

Directions:

Cut the broccoli into small florets and cook for 8 minutes. Cut the red onion into thin half rings. Halve the grapes. Mix coconut yogurt, water and mustard with a pinch of salt to make the dressing.
Drain the broccoli and rinse with ice-cold water to stop the cooking process.
Mix the broccoli with the carrot, onion and red grapes in a bowl. Serve the dressing separately on the side.

Nutrition Facts:

Calories: 230 Fat: 18g Carbohydrate: 35g Protein: 10g

Fresh Chicory Salad

Preparation Time: 10 minutes
Cooking Time: 0 minutes
Servings: 1
Ingredients:

½ medium red chicory 1 medium Orange
1 large Tomato
1/2 medium Cucumber
1/2 medium Red onion

Directions:

Cut off the hard stem of the chicory and remove the leaves. Peel the orange and cut the pulp into wedges.
Cut the tomatoes and cucumbers into small pieces. Cut the red onion into thin half rings. Place the chicory boats on a plate; spread the orange wedges, tomato, cucumber and red onion over the boats. Drizzle some olive oil and fresh lemon juice and serve.

Nutrition Facts:

Calories: 112 Fat: 11g Carbohydrate: 2g Protein: 0g

Steak Salad

Preparation Time: 90 minutes
Cooking Time: 30 minutes
Servings: 4
Ingredients:

2 4 oz. Beef steak
2 cloves Garlic
1-medium Red onion 2 Eggs
1 cup Cherry tomatoes 2 tbsp. olive oil
1-ripe Avocado 1/2 Cucumber
1 pinch Salt and pepper 1 tbsp. white vinegar

Directions:

Place the steaks in a flat bowl. Pour the olive oil over the steaks and crush the garlic over. Turn the steaks a few times so that they are covered with oil and garlic. Cover the meat and let it marinate for at least 1 hour. Boil eggs until done, rinse and let cool.

Heat a grill pan and fry the steaks. When done, let them rest 5 minutes wrapped in aluminum foil. Spread the lettuce on the plates. Cut the steaks into slices and place them in the middle of the salad.
Cut the eggs into wedges, the cucumber into half-moons, the red onion
into thin half-rings, the cherry tomatoes into halves and the avocado into slices.
Spread this around the steaks. Drizzle over the olive oil and white wine vinegar and season with a little salt and pepper.
Nutrition Facts:
Calories: 513 Fat: 15g Carbohydrate: 1g Protein: 47g

Zucchini Salad With Lemon Chicken

Preparation Time: 90 minutes
Cooking Time: 30 minutes
Servings: 1
Ingredients:
2 zucchini, sliced
4 oz. Cherry tomatoes 5 oz. Chicken breast 1 Lemon
2 tbsp. Olive oil 1 tbsp. rosemary
1 clove of garlic, crushed Salt and pepper to taste
Direction:
Use a meat mallet or a heavy pan to make the chicken fillets as thin as possible. Put the fillets in a bowl. Squeeze the lemon over the chicken and add the olive oil, salt, pepper, rosemary and garlic.
Cover it and let it marinate for at least 1 hour. Heat a pan over medium- high heat and fry the chicken until cooked through and browned.
Quarter the tomatoes and slice the zucchini and put everything in a serving plate. Slice the chicken fillets diagonally and place them on the salad.
Drizzle the salad with a little olive oil and season with salt and pepper.
Nutrition Facts:
Calories: 286kcal Fat: 8g Carbohydrate: 4g Protein: 0g

Tuna Salad and Red Chicory

Preparation Time: 20 minutes
Cooking Time: 0 minutes
Servings: 2
Ingredients:
4 pieces Red chicory 5 oz. Tuna
1- piece Orange
1 tbsp. fresh parsley, finely chopped 5 pieces Radish
1 tsp Olive oil
Directions:
Drain the tuna. Cut the orange into wedges and and then into small pieces. Cut radishes into small pieces too.
Mix all the ingredients (except the red chicory) in a small bowl. Season with salt and pepper
Spread the tuna mix on the red chicory leaves and enjoy!
Nutrition Facts:
Calories: 93 Fat: 6g Carbohydrate: 2g Protein: 9g

Salad With Bacon, Cranberries And Apple

Preparation Time: 40 minutes
Cooking Time: 10 minutes
Servings: 3
Ingredients:
½ cup Arugula 4 slices Bacon
1 / 2 pieces Apple
2 tbsp. Dried cranberries 1 / 2 pieces Red onion
1 / 2 pieces Red bell pepper
10 Walnuts

Ingredients dressing:
1 tsp Mustard yellow 1 tsp Honey
3 tbsp. Olive oil
Directions:
Heat a pan over medium heat and fry the bacon until crispy. Place the bacon on a piece of kitchen roll so that the excess fat is absorbed. Cut half the red onion into thin rings. Cut the bell pepper into small cubes. Cut the apple into four pieces and remove the core. Then cut into thin wedges. Drizzle some lemon juice on the apple wedges so that they do not change color.
Roughly chop walnuts. Mix the ingredients for the dressing in a bowl.
Season with salt and pepper. Spread the lettuce on a plate and season with red pepper, red onions, apple wedges and walnuts.
Sprinkle bacon and cranberries over the salad. Drizzle the dressing over the salad and serve.
Nutrition Facts:
Calories: 70 Fat: 3g Carbohydrate: 6g Protein: 7g

Hawaii Salad

Preparation Time: 25 minutes
Cooking Time: 0 minutes
Servings: 1
Ingredients:
½ cup rocket
1/2 pieces Red onion 1-piece winter carrot 1 cup Pineapple
3 oz. ham, diced 1 pinch Salt
1 pinch Black pepper
Directions:
Cut the red onion into thin half rings. Remove the peel and hard core from the pineapple and cut the pulp into thin pieces. Clean the carrot and use a spiralizer to make strings.
Mix rocket and carrot in a bowl. Spread this over a plate. Spread red onion, pineapple and diced ham over the rocket.
Drizzle the olive oil and balsamic vinegar on the salad to your taste. Season with salt and pepper.
Nutrition Facts:
Calories: 200kcal Fat: 6g Carbohydrate: 28g Protein: 8g

Rainbow Salad

Preparation Time: 10 minutes
Cooking Time: 0 minutes
Servings: 1
Ingredients:
1 cup lettuce
1/2 pieces Avocado
1 Egg
1/4 pieces green peppers 1/4 pieces Red bell pepper 2 large Tomato
1/2 pieces Red onion 4 tbsp. Carrot, grated 2 tbsp olive oil
1 tbsp white vinegar Salt
Pepper
Directions:
Boil the egg until done (6 minutes for soft boiled, 8 minutes for hard boiled). Cool it under running water, peel it and cut into slices.
Remove the seeds from the peppers and cut them into thin strips. Cut the tomatoes into small cubes. Cut the red onion into thin half rings.
Cut the avocado into thin slices.
Place the salad on a plate and distribute all the vegetables in colorful rows.
Drizzle the vegetables with olive oil and white wine vinegar. Season with salt and pepper.
Nutrition Facts:
Calories: 40kcal Fat: 1g Carbohydrate: 5g Protein: 2g

Mung Beans Snack Salad

Preparation Time: 10 minutes
Cooking Time: 0 minutes
Servings: 6
Ingredients:
2 cups tomatoes, chopped 2 cups cucumber, chopped 3 cups mixed greens
2 cups mung beans, sprouted 2 cups clover sprouts
For the dressing:
1 tbsp. cumin, ground 1 cup dill, chopped
4 tbsp. lemon juice
1 avocado, pitted and roughly chopped 1 cucumber, roughly chopped
Directions:
In a salad bowl, mix tomatoes with 2 cups cucumber, greens, clover and mung sprouts. In your blender, mix cumin with dill, lemon juice, 1 cucumber and avocado, blend really well, add this to your salad, toss well and serve.
Nutrition Facts:
Calories 120 kcal, Fat 3g, Carbohydrate 10g, Protein 6g

Sprouts And Apples Snack Salad

Preparation Time: 10 minutes
Cooking Time: 0 minutes
Servings: 4
Ingredients: 1 lb. Brussels sprouts, shredded
1 cup walnuts, chopped
1 apple, cored and cubed
1 red onion, chopped 3 tbsp. red vinegar
1 tbsp. mustard - ½ cup olive oil
1 garlic clove, crushed Black pepper to the taste
Directions:
In a salad bowl, mix sprouts with apple, onion and walnuts. In another bowl, mix vinegar with mustard, oil, garlic and pepper, whisk really well, add this to your salad, toss well and serve as a snack.
Nutrition Facts:
Calories 120 kcal, Fat 2g, Carbohydrate 8g, Protein 6g

Moroccan Leeks Snack Salad

Preparation Time: 10 minutes
Cooking Time: 0 minutes
Servings: 4
Ingredients:
1 bunch radishes, sliced 3 cups leeks, chopped
1 and ½ cups olives, pitted and sliced
A pinch of turmeric powder 1 cup cilantro, chopped Salt to taste
Black pepper to taste 2 tbsp. olive oil
Directions:
In a bowl, mix radishes with leeks, olives and cilantro. Add black pepper, oil and turmeric, toss to coat and serve.
Nutrition Facts:
Calories 135kcal, Fat 1g, Carbohydrate18g, Protein 9g

Celery And Raisins Snack Salad

Preparation Time: 10 minutes
Cooking Time: 0 minutes
Servings: 4
Ingredients:
½ cup raisins
4 cups celery, sliced
¼ cup parsley, chopped
½ cup walnuts, chopped Juice of ½ lemon
2 tbsp. olive oil
Salt and black pepper to taste
Directions:
In a salad bowl, mix celery with raisins, walnuts, parsley, lemon juice, oil and black pepper, toss, divide into small cups and serve as a snack.
Nutrition Facts:
Calories 120 kcal, Fat 1g, Carbohydrate 6g, Protein 5g

Dijon Celery Salad

Preparation Time: 10 minutes
Cooking Time: 0 minutes
Servings: 4
Ingredients:
½ cup lemon juice
1/3 cup Dijon mustard 2/3 cup olive oil Black pepper to taste
2 apples, cored, peeled and cubed 1 bunch celery roughly chopped
¾ cup walnuts, chopped
Directions:
In a salad bowl, mix celery and its leaves with apple pieces and walnuts.
Add black pepper, lemon juice, mustard and olive oil, whisk well, add to your salad, toss, divide into small cups and serve.
Nutrition Facts:
Calories 125 kcal, Fat 2g, Carbohydrate 7g, Protein 7g

CHAPTER 13:

VEGETARIAN RECIPES

Classic pasta sauce

Ingredients:

3 onions
3 garlic cloves
4 stems basil
2 tbsp oil
175 ml wine or vegetable stock
850 g stripped tomatoes (can)
Salt
Pepper
1 tsp agave syrup

Planning Steps

Peel and finely slash onions and garlic. Wash the basil and shake dry.

Heat oil during a pot. Braise the onions and garlic during a refined warmth for 4–5 minutes. Include the basil and braise quickly.

Add wine or stock and let it come down totally

Chop the canned tomatoes generally with a blade. Put within the pot with tomato fluid and convey it to the bubble. Cook over medium warmth for 25-30 minutes. Expel the basil. Season the sauce with salt, pepper, and agave syrup and use it promptly if vital. Something else, refrigerate and store within the cooler; it remains there for as long as 3 days.

You'll likewise save the sauce. To undertake to the present, pour the fluid at bubbling temperature into 2 glasses with a cover (each containing 300 ml) that are flushed with bubbling water. Close containers promptly and flip around them for five minutes, at that point stand upstanding and keep cool. The timeframe of realistic usability for around 3 months.

Colorful Vegetable Noodles

Ingredients:

200 g little carrots (3 little carrots)
200 g little zucchini (1 little zucchini)
125 g leek (1 stick)
150 g linguine wholegrain pasta
2 tbsp oil
Salt
Pepper
125 ml exemplary vegetable stock
150 ml soy cream
1 squeeze saffron strings
Chervil freely

Arrangement Steps

Peel and clean carrots, wash zucchini, rub dry, and clean. Cut both lengthways into slim strips utilizing a peeler or a vegetable slicer.

Clean the leek, split lengthways, wash, and separate the individual leaves.

Within the interim, heat oil during a skillet. Braise the carrots and zucchini in it over medium warmth for 1 moment, mixing.

Add the leek and braise for an extra 1 moment. Season everything with salt and pepper.

Add the vegetable stock, soy cream, and thus the saffron strings and convey them to the bubble. Cook until velvety over medium warmth for 2-3 minutes.

Drain the pasta during a strainer, a channel well, and increase the skillet.

Mix the pasta with the vegetables. Season once more. Placed on plates and serve sprinkled with chervil as you would like.

Shrimp Arugula Salad

Ingredients:

10 cups of arugula (baby)
One large-sized avocado (cubed)
Two large lemons (one for juice and therefore the other for wedges)
Five tbsps. of oil or vegetable oil
Half pound large shrimp (cooked)
Salt for taste
Fresh pepper (cracked)

Method:

Take a bowl and add arugula, avocado, and cooked shrimp. Mix the ingredients and add pepper, two tbsps. of vegetable oil , lemon, and salt consistent with taste. Give the ingredients a correct mix.

Add the remainder of the vegetable oil if you would like to toss the salad again or for coating the arugula.

Taste the salad and adjust the seasoning.

Serve the salad on a plate by adding wedges of lemon by the side.

Cucumber, Tomato, And tuna fish salad

Ingredients:

Four tbsps. Of peppercorns (fresh, ground)
One and a half cup of tomatoes (cherry variety, add more consistent with your need)
8 oz. of tuna
One small lemon
Salad greens or arugula (any kind that you simply like)
Two medium-sized cucumbers

Method:

Remove the stems from the cherry tomatoes and wash them properly under running water. Confirm that they're absolutely clean. Clean the tomatoes then dry them by employing a towel or kitchen towel.

Slice the washed tomatoes into half and keep them aside during a bowl.

an equivalent guidelines will got to be followed for cucumbers also . Wash them under cold running water and make them dry by employing a kitchen towel. Cleaning the veggies is extremely important as they're going to be consumed raw within the sort of salad.

Cut the cucumbers consistent with your preferred size and keep them with the tomatoes.

Mix the tomatoes and cucumber together.

The animal oil also will be utilized in this salad alongside the fish.

Add the tuna chunks and blend everything gently in order that you are doing not break the fish chunks.

Add juice alongside ground pepper and blend well.

Add salad greens to a plate and top it with tuna fish salad.

May Beet Salad with Cucumber

Ingredients:

3 May turnips
1 cucumber
1 onion
2 stems parsley
150 g Greek yogurt
1 tbsp fruit crush vinegar
1 tsp nectar
1 tsp mustard
Sea-salt
Cayenne pepper
Pepper

Planning Steps

Clean, strip, and cut the turnips. Clean and wash the cucumber and furthermore slicer. Clean, wash and cut the spring onions into

rings. Put everything during a serving of mixed greens bowl and blend.
Wash parsley shake dry and slash finely. Combine dressing with yogurt, fruit crush vinegar, nectar, mustard, and 2–3 tbsp water. Season with salt and cayenne pepper.
Mix the plate of mixed greens dressing with the mayonnaise and cucumber and let it steep for around 10 minutes, at that point crush it with pepper and serve.

Ricotta Pancakes with Apricots

Ingredients:
80 g ricotta
1 egg
3 tbsp juice
1 tsp nectar
40 g buckwheat flour
½ tsp preparing powder
1 tsp coconut oil
2 apricots
3 tbsp yogurt (3.5% fat)
1 stem mint

Arrangement Steps

Mix the ricotta with the egg, lemon squeeze, and nectar until smooth. Include buckwheat flour and preparing powder and blend into a gooey mixture. Warmth coconut oil during a container and include a huge tablespoon of hitter to the dish, steel oneself against 1 moment over medium warmth, divert, and keep heating from the opposite side. Do likewise for around 5 flapjacks.
Within the interim wash, split, and cut apricots. Blend the yogurt until velvety. Wash mint, shake dry, and pluck leaves. Stack the flapjacks on a plate, including the yogurt and apricot wedges, and serve improved with mint.

Buddha Bowl with Green Asparagus and Soba Noodles

Ingredients:
125 g soba noodle (buckwheat noodles)
Salt
2 bunches child spinach (40 g)
½ pack youthful radishes
100 g sugar snap
200 g green asparagus
1 tbsp oil
1 tbsp tahini (15 g)
2 tbsp juice
Pepper
1 nectarine
75 g feta
2 tsp dark sesame (10 g)

Directions:

Cook soba noodles in bubbling salted water in 4–5 minutes, channel, extinguish with cold water and channel. Clean and wash infant spinach, radishes, and sugar snap peas. Cut the sugar snap unit lengthways.
Clean, wash, and cut green asparagus. Warmth 1 tablespoon of oil during a container and fry the asparagus in it over medium warmth for five minutes. Meanwhile, mix the tahini with juice until smooth and blend in enough water until the consistency is adequate fluid. Season the sauce with salt and pepper.
Wash, divide, expel the center and cut the nectarine into wedges. Disintegrate the feta. Spread the soba noodles, all vegetables and nectarine cuts on two dishes, and serve beat with tahini sauce, feta, and dark sesame.

Chia Pudding with Yogurt and Strawberry Puree

Ingredients:
200 g strawberries (new or solidified)
2 tbsp chia seeds
350 g yogurt (3.5% fat)

1 tsp nectar
1 squeeze Tonka bean
50 g almond pieces
20 g dull chocolate (at any rate 70% cocoa

Arrangement Steps

Put the strawberries during a pot with slightly water and cook tenderly on medium warmth in around 7 minutes and crush them if vital. Meanwhile, blend the chia seeds well with yogurt and nectar and season with Tonka beans.

Roughly cleave the almonds and chocolate. On the other hand layer chia yogurt and strawberry puree in glasses and serve sprinkled with almonds and chocolate.

Lentil Salad with Spinach, Rhubarb, and Asparagus

Ingredients:

100 g beluga lentils
2 tbsp oil
Salt
250 g white asparagus
100 g rhubarb
1 tsp nectar
50 g infant spinach (2 bunches)
20 g pumpkin seeds

Directions:

Bring the beluga lentils to the overflow with multiple times the measure of water. Cook over medium warmth for around 25 minutes. Channel, flush, and channel. Blend in with 1 tablespoon of oil and a spot of salt. Meanwhile, wash, clean, strip, and cut asparagus into pieces. Wash, clean, and cut the rhubarb into pieces.

Heat 1 tablespoon of oil during a skillet and fry the asparagus in it for around 8 minutes over medium warmth, turning infrequently. At that point include rhubarb and nectar and fry and salt for an extra 5 minutes. Wash spinach and switch dry. Generally, hack the pumpkin seeds.Arrange spinach with lentils, asparagus, and rhubarb on two plates and serve sprinkled with pumpkin seeds.

Lentil Salad with Spinach, Rhubarb, and Asparagus

Ingredients:

100 g beluga lentils
2 tbsp vegetable oil
Salt
250 g white asparagus
100 g rhubarb
1 tsp nectar
50 g infant spinach (2 bunches)
20 g pumpkin seeds

Directions:

Bring the beluga lentils to the overflow with many times the measure of water. Cook over average warmth for about 25 minutes. Channel, flush, and channel. Blend in with 1 tablespoon of vegetable oil and a spot of salt. Meanwhile, wash, clean, strip, and chopped asparagus into pieces. Wash, clean, and cut the rhubarb into pieces.

Heat 1 tablespoon of vegetable oil through a skillet and fry the asparagus in it for about 8 minutes over average warmth, turning infrequently. At that time include rhubarb and nectar and fry and salt for an additional 5 minutes. Wash spinach and switch dry. Generally, hack the pumpkin seeds.

Prepare spinach with lentils, asparagus, and rhubarb on two plates and serve sprinkled with pumpkin seeds.

Sweet Potatoes with Asparagus, Eggplant and Halloumi

Ingredients:

1 aborigine
9 tbsp oil bean stew drops
Salt
Pepper

2 yams
1 red bean stew pepper
2 tbsp sunflower seeds
1 bundle green asparagus
4 tbsp juice
200 g chickpeas (can; trickle weight)
½ group basil
½ group lemon demulcent
1 tsp mustard
½ tsp turmeric powder
1 tsp nectar
300 g halloumi

Planning Steps

Clean, wash and cut the eggplant. Warmth 2 tablespoons of oil during a dish and sauté the aborigine cuts in medium warmth on the two sides for 5–7 minutes until brilliant earthy colored and
season with bean stew drops, salt, and pepper. Expel from the skillet and put it during a secure spot.

Within the interim, strip the yam and cut it into 3D squares. Split the stew lengthways, expel the stones, wash and dig cuts. Warmth 1 tablespoon of oil within the dish, fry the yam 3D squares in it for 10 minutes. Include 1 tbsp sunflower seeds and stew cuts and season with salt and pepper.

Wash asparagus as an afterthought, remove the woody closures, and strip the lower third of the stalks if essential. Warmth 1 tablespoon of oil within the skillet, fry the asparagus in it for five minutes over medium warmth. Deglaze with 1 tablespoon of juice, pour in 2 tablespoons of water and spread and cook for an extra 3 minutes.

Rinse the chickpeas and permit them to channel. Wash the basil and lemon emollient, shake dry and slash. Blend chickpeas in with half the herbs and 1 tablespoon of oil and season with salt and pepper.

Whisk the rest of the oil with the remainder of juice, mustard, turmeric and nectar, season with salt and pepper, and blend within the rest of the herbs.

Cut the halloumi and cut during a hot container on the two sides for five minutes over medium warmth until brilliant yellow.

Arrange yams, aubergine cuts on plates, present with chickpeas, asparagus, and halloumi and shower with the dressing. Sprinkle with the rest of the sunflower seeds.

Vegetarian Bolognese with Fusilli

Ingredients:

3 enormous onions
3 cloves of garlic
2 tbsp tomato glue
1 eggplant
1 zucchini, medium size
3 carrots
3 enormous hamburger tomatoes
1 ringer pepper
500 ml of passed tomatoes
375 ml water (approx.)
100 g couscous
500 g fusilli
Vegetable oil
Fresh parmesan

Planning Steps

Peel the onions, slash them finely, and afterward earthy colored them in hot oil or vegetable margarine during an enormous container until brilliant earthy colored.

Finely slash the cloves of garlic and dish them with

Then blend within the tomato glue.

Meanwhile, clean the vegetables, cut everything into fine solid shapes, and add them to the dish.

Add the pasta sauce and pour around 1/4 liter of water.

Season and let stew slightly.

Then refine the consistency of the sauce with a hand blender, puree almost relying upon the taste.

Pour some water (approx. 1/8 L) if fundamental, therefore the sauce seems to be increasingly liquid.

Then cut the oven, add the couscous to the sauce, mix well and let it stand. The couscous ingests the fluid well and thus the sauce gets a smooth consistency.

Cook the fusilli or other durum semolina cake as per the bundle guidelines and present with the sauce. 11. If you would like, you'll rub the new Parmesan over it.

Fermented Pumpkin Vegetables

Ingredients:

1 little pumpkin

Spices of your decision, for instance, B. mustard seeds and curry

1-2 tablespoons of salt

Directions:

Cut the pumpkin into the tiniest potential cuts or pieces.

Mix the cut pumpkin with salt and flavors.

Stir the blend appropriately, applying some weight until fluid

departures. On the off chance that it doesn't, include some spring water.

Now the vegetables including the next brackish water are layered in an inventive pot. Continuously leave some space within the compartment and do not top it off to the highest. Spread the vegetables with a plate, which you likewise burden. This assists with crushing out the overabundance air.

Set the container aside for seven days at temperature. You'll likewise stand by longer and strengthen the taste.

Your tolerance has paid off, you'd now be ready to eat your first self-aged vegetables.

Tomato Cream of Red Lentils

Fixing

¾ cup dry red lentils

1-2 canned tomatoes plate (in season 2-4 cups of cut new)

1 white onion

1 clove of garlic

1 huge carrot

1 tablespoon oil rapeseed

1-2 tablespoons of juice of a lemon

1 - 2 teaspoon cumin

1 teaspoon smoked pepper (ideally intense)

1 teaspoon appetizing or lovage

Teaspoon thyme

Decoction vegetable or water

Salt, pepper

To serve: buckwheat, parsley, coriander

Arrangement Steps

During a thick-bottomed pot or profound pan, heat the oil and fry the finely cleaved onion, at that point include garlic.

Then include the diced carrot and thus the washed lentils and pour the vegetable stock with the goal that it completely covers all Ingredients: to the tallness of 2-3 cm. Cook until carrots and lentils are delicate.

When the vegetables mellow, include canned tomatoes and flavors. Bubble for a further 10-15 minutes, at that point mix with a hand blender, add lemon squeeze, and season to tastė. Present with buckwheat and new herbs.

Chickpeas Meatballs - like from a Swedish Buffet

Ingredients:

1 cup chickpea flour

1 red pepper

1 cup canned corn (in the season from the cob, unavailable from the container)

1 cup of solidified green peas

1 tsp curry flavor

2 tbsp yeast pieces (discretionary)

2 tbsp soy
2 tbsp oil
Water
Salt, pepper

Directions:

Sieve chickpea flour through a sifter into an enormous bowl, include flavors and blend. Cut the peppers into little shapes, pour the sweetcorn and peas with warm water.

Add ½ cup of tepid water and each one vegetables, soy sauce, and oil to the bowl. Combine the Ingredients: and include more water if important until a cement mass structures. Represent a few of minutes.

The mass for meatballs got to be thick, however, it must not be excessively dry - it alright could even be effectively framed. Structure balls with wet hands and spot them on a heating plate fixed with preparing the paper. Place the meatballs within the broiler preheated to 190 ° C and prepared for around half-hour until firm and caramelized.

Marinated Portobello Steaks

Ingredients:

3 tbsp balsamic vinegar
2 tbsp soy
2 tbsp syrup
1 tsp mustard
2 cloves garlic
1 bean stew pepper
Salt, pepper
5 portobello mushrooms or twelve standard mushrooms
Favorite vegetables to serve
Oil for singing

Planning Steps

Peel the garlic and cut the bean stew pepper into little pieces, and alternatively expel the seeds from it (in the event that you simply don't take care of zesty nourishments). Blend all marinade Ingredients: altogether with a blender or ply during a mortar. Wash Portobello mushrooms and deduct their stems. during a huge bowl, rub them well with the marinade (ideally with gloved hands) and put during a secure spot for a minimum of quarter- hour , ideally a couple of hours (you can acknowledged the entire day the day preceding and fry the next day). Fry marinated mushrooms during a flame broil skillet or common dish squeezing the mushrooms until they're for the foremost part delicate. You'll likewise organize them on the flame broil or significantly over the fireside.

Serve prepared mushrooms alongside your preferred vegetables, pour the remainder of the marinade and eat with a fresh loaf.

Garden pea Pasta with Arugula

Ingredients:

Salt
250 g penne from green peas
90 g arugula
5 tbsp pitted dark olives
125 g mozzarella - 2 tbsp oil
1 tbsp balsamic vinegar
1 tsp Aglio-e-olio zest blend
Pepper
Hot paprika powder
2 tbsp center blend

Planning Steps

Bring 2 liters of water to a bubble, salt and cook pea peas in it for 6 minutes. At that point channel, channel and let cool.

Within the interim, clean the arugula, wash, and shake dry. Cut olives. Channel the mozzarella and cut it into 3D squares.

Mix dressing with oil, vinegar, salt, Aglio-e-olio, pepper, and paprika powder. Include some water within the event that you simply like. Mix penne with arugula, sprinkle with olives, mozzarella, and piece blend and shower with the dressing.

CHAPTER 14:

JUICES AND SMOOTHIES

Celery Juice

Preparation Time: 10 minutes
Servings: 2
Ingredients:
8 celery stalks with leaves 2 tbsp. fresh ginger, peeled 1 lemon, peeled
½ cup filtered water Pinch of salt
Directions:
Add all ingredients into a juicer and extract the juice according to the manufacturer's method.
In case you don't have one, add all the ingredients in a blender and pulse until well combined.
Filter the juice through a fine mesh strainer and transfer into two glasses. Serve immediately.
Nutrition Facts:
Calories 32kcal, Fat 0.5 g, Carbohydrate 6.5 g, Protein 1 g

Orange & Kale Juice

Preparation Time: 10 minutes
Servings: 2
Ingredients:
5 oranges, peeled 2 cups fresh kale
Directions:
Add all ingredients into a juicer and extract the juice according to the manufacturer's method.
In case you don't have one, add all the ingredients in a blender and pulse until well combined.
Filter the juice through a fine mesh strainer and transfer into two glasses. Serve immediately.
Nutrition Facts:
Calories 52 kcal, Fat 0.7 g, Carbohydrate 8.5 g, Protein 1.5 g

Apple, Cucumber & Celery Juice

Preparation Time: 10 minutes
Servings: 2
Ingredients:
3 apples, cored and sliced 2 cucumbers, sliced 4 celery stalks
1 1-inch piece fresh ginger, peeled 1 lemon, peeled
Directions:
Add all ingredients into a juicer and extract the juice according to the manufacturer's method.
In case you don't have one, add all the ingredients in a blender and pulse until well combined.
Filter the juice through a fine mesh strainer and transfer into two glasses. Serve immediately.
Nutrition Facts:
Calories 71kcal, Fat 0.7 g, Carbohydrate 9.2 g, Protein 1.3 g

Lemony Apple & Kale Juice

Preparation Time: 10 minutes
Servings: 2
Ingredients:
2 green apples, cored and sliced 4 cups fresh kale leaves
4 tbsp. fresh parsley leaves 1 tbsp. fresh ginger, peeled 1 lemon, peeled
½ cup filtered water Pinch of salt
Directions:
Add all ingredients into a juicer and extract the juice according to the manufacturer's method.
In case you don't have one, add all the ingredients in a blender and pulse until well combined.
Filter the juice through a fine mesh strainer and transfer into two glasses. Serve immediately.
Nutrition Facts:
Calories 55kcal, Fat 0.3 g, Carbohydrate 6.9 g, Protein 1.2 g

Apple & Celery Juice

Preparation Time: 10 minutes
Servings: 2
Ingredients:
4 large green apples, cored and sliced 4 large celery stalks
1 lemon, peeled
Directions:
Add all ingredients into a juicer and extract the juice according to the manufacturer's method.
In case you don't have one, add all the ingredients in a blender and pulse until well combined. Filter the juice through a fine mesh strainer and transfer into two glasses. Serve immediately.
Nutrition Facts:
Calories 62kcal, Fat 0.6 g, Carbohydrate 6.7 g, Protein 1.8 g

Apple, Orange & Broccoli Juice

Preparation Time: 10 minutes
Servings: 2
Ingredients:
2 broccoli stalks, chopped
2 large green apples, cored and sliced 3 oranges, peeled - 4 tbsp. fresh parsley
Directions:
Add all ingredients into a juicer and extract the juice according to the manufacturer's method.
In case you don't have one, add all the ingredients in a blender and pulse until well combined.
Filter the juice through a fine mesh strainer and transfer into two glasses. Serve immediately.
Nutrition Facts:
Calories 82kcal, Fat 0.3 g, Carbohydrate 8.5 g, Protein 2 g

Apple, Grapefruit & Carrot Juice

Preparation Time: 10 minutes
Servings: 2
Ingredients:
3 cups fresh kale
2 large apples, cored and sliced
2 medium carrots, peeled and chopped
2 medium grapefruit, peeled and sectioned 1 tsp fresh lemon juice
½ cup filtered water
Directions:
Add all ingredients into a juicer and extract the juice according to the manufacturer's method. In case you don't have one, add all the ingredients in a blender and pulse until well combined. Filter the juice through a fine mesh strainer and transfer into two glasses. Serve immediately.
Nutrition Facts:
Calories 67kcal, Fat 0.2 g, Carbohydrate 8 g, Protein 0.8 g

Fruity Kale Juice

Preparation Time: 10 minutes
Servings: 2
Ingredients:
2 large green apples, cored and sliced 2 large pears, cored and sliced
3 cups fresh kale leaves 3 celery stalks
1 lemon, peeled
½ cup filtered water
Directions:
Add all ingredients into a juicer and extract the juice according to the manufacturer's method.
In case you don't have one, add all the ingredients in a blender and pulse until well combined.
Filter the juice through a fine mesh strainer and transfer into two glasses. Serve immediately.
Nutrition Facts:
Calories 65kcal, Fat 0.3 g, Carbohydrate 5.9 g, Protein 2.5 g

Green Fruit Juice

Preparation Time: 10 minutes
Servings: 2
Ingredients:
3 large kiwis, peeled and chopped
3 large green apples, cored and sliced 2 cups seedless green grapes
2 tsp fresh lime juice
½ cup filtered water
Directions:
Add all ingredients into a juicer and extract the juice according to the manufacturer's method.
In case you don't have one, add all the ingredients in a blender and pulse until well combined.
Filter the juice through a fine mesh strainer and transfer into two glasses. Serve immediately.
Nutrition Facts:
Calories 105kcal, Fat 0.5 g, Carbohydrate 12.5 g, Protein 1 g

Apple & Carrot Juice

Preparation Time: 10 minutes
Servings: 2
Ingredients:
5 carrots, peeled and chopped
1 large apple, cored and chopped
1 ½-inch piece fresh ginger, peeled and chopped
½ of lemon
½ cup filtered water
Directions:
Add all ingredients into a juicer and extract the juice according to the manufacturer's method.
In case you don't have one, add all the ingredients in a blender and pulse until well combined.
Filter the juice through a fine mesh strainer and transfer into two glasses. Serve immediately.
Nutrition Facts:
Calories 125kcal, Fat 0.3 g, Carbohydrate 21.4 g Protein 1.7 g

Strawberry Juice

Preparation Time: 10 minutes
Servings: 2
Ingredients:
2½ cups fresh ripe strawberries, hulled 1 apple, cored and chopped
1 lime, peeled
Directions:
Add all ingredients into a juicer and extract the juice according to the manufacturer's method.
In case you don't have one, add all the ingredients in a blender and pulse until well combined.

Filter the juice through a fine mesh strainer and transfer into two glasses.
Serve immediately. It can be stored in the fridge in a proper container up to 3 days.
Nutrition Facts:
Calories 108kcal, Fat 0.8 g, Carbohydrate 18.5 g, Protein 1.6 g

Chocolate and Date Smoothie

Preparation Time: 10 minutes
Servings: 2
Ingredients:
4 Medjool dates, pitted 2 tbsp. cacao powder
2 tbsp. flaxseed
1 tbsp. almond butter 1 tsp vanilla extract
¼ tsp ground cinnamon
1½ cups almond milk, unsweetened 4 ice cubes
Directions:
Add all ingredients in a high-power blender and pulse until smooth. Pour into two glasses and serve immediately.
It can be stored in the fridge in a proper container up to 3 days.
Nutrition Facts:
Calories 234kcal, Fat 5 g, Carbohydrate 25.5 g, Protein 6 g

Blueberry & Kale Smoothie

Preparation Time: 10 minutes
Servings: 2
Ingredients:
2 cups frozen blueberries 2 cups fresh kale leaves 2 Medjool dates, pitted
1 tbsp. chia seeds
1 ½-inch piece fresh ginger, peeled and chopped 1½ cups almond milk, unsweetened
Directions:
Add all ingredients in a high-power blender and pulse until smooth. Pour the smoothie into two glasses and serve immediately.
It can be stored in the fridge in a proper container up to 3 days.
Nutrition Facts:
Calories 230kcal, Fat 4.5 g, Carbohydrate 28.8 g, Protein 5.6 g

Strawberry & Beet Smoothie

Preparation Time: 10 minutes
Servings: 2
Ingredients:
2 cups frozen strawberries, pitted and chopped 2/3 cup frozen beets, chopped
1 ½-inch piece ginger, chopped
1 ½-inch piece fresh turmeric, chopped (or 1 tsp turmeric powder)
½ cup fresh orange juice
1 cup almond milk, unsweetened
Directions:
Add all ingredients in a high-power blender and pulse until smooth. Pour the smoothie into two glasses and serve immediately.
It can be stored in the fridge in a proper container up to 3 days.
Nutrition Facts:
Calories 130kcal, Fat 0.2g, Carbohydrate 22.5 g, Protein 2 g

Green Pineapple Smoothie

Preparation Time: 5 minutes
Servings: 1
Ingredients:
1 cup spinach
1 apple
1 cup pineapple 1tsp. of flax seeds
½ cup filtered water
Directions:
Add all ingredients in a high-power blender and pulse until smooth. Pour the smoothie into two glasses and serve immediately.
Nutrition Facts:
Calories 102kcal, Fat 0.3 g, Carbohydrate 18.5 g, Protein 1 g

Spinach Smoothie

Preparation Time: 5 minutes
Servings: 1
Ingredients:
1 cup spinach
1 pear
½ bananas
¼ zucchini
½ cup almond milk, unsweetened
Directions:
Add all ingredients in a high-power blender and pulse until smooth. Pour the smoothie into two glasses and serve immediately.
Nutrition Facts:
Calories 123kcal, Fat 0.9 g, Carbohydrate 18.5 g, Protein 2.4 g

Kale Smoothie

Preparation Time: 5 minutes
Servings: 1
Ingredients:
1 cup kale
½ mango
½ banana
1 tbsp. chia seeds
¼ cup coconut milk, unsweetened
½ cup filtered water
Directions:
Add all ingredients in a high-power blender and pulse until smooth. Pour the smoothie into two glasses and serve immediately
Nutrition Facts:
Calories 156kcal, Fat 4.5 g, Carbohydrate 20.5 g, Protein 3.2 g

Avocado Smoothie

Preparation Time: 5 minutes
Cooking Time: 0 minutes
Servings: 1
Ingredients:
½ avocado 1 banana
1 cup spinach
1 tbsp. linseed
¼ cup almond milk, unsweetened
½ cup filtered water
Directions:
Add all ingredients in a high-power blender and pulse until smooth. Pour the smoothie into two glasses and serve immediately
Nutrition Facts:
Calories 161kcal, Fat 5.5 g, Carbohydrate 29.5 g, Protein 1 g

Lettuce Smoothie

Preparation Time: 5 minutes
Servings: 1
Ingredients:
½ small head of lettuce 3 fresh plums, seeded
½ banana
1 tbsp. linseed
½ cucumber
½ cup almond milk, unsweetened
Directions:
Add all ingredients in a high-power blender and pulse until smooth. Pour the smoothie into two glasses and serve immediately.
Nutrition Facts: C
alories 138kcal, Fat 2.5 g, Carbohydrate 19.8 g, Protein 3g

Apple and Cinnamon Smoothie

Preparation Time: 5 minutes
Servings: 2
Ingredients:
2 apples, peeled, cored, sliced 4 tbsp. pecans
4 Medjool dates, pitted
½ tsp vanilla extract, unsweetened 2 cups almond milk, unsweetened 1 ½ tbsp. ground cinnamon
Directions:
Add all ingredients in a high-power blender and pulse until smooth. Pour the smoothie into two glasses and serve immediately.

It can be stored in the fridge in a proper container up to 3 days.

Nutrition Facts:

Calories 183kcal, Fat 5.5 g, Carbohydrate 12.8 g, Protein 4.5g

Strawberry, Mango and Yogurt Smoothie

Preparation Time: 5 minutes

Servings: 2

Ingredients

1 mango, destoned, peeled, diced 4 oz. strawberries

1.3 oz. yogurt

2 cups almond milk, unsweetened

Directions

Add all ingredients in a high-power blender and pulse until smooth. Pour the smoothie into two glasses and serve immediately.

It can be stored in the fridge in a proper container up to 3 days.

Nutrition Facts:

Calories 166kcal, Fat 3.7 g, Carbohydrate 27 g, Protein 3.5g

Berries Vanilla Protein Smoothie

Preparation Time: 5 minutes

Servings: 2

Ingredients:

2 oz. blackberries - 2 oz. strawberries

2 oz. raspberries

2 scoops of vanilla protein powder 1 ½ cup almond milk, unsweetened

Directions:

Add all ingredients in a high-power blender and pulse until smooth. Pour the smoothie into two glasses and serve immediately.

It can be stored in the fridge in a proper container up to 3 days.

Nutrition Facts:

Calories 151kcal, Fat 2.8 g, Carbohydrate 10.9 g, Protein 20.3g

Sirtfood Green Juice

Ingredients::

1/3 cup rocket (rocket)

two cups kale

one tablespoon lovage leaves

one tablespoon level leaf parsley

½ teaspoon matcha tea

½ lemon, squeezed

½ apple

Giant stems inexperienced celery, as well as leaves

Bearings:

Combine the greens (rocket, kale, parsley, and lovage leaves) along, at that point juice them to urge 50ml of juice from the inexperienced. Juice the apple and so the celery.

You'll strip the lemon and place it through the juicer, or primarily press the lemon by hand into the juice. You would like to possess 250ml of juice altogether by this stage.

Once the juice is made and prepared to serve, as well as the matcha tea. Pour a modest amount of juice into a glass, at that point embrace the matcha and mix vivaciously with a fork or a teaspoon. (Use matcha simply at intervals the initial 2 beverages of the day as a result of it contains a moderate live of caffeine)

Once the match is stormy embrace the rest of the juice. Provides it a final combine.

Enjoy!

Lime and Ginger Smoothie

Ingredients::

½ cup while not farm milk

½ cup of water

½ teaspoon new ginger

½ cup mango items

Juice from one lime

one tablespoon dried destroyed coconut

one tablespoon flaxseeds

one cup spinach

Bearings:
Mix along all the Ingredients: till swish.
Serve and appreciate it!
Dietary information per serving:
Calories 178,
Fat 1g,
Carbohydrates 7g,
Macromolecule 4g

Turmeric Strawberry Smoothie

This simple smoothie can support your assimilation! Too nice to not try it!
Ingredients:: one serving
one cup kale, stalks exhausted
one teaspoon turmeric
one cup strawberries
½ cup coconut yoghurt
Six pecan components
one tablespoon crude angiospermous tree powder
1-2 metric linear unit cut of superior stew
one cup nonsweet almond milk
One faveolate Medjool date
Headings:
Mix along all the Ingredients: and appreciate right away!
Watch out regarding what proportion almond milk you embrace thus you will choose your most well-liked consistency.

Sirtfood marvel Smoothie

Ingredients::
one cup rocket (rocket)
two cups natural strawberries or blueberries
one cup kale
½ teaspoon matcha tea
Juice of ½ lemon or lime
Three twigs of parsley
½ cup of watercress
¾ cup of water
Bearings:
Add all the Ingredients: with the exception of matcha to a liquidiser and whizz up till swish.
Add the matcha tea powder and provides it a final rush till significantly intermingled.
Enjoy!

Strawberry Spinach Smoothie

Ingredients:: one serving
one cup entire solid strawberries
three cups ironed spinach
¼ cup solid pineapple lumps
One medium prepared banana, dig lumps and solid
one cup nonsweet milk
one tablespoon chia seeds
Headings:
Place all the Ingredients: throughout a strong liquidiser.
Mix till swish.
Enjoy!

Berry Turmeric Smoothie

Ingredients:: one serving
One ½ cups solid intermingled berries • ½ teaspoon ground turmeric
two cups babe spinach
¾ cup no sweet vanilla almond milk, or milk of call
½ cup non-fat plain Greek yoghurt, or yoghurt of call
¼ teaspoon ground ginger
2-3 teaspoons nectar
three tablespoons old rapt oats
Bearings:
Place all the Ingredients: throughout a strong liquidiser.
Mix till swish.
Style and alter pleasantness as wished.
Get pleasure from right away!

Mango inexperienced Smoothie

Ingredients:: one serving
One ½ cups solid mango items
one cup stuffed kid spinach leaves
One prepared banana
¾ cup nonsweet vanilla almond milk
Bearings:
Place all the Ingredients: throughout a liquidizer.
Mix till swish.
Enjoy!

Apple Avocado Smoothie

Ingredients:: one serving
two cups stuffed spinach
½ medium avocado
One medium apple, stripped and quartered
½ medium banana, dig items and solid
½ cup no sweet almond milk
one teaspoon nectar
¼ teaspoon ground ginger
Little bunch of ice 3D shapes
Bearings:
At intervals the organized summing up, as well as the almond milk, spinach, avocado, banana, apples, nectar, ginger, and ice to a powerful liquidiser.
Mix till swish.
Style and alter pleasantness and flavors as wished.
Get pleasure from right away!

Kale Pineapple Smoothie

A delightful and velvety inexperienced kale pineapple smoothie with banana and Greek yoghurt. This smoothie can keep you full for quite long time!
Ingredients:: one serving
two cups softly ironed cleaved kale leaves, stems exhausted
¼ cup solid pineapple items
One solid medium banana, dig lumps
¼ cup non-fat Greek yoghurt
two teaspoons nectar
¾ cup nonsweet vanilla almond milk, or any milk of call
two tablespoons nutty unfold, swish or crisp
Bearings:
Place all the Ingredients: throughout a liquidiser.
Mix till swish.
Add additional milk varied to achieve wished consistency.
Get pleasure from right away!

Blueberry Banana Avocado Smoothie

Ingredients:: one serving
One medium prepared banana, stripped
two cups solid blueberries
one cup new spinach
one tablespoon ground linseed dinner
½ prepared avocado
one tablespoon almond unfold
¼ teaspoon cinnamon
½ cup no sweet vanilla almond milk
Bearings:
Place all the Ingredients: in your liquidizer at intervals the organized rundown: vanilla almond milk, spinach, banana, avocado, blueberries, linseed supper, and almond unfold.
Mix till swish.
If you want a thicker smoothie, embrace barely bunch of ice.
Get pleasure from right away!

Carrot Smoothie

Ingredients:: one serving
one cup cleaved carrots
¼ cup solid diced pineapple
½ cup solid cut banana
¼ teaspoon cinnamon
one tablespoon shredded coconut

½ cup Greek yoghurt
two tablespoons cooked pecans
Pinch nutmeg
½ cup no sweet vanilla almond milk, or milk of call
For the garnish: destroyed carrots, coconut, press pecans
Headings:
Add all the Ingredients: into a liquidizer. Blend till swish.
Get pleasure from quickly, beat with further destroyed carrots, coconut, and press pecans as wanted!

Matcha Berry Smoothie

This sparkling Matcha Berry Smoothie is made with tea powder, berries, and all-normal plant-based
Ingredients:: one serving
½ banana
½-tablespoon matcha powder
one cup almond milk
one cup solid blueberries
¼ teaspoon ground ginger
½ tablespoon chia seeds
¼ teaspoon ground cinnamon
Bearings:
Throughout a liquidizer, combine the almond milk, banana, blueberries, matcha powder, chia seeds, cinnamon, and ginger till swish.
Get pleasure from right away!

Grape Smoothie

Ingredients:
Two tsp. of any natural sweetener or honey
One cup of fresh green grapes (seedless)
1 ½ cup almond milk (sweetened)
One stalk of huge celery (with leaves)
One large cucumber (thinly sliced and peeled)
Method:
Start by taking a blender and add altogether the listed ingredients. You'll got to make sure that you begin with liquid first. So, during this case, you'll got to add almond milk first, followed by the opposite ingredients. Start blending the ingredients until the mixture is frothy and smooth.
Pour the smoothie into two smoothie glasses. Serve and enjoy!

Mixed Berry Summer Smoothie

Ingredients:
One cup of yogurt (Greek)
2 ½ cups fresh fruit juice (you can use canned juice as well)
Two cups berries (mixed, frozen)
One medium-sized banana (fresh, sliced)
One tsp. honey (optional)
Fresh berries and mint (for garnishing, optional)
Method:
Add yogurt, fruit juice, banana, and berries to a blender. Start blending the ingredients until frothy and smooth. If the smoothie seems to be a touch thick, you'll change the consistency adding some more liquid.
Blend the smoothie once more. Taste it and add the honey if you would like more sweetness.
Pour the smoothie in glasses and garnish it with fresh berries and mint.

Strawberry and Cherry Smoothie

Ingredients:
One large cup of water
Two cups fresh or frozen sweet cherries
One cup fresh or frozen strawberries
One large peeled orange (fresh, wedges separated)
1 ½ tbsp. chia seeds
One medium-sized banana
Honey or the other natural sweetener (optional)

Method:

Take a blender and begin adding all the ingredients thereto. Confirm to feature the ingredients within the proper order as they're listed. Because the general rule, you ought to always add ingredients that are frozen eventually with the liquid ingredients first. The remainder of the ingredients are often added in between.

Blend the ingredients until it turns frothy and smooth.

If you would like the smoothie to be a touch sweet, you'll add honey or the other natural sweetener.

Just in case you're adding honey, blend the smoothie another time before pouring in glasses.

Kale Ginger Mango Smoothie

Ingredients:

One tbsp. fresh ginger (minced)
Two cups of every
Ripe peaches (frozen)
Ripe mango (cubed, frozen)
Half cup ice
Two cups fresh kale
One and a half cup of water
Two small lemons or lime (juiced)
One and a half tbsp. syrup (optional)

Method:

Crush the ice by adding it to a kitchen appliance or blender.

Start adding peach, mango cubes, ginger, juice, kale, and water to the blender. The quantity of water that you simply are going to be using within the smoothie will believe the amount of frozen items.

Blend all the ingredients properly until the mixture is frothy and smooth.

You'll adjust the consistency of the smoothie by adding water thereto

Confirm that you simply scrape the blender walls in between blending.

Once the ingredients are blended, taste it and you'll add more seasonings if you would like.

If the smoothie is just too tart, you'll add in syrup or more fruits. Ginger are often added for adding zing to the smoothie. You'll use juice to extend the acidity. You'll add more crushed ice to extend the consistency of the smoothie.

After you're through with blending, serve the smoothie immediately.

Kale and Melon Smoothie

Ingredients:

One large apple (properly peeled, cubed)
Half cup ice
Two cups chopped kale (fresh)
One and a half cup of honeydew melon (cut into cubes)
Two tbsps. Juice (fresh)

Method:

Start by adding ice and melon to a kitchen appliance. Turn it into a smooth puree.

Now add juice, kale, and cubed apples to the mixture.

Start blending all the ingredients until frothy and smooth. If you would like to vary the consistency of the smoothie, you'll add water.

If you're adding water, blend the smoothie another time.

Divide the smoothie into smoothie glasses and luxuriate in.

Zingy Green Juice

Ingredients:

One medium-sized lemon (juiced)
80 g kale (fresh)
6 g parsley (fresh)
One green apple (cubed)
40 g arugula (rocket variety)
Three medium celery sticks

Half centimeter fresh ginger
One tsp. tea (matcha variety)
Method:
Start by lowering all the listed ingredients apart from the lemon and tea.
Confirm to chop all the ingredients in proper size in order that they will be accommodated within the juicer.
Juice the ingredients.
Add a couple of drops of juice to the juice and blend it with a spoon.
Now pour a number of the juice during a glass and add the matcha tea thereto. Stir the mixture properly.
Add the remainder of the juice to the glass and blend properly for getting all the flavors.
Consume immediately.

Matcha Green Smoothie

Ingredients:
One large ripe mango (fresh or frozen)
One frozen banana
Two cups spinach
Two tbsps. Tea powder (matcha)
Half cup unsweetened almond milk
One tsp. honey
One cup of almonds (chopped)
Half cup yogurt (Greek)
Method:
Start by adding all the ingredients to a blender.
Blend for one minute until the mixture turns frothy and smooth.
If you would like the smoothie a touch thick, you'll add ice cubes.
For reducing the consistency, add almond milk and blend again.
Divide the smoothie in glasses and serve chilled.

Tropical Kale juice

Ingredients:
One few fresh kale
One large orange
Eight carrots
One medium-sized apple
Three rounds of pineapple (one-inch)
Method:
Start by washing the ingredients and dry them.
Cut the ingredients within the proper size for accommodating them within the juicer.
Juice all the ingredients properly by employing a juicer.
You'll got to mix the juice with the assistance of a spoon in order that all the flavors can get mixed.
Divide the juice into three glasses and serve.

Orange and Celery Juice

Ingredients:
Four large sticks of celery (chopped)
800 ml of fruit juice (fresh)
Five large carrots (cubed and peeled)
For garnishing
Leaves of celery
Two celery sticks (halved, peeled)
Method:
Add carrots, fruit juice, and celery to a blender. Blend all the ingredients properly until frothy and smooth.
You'll got to check the consistency of the juice and keep it up adding fruit juice consistent with your required consistency.
Blend the juice another time.
Let the juice sit within the blender for a few time.
Pour the juice into tall glasses and serve with celery sticks and leaves from the highest.

Kale Blackcurrant Smoothie

Ingredients:

Three tbsps. Of each
Honey or the other sweetener
Wheatgrass
One medium avocado (peeled and chopped)
One few kale (lightly steamed)
Two cups of ice cubes
Five hundred ml of coconut milk (fresh)
Two hundred grams blackcurrant (fresh or thawed)
One green apple (cored, chopped)

Method:

Start by taking a blender and add in avocado, kale, apple, coconut milk, and blackcurrant thereto. Blend the mixture until smooth.
Add honey to the mixture.
Add ice cubes to the blender and whizz the mixture once more.
Pour the smoothie in smoothie glasses.
Serve immediately and garnish with green apple at the highest.
Dust wheatgrass consistent with your need.

Grapefruit Celery Juice

Ingredients:

Half cup ice cubes
One large apple (cubed)
One small lime
One large-sized cucumber
Half portion of pomelo grapefruit
One stalk of celery

Method:

Wash all the ingredients under running water properly.
Remove the outer skin of pomelo grapefruit and lime.
Just in case you would like the taste to be less bitter, you'll leave the outer skin intact.
Now it's time to require a juicer and begin juicing all the related ingredients.
For crushing the ice, use a blender.
Pour the juice in glasses and add crushed ice to an equivalent.
Serve immediately.

Summer Blackcurrant Smoothie

Ingredients:

One cup of every
Fresh or frozen blackcurrant
Water
One full cup strawberries (fresh or frozen)
Half cup of coconut milk
Three tbsps. Chia seeds (whole or powdered)
Liquid stevia (for sweetness, optional)
One tsp. vanilla

Method:

Start by putting all the ingredients during a blender. Pulse the ingredients to form the mixture frothy and smooth.
Leave the smoothie within the blender for about five minutes.
Add the vanilla to the smoothie and pulse once more.
Serve the smoothie in tall glasses and luxuriate in.

Pineapple and Cucumber Juice

Ingredients:

Two large cucumbers
Three inches of ginger (you can add more for improving the zing)
Six stalks of celery (fresh)
Half of a pineapple (remove the outer skin)
One small lemon

Method:

Start by adding all the listed ingredients during a juicer. Blend everything properly until smooth and frothy.
cut the cucumbers and lemon into cubes in order that they will be fitted within the juicer. Cutting the ingredients into smaller size will make the task of blending much easier. It'll be taking less time also.

As you juice the ingredients, check the consistency in between. If you would like to scale back the consistency, add water.
Mix the juice properly and serve in tall glasses.

Spinach, Date, and Vanilla Smoothie

Ingredients:

One large-sized banana (frozen or fresh)
Two and a half cup of vanilla almond milk (unsweetened)
Three cups of fresh spinach
5 dates (Medjool dates is preferred, pitted, chopped)

Method:

Start by taking a blender and add altogether the listed ingredients. Blend the mixture turns frothy and smooth. Confirm that there are not any remaining spinach flecks or date pieces within the mixture. Blend the mixture properly for the right mixing of all the flavors. Divide the smoothie in smoothie glasses and serve immediately.

Simple Cucumber Celery Green Juice

Ingredients:

Four stalks of fresh celery (trim the ends)
One large cucumber
One few kale (fresh)
One cup fresh parsley (chopped)
One medium-sized apple
Two inches of fresh ginger (peeled)

Method:

Wash all the ingredients in cold water and dry them employing a kitchen towel. Cut the ingredients in cubes in order that they will be accommodated within the juicer. Add the veggies following this order- kale, ginger, apple, cucumber, and parsley.
Juice the ingredients properly and confirm there are not any leftover chunks. Attempt to make the juice as smooth as possible.
Pour the juice in juice glasses. Serve with honey from the highest (optional).

Cranberry Kale Smoothie

Ingredients:

One few fresh kale - One large orange
One cup of every
Cranberries (frozen or fresh)
Water - One large banana (frozen)

Method:

First, confirm that you simply have arranged all the listed ingredients in one place in order that you don't have to rush for them while blending the smoothie. You will got to hamper the ingredients to a convenient size in order that they will be fitted within the blender with no problem. Blend the listed ingredients. Continue blending until the smoothie is frothy and smooth. Confirm that each one the ingredients get mixed properly.
Pour the blended in smoothie glasses and enjoy!

Banana Matcha Smoothie

Ingredients:

One and a half cup of fresh spinach
Two cups banana (frozen, sliced)
Half tsp. tea powder (matcha)
One and a half tsp. flax seed
Two tsp. vanilla
Two cups of almond milk (preferably unsweetened)

Method:

Start by taking a blender and add all the listed ingredients. Blend the smoothie until smooth and frothy. You'll got to make sure that all the flavors and ingredients get mixed properly.
Divide the smoothie in glasses. Serve immediately.

CHAPTER 15:

DESSERT

Snowflakes

Preparation time: 15 minutes
Cooking time: 10 minutes
Servings: 1
Ingredients:

Won ton wrappers Oil to frying Powdered sugar

Directions:

Cut won ton wrappers just like you'd a snowflake

Heat oil. When hot, add wonton, fry for approximately 30 seconds then flip over.

Drain on a paper towel and dust with powdered sugar.

Nutrition:

Calories: 96 Net carbs: 24.1g Fat: 0.6g Fiber: 5.3g Protein: 2.8g

Home-Made Marshmallow Fluff

Preparation time: 15 minutes
Cooking time: 20 minutes
Servings: 4
Ingredients:

3/4 cup sugar

1/2 cup light corn syrup 1/4 cup water

⅛ Teaspoon salt 3 little egg whites

1/4 teaspoon cream of tartar

1 teaspoon 1/2 teaspoon vanilla extract

Directions:

In a little pan, mix together sugar, corn syrup, salt and water. Attach a candy thermometer into the side of this pan, but make sure it will not touch the underside of the pan.

From the bowl of a stand mixer, combine egg whites and cream of tartar. Begin to whip on medium speed with the whisk attachment.

Meanwhile, turn a burner on top and place the pan with the sugar mix onto heat. Pout mix into a boil and heat to 240 degrees, stirring periodically.

The aim is to have the egg whites whipped to soft peaks and also the sugar

heated to 240 degrees at near the same moment. Simply stop stirring the egg whites once they hit soft peaks.

Once the sugar has already reached 240 amounts, turn heat low allowing it to reduce. Insert a little quantity of the popular sugar mix and let it mix. Insert still another little sum of the sugar mix. Add mix slowly and that means you never scramble the egg whites.

After all of the sugar was added into the egg whites, then decrease the speed of the mixer and also keep mixing concoction for around 7- 9 minutes until the fluff remains glossy and stiff. At roughly the 5-minute mark, then add the vanilla extract.

Use fluff immediately or store in an airtight container in the fridge for around two weeks.

Nutrition:

Calories: 23 Net carbs: 5.8g Protein: 0.1g

Guilt Totally Free Banana Ice-Cream

Preparation time: 15 minutes
Cooking time: 0 minutes
Servings: 3
Ingredients:

3 quite ripe banana - peeled and chopped A couple of chocolate chips
Two skim milk

Directions:

Throw all ingredients into a food processor and blend until creamy. Eat: freeze and appreciate afterward.

Nutrition:

Calories: 387 Net carbs: 47.3g Fat: 19.5g Fiber: 1g Protein: 6.3g

Perfect Little PB Snack Balls

Preparation time: 15 minutes
Cooking time: 0 minutes
Servings: 1
Ingredients:

1/2 cup chunky peanut butter 3 flax seeds
3 wheat germ
1 honey or agave
1/4 cup powdered sugar

Directions:

Blend dry ingredients and adding from the honey and peanut butter.
Mix well and roll into chunks and then conclude by rolling into wheat germ.

Nutrition:

Calories: 95 Net carbs: 6.6g Fat: 5.6g Fiber: 1.2g Protein: 5.7g

Dark Chocolate Pretzel Cookies

Preparation time: 15 minutes
Cooking time: 20 minutes
Servings: 4
Ingredients:

1 cup yogurt
1/2 teaspoon baking soda 1/4 teaspoon salt
1/4 teaspoon cinnamon 4 butter (softened/0
1/3 cup brown sugar
1 egg
1/2 teaspoon vanilla
1/2 cup dark chocolate chips 1/2 cup pretzels, chopped

Directions:

Preheat oven to 350 degrees.
In a medium bowl whisk together the sugar, butter, vanilla and egg. In another bowl, stir together the flour, baking soda, and salt.
Stir the bread mixture in, using all the wet components, along with the chocolate chips and pretzels until just blended.
Drop large spoonful of dough on an unlined baking sheet.
Bake for 15-17 minutes, or until the bottoms are somewhat all crispy.
Allow cooling on a wire rack.

Nutrition:

Calories: 300 Net carbs: 44.3g Fat: 11.2g Fiber: 1.3g Protein: 3.8g

Marshmallow Popcorn Balls

Preparation time: 5 minutes
Cooking time: 20 minutes
Servings: 6
Ingredients:

2 bag of microwave popcorn 1 12.6 ounces. Tote M&M's
3 cups honey roasted peanuts
1 pkg. 16 ounce. Massive marshmallows 1 cup butter, cubed

Directions:

In a bowl, blend the popcorn, peanuts and M&M's. In a big pot, combine marshmallows and butter. Cook using medium-low heat. Insert popcorn mix, blend thoroughly Spray muffin tins with non-stick cooking spray.
When cool enough to handle, spray hands together with non-stick cooking spray and then shape into chunks and put into the

muffin tin to shape. Add Popsicle stick into each chunk and then let cool.
Wrap each serving in vinyl when chilled.
Nutrition:
Calories: 36 Net carbs: 7.4g Fat: 0.2g Fiber: 0.3g Protein: 0.9g

Home-Made Ice-Cream Drumsticks

Preparation time: 15 minutes
Cooking time: 0 minutes
Servings: 4
Ingredients:
Vanilla ice cream
Two Lindt hazelnut chunks Magical shell - out chocolate Sugar levels
Nuts (I mixed crushed peppers and unsalted peanuts) Parchment paper
Directions:
Soften ice cream and mixing topping - I had two sliced Lindt hazelnut balls. Fill underside of Magic shell with sugar and nuts and top with ice-cream.
Wrap parchment paper round cone and then fill cone over about 1.5 inches across the cap of the cone (the paper can help to carry its shape).
Sprinkle with magical nuts and shells.
Freeze for about 20 minutes, before the ice cream is eaten.
Nutrition:
Calories: 267 Net carbs: 32.4g Fat: 14.2g Fiber: 0.9g Protein: 4.6g

Ultimate Chocolate Chip Cookie N' Oreo Fudge Brownie Bar

Preparation time: 20 minutes
Cooking time: 70 minutes
Servings: 4
Ingredients:
1 cup (2 sticks) butter, softened 1 cup granulated sugar
3/4 cup light brown sugar 2 large egg
1 pure vanilla extract
2 ½ cups all-purpose flour 1 teaspoon baking soda
1 teaspoon lemon
2 cups (12 Oz) milk chocolate chips 1 package double stuffed Oreo
1 family-size (9×1 3) brownie mixture 1/4 cup hot fudge topping
Directions:
Preheat oven to 350 degrees F.
Cream the butter and sugars in a large bowl using an electric mixer at medium speed for 35 minutes.
Add the vanilla and eggs and mix well to combine thoroughly. In another bowl, whisk together the flour, baking soda and salt, and slowly incorporate in the mixer everything is combined.
Stir in chocolate chips.
Spread the cookie dough at the bottom of a 9×1-3 baking dish that is wrapped with wax paper and then coated with cooking spray.
Shirt with a coating of Oreos. Mix together brownie mix, adding an optional
1/4 cup of hot fudge directly into the mixture. Stir the brownie batter within the cookie-dough and Oreos. Cover with foil and bake at 350 degrees F for 30 minutes. Remove foil and continue baking for another 15 25 minutes.
Let cool before cutting on brownies. They may be gooey at the while warm but will also set up perfectly once chilled.
Nutrition:
Calories: 181 Net carbs: 30g Fat: 5.4g Fiber: 1.1g Protein: 3g

Crunchy Chocolate Chip Coconut Macadamia Nut Cookies

Preparation time: 15 minutes
Cooking time: 5 minutes
Servings: 5
Ingredients:

1 cup yogurt 1 cup yogurt 1/2 teaspoon baking soda 1/2 teaspoon salt
1 of butter, softened
1 cup firmly packed brown sugar 1/2 cup sugar
1 large egg
1/2 cup semi-sweet chocolate chips 1/2 cup sweetened flaked coconut
1/2 cup coarsely chopped dry-roasted macadamia nuts 1/2 cup raisins

Directions:

Preheat the oven to 325°f.
In a little bowl, whisk together the flour, oats and baking soda and salt; then place aside.
In your mixer bowl, mix together the butter/sugar/egg mix.
Mix in the flour/oats mix until just combined and stir into the chocolate chips, raisins, nuts, and coconut.
Place outsized bits on a parchment-lined cookie sheet.
Bake for 1-3 minutes, before biscuits are only barely golden brown.
Remove from the oven and then leave the cookie sheets to cool at least 10 minutes.

Nutrition:

Calories: 317 Net carbs: 20.5g Fat: 9.9g Fiber: 2.3g Protein: 35.2g

Peach and Blueberry Pie

Preparation time: 20 minutes
Cooking time: 60 minutes
Servings: 4
Ingredients:

1 box of noodle dough Filling:
5 peaches, peeled and chopped (I used roasted peaches) 3 cups strawberries
3/4 cup sugar 1/4 cup bread
Juice of 1/2 lemon 1 egg yolk, beaten

Directions:

Preheat oven to 400 degrees. Place dough to a 9-inch pie plate
In a big bowl, combine tomatoes, sugar, bread, and lemon juice, then toss to combine. Pour into the pie plate, mounding at the center.
Simply take some of bread and then cut into bits, then put a pie shirt and put the dough in addition to pressing on edges.
Brush crust with egg wash then sprinkles with sugar. Set onto a parchment paper-lined baking sheet. Bake at 400 for about 20 minutes, until crust is browned at borders.
Turn oven down to 350, bake for another 40 minutes. Remove and let sit at least 30minutes.
Have with vanilla ice-cream.

Nutrition:

Calories: 360 Net carbs: 49.2g Fat: 17.4g Protein: 3.9g

Pear, Cranberry And Chocolate Crisp

Preparation time: 15 minutes
Cooking time: 40 minutes
Servings: 4
Ingredients:

Crumble topping: 1/2 cup flour
1/2 cup brown sugar 1 teaspoon cinnamon
⅛ Teaspoon salt 3/4 cup yogurt
1/4 cup sliced peppers 1/3 cup butter, melted
1 teaspoon vanilla Filling:
1 brown sugar
3 teaspoon, cut into balls 1/4 cup dried cranberries 1 teaspoon lemon juice
Two handfuls of milk chocolate chips

Directions:
Preheat oven to 375.
Spray a casserole dish with a butter spray.
Put all of the topping ingredients - flour, sugar, cinnamon, salt, nuts, legumes and dried Butter a bowl and then mix. Set aside.
In a large bowl combine the sugar, lemon juice, pears, and cranberries. Once the fully blended move to the prepared baking dish.
Spread the topping evenly over the fruit. Bake for about half an hour.
Disperse chocolate chips out at the top. Cook for another 10 minutes.
Have with ice cream.
Nutrition:
Calories: 418 Net carbs: 107.7g Fat: 0.4g Fiber: 2.8g Protein: 0.5g

Apricot Oatmeal Cookies

Preparation time: 10 minutes
Cooking time: 40 minutes
Servings: 7
Ingredients:
1/2 cup (1 stick) butter, softened
2/3 cup light brown sugar packed 1 egg 3/4 cup all-purpose flour
1/2 teaspoon baking soda 1/2 teaspoon vanilla extract
1/2 teaspoon cinnamon 1/4 teaspoon salt 1 teaspoon 1/2 cups chopped oats
3/4 cup yolks 1/4 cup sliced apricots 1/3 cup slivered almonds
Directions:
Preheat oven to 350°. In a big bowl combine with the butter, sugar, and egg until smooth. In another bowl whisk the flour, baking soda, cinnamon, and salt together. Stir the dry ingredients to the butter-sugar bowl. Now stir in the oats, raisins, apricots, and almonds.
I heard on the web that in this time, it's much better to cool with the dough (therefore, your biscuits are thicker)
Nutrition:
Calories: 196 Net carbs: 30g Fat: 8.1g Fiber: 0.5g Protein: 3g

Raw Vegan Reese's Cups

Preparation time: 10 minutes
Cooking time: 35 minutes
Servings: 4
Ingredients:
"Peanut" butter filling
½ cup sunflower seeds butter
½ cup almond butter 1 raw honey
2 melted coconut oil
Super foods chocolate part:
½ cup cacao powder 2 raw honey
1/3 cup of coconut oil (melted)
Directions:
Mix the "peanut" butter filling ingredients.
Put a spoonful of the mixture into each muffin cup. Refrigerate.
Mix super foods chocolate ingredients.
Put a spoonful of the super foods chocolate mixture over the "peanut" butter mixture. Freeze!
Nutrition:
Calories: 549 Net carbs: 54g Fat: 31.7g Fiber: 2.1g Protein: 11.8g

Raw Vegan Coffee Cashew Cream Cake

Preparation time: 10 minutes
Cooking time: 35 minutes
Servings: 4
Ingredients:
Coffee cashew cream 2 cups raw cashews
1 teaspoon of ground vanilla bean 3 melted coconut oil
¼ cup raw honey
1/3 cup very strong coffee or triple espresso shot

Directions:
Blend all ingredients for the cream, pour it onto the crust and refrigerate. Garnish with coffee beans.
Nutrition:
Calories: 94 Net carbs: 4.4g Fat: 7.9g Fiber: 0.3g Protein: 2.8g

Raw Vegan Chocolate Cashew Truffles

Preparation time: 10 minutes
Cooking time: 35 minutes
Servings: 4
Ingredients: 1 cup ground cashews
1 teaspoon of ground vanilla bean
½ cup of coconut oil
¼ cup raw honey 2 flax meal
2 hemp hearts
2 cacao powder
Directions:
Mix all ingredients and make truffles. Sprinkle coconut flakes on top.
Nutrition:
Calories: 87 Net carbs: 6g Fat: 6.5g Fiber: 0.5g Protein: 2.3g

Raw Vegan Double Almond Raw Chocolate Tart

Preparation time: 10 minutes
Cooking time: 35 minutes
Servings: 4
Ingredients:
1½ cups of raw almonds
¼ cup of coconut oil, melted 1 raw honey or royal jelly
8 ounces dark chocolate, chopped 1 cup of coconut milk
½ cup unsweetened shredded coconut
Directions:
Crust: Ground almonds and add melted coconut oil, raw honey and combine. Using a spatula, spread this mixture into the tart or pie pan.
Filling:
Put the chopped chocolate in a bowl, heat coconut milk and pour over chocolate and whisk together. Pour filling into tart shell.
Refrigerate.
Toast almond slivers chips and sprinkle over tart.
Nutrition:
Calories: 101 Net carbs: 3.4g Fat: 9.4g Fiber: 0.6g Protein: 2.4g

Raw Vegan Bounty Bars

Preparation time: 10 minutes
Cooking time: 35 minutes
Servings: 4
Ingredients:
"Peanut" butter filling
2 cups desiccated coconut 3 coconut oil - melted
1 cup of coconut cream - full fat 4 of raw honey
1 teaspoon ground vanilla bean Pinch of sea salt
Super foods chocolate part:
½ cup cacao powder 2 raw honey 1/3 cup of coconut oil (melted)
Directions:
Mix coconut oil, coconut cream, and honey, vanilla and salt. Pour over desiccated coconut and mix well.
Mold coconut mixture into balls, small bars similar to bounty and freeze.
Or pour the whole mixture into a tray, freeze and cut into small bars. Make super foods chocolate mixture, warm it up and dip frozen coconut into the chocolate and put on a tray and freeze again.
Nutrition:
Calories: 70 Net carbs: 6.7g Fat: 4.3g Fiber: 0.2g Protein: 1g

Raw Vegan Tartlets with Coconut Cream

Preparation time: 10 minutes
Cooking time: 35 minutes
Servings: 4
Ingredients:
Pudding:
1 avocado
2 coconut oil
2 raw honey
2 cacao powder
1 teaspoon ground vanilla bean Pinch of salt
¼ cup almond milk, as needed
Directions:
Blend all the ingredients in the food processor until smooth and thick. Spread evenly into tartlet crusts.
Optionally, put some goji berries on top of the pudding layer.
Make the coconut cream, spread it on top of the pudding layer, and put back in the fridge overnight.
Serve with one blueberry on top of each tartlet.
Nutrition:
Calories: 200 Net carbs: 25.2g Fat: 4.3g Fiber: 4.6g Protein: 12.8g

Raw Vegan "Peanut" Butter Truffles

Preparation time: 10 minutes
Cooking time: 30 minutes
Servings: 4
Ingredients:
5 sunflower seed butter 1 coconut oil
1 raw honey
1 teaspoon ground vanilla bean
¾ cup almond flour 1 flaxseed meal Pinch of salt
1 cacao butter
Hemp hearts (optional)
¼ cup super-foods chocolate
Directions:
Mix until all ingredients are incorporated.
Roll the dough into 1-inch balls, place them on parchment paper and refrigerate for half an hour (yield about 14 truffles).
Dip each truffle in the melted super foods chocolate, one at the time. Place them back on the pan with parchment paper or coat them in cocoa powder or coconut flakes.
Nutrition:
Calories: 94 Net carbs: 3.1g Fat: 8g Fiber: 1g Protein: 4g

Raw Vegan Chocolate Pie

Preparation time: 10 minutes
Cooking time: 25 minutes
Servings: 4
Ingredients: Crust:
2 cups almonds, soaked overnight and drained
1 cup pitted dates, soaked overnight and drained 1 cup chopped dried apricots
1½ teaspoon ground vanilla bean 2 teaspoon chia seeds 1 banana Filling:
4 raw cacao powder 3 raw honey
2 ripe avocados 2 organic coconut oil
2 almond milk (if needed, check for consistency first)
Directions:
Add almonds and banana to a food processor or blender. Mix until it forms a thick ball.
Add the vanilla, dates, and apricot chunks to the blender.
Mix well and optionally add a couple of drops of water at a time to make the mixture stick together. Spread in a 10-inch dis.
Mix filling ingredients in a blender and add almond milk if necessary. Add filling to the crust and refrigerate.
Nutrition:
Calories: 380 Net carbs: 50.2g Fat: 18.4g Fiber: 2.2g Protein: 7.2g

Raw Vegan Chocolate Walnut Truffles

Preparation time: 10 minutes
Cooking time: 35 minutes
Servings: 4
Ingredients:

1 cup ground walnuts 1 teaspoon cinnamon
½ cup of coconut oil
¼ cup raw honey 2 chia seeds
2 cacao powder

Directions:

Mix all ingredients and make truffles.
Coat with cinnamon, coconut flakes or chopped almonds.

Nutrition:

Calories: 120 Fat: 13.6g

Raw Vegan Carrot Cake

Preparation time: 10 minutes
Cooking time: 35 minutes
Servings: 4
Ingredients: Crust:

4 carrots, chopped 1½ cups oats
½ cup dried coconut 2 cups dates
1 teaspoon cinnamon ½ teaspoon nutmeg 1½ cups cashews 2 coconut oil
Juice from 1 lemon 2 raw honey 1 teaspoon ground vanilla bean Water, as needed

Directions:

Add all crust ingredients to the blender.
Mix well and optionally add a couple of drops of water at a time to make the mixture stick together.
Press in a small pan.
Take it out and put on a plate and freeze.
Mix frosting ingredients in a blender and add water if necessary. Add frosting to the crust and refrigerate.

Nutrition:

Calories: 241 Net carbs: 28.4g Fat: 13.4g Fiber: 0.8g Protein: 2.4g

Frozen Raw Blackberry Cake

Preparation time: 10 minutes
Cooking time: 45 minutes
Servings: 4
Ingredients: Crust:

3⁄4 cup shredded coconut
15 dried dates soaked in hot water and drained 1/3 cup pumpkin seeds 1/4 cup of coconut oil Middle filling Coconut whipped cream
Top filling:
1 pound of frozen blackberries
3-4 raw honey 1/4 cup of coconut cream 2 egg whites

Directions:

Grease the cake tin with coconut oil and mix all base ingredients in the blender until you get a sticky ball. Press the base mixture in a cake tin. Freeze. Make Coconut Whipped Cream. Process berries and add honey, coconut cream and egg whites. Pour middle filling - Coconut Whipped Cream in the tin and spread evenly. Freeze. Pour top filling - berries mixture- in the tin, spread, decorate with blueberries and almonds and return to freezer.

Nutrition:

Calories: 472 Net carbs: 15.8g Fat: 18g Fiber: 16.8g Protein: 33.3g

Raw Vegan Chocolate Hazelnuts Truffles

Preparation time: 10 minutes
Cooking time: 30 minutes
Servings: 4
Ingredients:

1 cup ground almonds
1 teaspoon ground vanilla bean
½ cup of coconut oil
½ cup mashed pitted dates 12 whole hazelnuts
2 cacao powder

Directions:
Mix all ingredients and make truffles with one whole hazelnut in the middle.
Nutrition:
Calories: 370 Net carbs: 66.9g Fat: 11.8g Fiber: 2.6g Protein: 4.2g

Raw Vegan Chocolate Cream Fruity Cake

Preparation time: 10 minutes
Cooking time: 45 minutes
Servings: 4
Ingredients:
Chocolate cream
1 avocado 2 raw honey 2 coconut oil
2 cacao powder
1 teaspoon ground vanilla bean Pinch of sea salt
¼ cup of coconut milk 1 coconut flakes
Fruits:
1 chopped banana
1 cup pitted cherries
Directions:
Prepare the crust and press it at the bottom of the pan.
Blend all chocolate cream ingredients, fold in the fruits and pour in the crust. Whip the top layer, spread and sprinkle with cacao powder. Refrigerate.
Nutrition:
Calories: 106 Net carbs: 0.4g Fat: 5g Fiber: 0.1g Protein: 14g

Jerusalem Artichoke Gratin

Preparation time: 10 minutes
Cooking time: 45 minutes
Servings: 3
Ingredients:
600g Jerusalem artichoke 250ml of milk
2 grated cheese
1 crème fraiche
1 butter
Curry, paprika powder, nutmeg, salt, pepper
Directions:
Wash and peel the Jerusalem artichoke tubers and slice them into approx. 3 mm thick slices. Bring them to a boil with the milk in a saucepan. Then stir in the spices and crème fraiche.
Grease a baking dish with butter and add the Jerusalem artichoke and milk mixture. Bake on the middle shelf in the oven for about half an hour at 160 °
C. Sprinkle with grated cheese and bake five minutes before the end of the baking time. Gorgeous!
Nutrition:
Calories: 133 Net carbs: 9.9g Fat: 8.1g Fiber: 1.1g Protein: 4.7g

Baked Quinces With A Cream Crown

Preparation time: 20 minutes
Cooking time: 90 minutes
Servings: 1
Ingredients:
1-2 quinces
70-80 g whipped cream 1 teaspoon sugar
1 teaspoon vanilla sugar
Directions:
After you have freed the quince from its fluff, you wrap it loosely in aluminum foil and put it in the oven at 200 ° C for 60 to 90 minutes, the thicker the fruit, the longer the baking time.
Spend the wait waiting to whip the cream stiff and sweeten it.
When the quinces have softened, halve them, remove the core with a small spoon and then pour the sweet whipped cream into this trough.
Nutrition:
Calories: 52 Net carbs: 14g Fiber: 1.7g Protein: 0.3g

Apple And Pear Jam With Tarragon

Preparation time: 15 minutes
Cooking time: 0 minutes
Servings: 3
Ingredients:

500g juicy pears 500g sour apples 1 large lemon

2 sprigs of tarragon 500g jam sugar 2: 1

Directions:

Peel and quarter apples and pears, remove the core and dice or grate very, very finely.

Squeeze the lemon and add to the fruit with the gelling sugar. Let the juice soak overnight!

Wash and dry the tarragon. Finely chop the leaves and add to the fruit mix.

Nutrition:

Calories: 242 Net carbs: 15g Fat: 20.5g Fiber: 3.2g Protein: 2g

Apple Jam With Honey And Cinnamon

Preparation time: 10 minutes
Cooking time: 15 minutes
Servings: 2
Ingredients:

300g apples 6 lemon juice

2 sticks of cinnamon 50 g liquid honey, 500g jam sugar 2: 1

Directions:

Peel and quarter the apples and remove the core.

Weigh 1 kg of pulp. Dice this finely and drizzle with lemon juice.

Mix the pulp, gelling sugar and cinnamon sticks well in a large saucepan. After cooking remove the cinnamon sticks and stir in the honey.

Nutrition:

Calories: 193 Net carbs: 38g Fat: 4.5g Fiber: 1.8g Protein: 1.8g

Plum Chutney

Preparation time: 5 minutes
Cooking time: 50 minutes
Servings: 4
Ingredients:

500 g pitted prunes 50 g ginger

350 g onions

2 s vegetable oil 250g brown sugar

300ml balsamic vinegar Salt, pepper

Directions:

Quarter the washed and pitted plums. Finely dice the ginger and onions and braise in 2 s of oil. Add the plums and steam briefly.

Add the brown sugar and let it melt while stirring. Then pour balsamic vinegar over it and let it boil for about 40 minutes on a low flame.

Season with salt and pepper and pour into boiled glasses.

Nutrition:

Calories: 125 Net carbs: 19.6g Fat: 4.9g Fiber: 0.8g Protein: 1.7g

Chocolate Chip Gelato

Preparation time: 30 minutes
Cooking time: 0 minutes
Servings: 4
Ingredients:

2 cups dairy-free milk

¾ cup pure maple syrup 1 pure vanilla extract

⅓ Semi-sweet vegan chocolate chips, finely chopped or flaked

Directions:

Beat dairy-free milk, maple syrup, and vanilla together in a large bowl until well combined.

Pour the mixture carefully into the container of an automatic ice cream maker and process it according to the manufacturer's instructions.

During the last 10 or 15 minutes, add the chopped chocolate and continue processing until the desired texture is achieved. Enjoy the gelato immediately, or let it harden further in the freezer for an hour or more.

Nutrition:

Calories: 94 Net carbs: 14.9g Fat: 3.4g Fiber: 0.5g Protein: 0.8g

Peanut Butter And Jelly Ice Cream

Preparation time: 40 minutes

Cooking time: 0 minutes

Servings: 6

Ingredients:

2 cups dairy-free milk, simple, sugar-free

⅔ Cup maple syrup

3 s creamy natural peanut butter

½ teaspoon ground ginger

2 teaspoons pure vanilla extract 6 spoons canned fruits

Directions:

Beat the milk without milk, maple syrup, peanut butter, and vanilla in a large bowl until well combined. Pour the mixture carefully into the container of an automatic ice cream maker and process it according to the manufacturer's instructions.

Add canned fruits for the last 10 minutes, and let them combine with the ice cream until the desired texture is achieved. Enjoy the ice cream immediately, or let it harden further in the freezer for an hour or more.

Nutrition:

Calories: 189 Net carbs: 33.8g Fat: 4.1g Fiber: 0.7g Protein: 5.6g

Watermelon Gazpacho In A Jar

Preparation time: 20 minutes

Cooking time: 0 minutes

Servings: 8

Ingredients:

1kg of ripe, aromatic tomatoes Half a red pepper +

Half a small chili pepper 3 ground cucumbers 1 onion

1 clove of garlic (optional) 2 cups cubed watermelon Juice of 1 lemon

A handful of leaves basil A handful of mint leaves 1 - 2 s olive oil

Salt, pepper

Directions:

Tomato peel slightly cut in several places, then transfer the tomatoes to a deep pot and pour boiling water, let stand for a few minutes. Drain the water and peel the tomatoes from the skin, but this is not a necessary stage if the skin does not bother you.

Peeled tomatoes in half and put in a blender cup or larger bowl. Add chopped onion, garlic, diced peppers, cucumbers, chili peppers, and lemon juice. Also, add basil and mint leaves. All mix well in a blender or using a hand blender, finally adding olive oil.

Then add chopped pieces of watermelon and mix only for a moment, so that the remaining watermelon particles can be felt. Season with salt and pepper to taste.

Serve well chilled with diced paprika, lemon juice, stale bread, and a large dose of fresh, chopped basil.

Nutrition:

Calories: 46 Net carbs: 4.3g Fat: 0.2g Fiber: 0.5g

CHAPTER 16:

DESSERT RECIPES

Fruit Cake without Sugar

Ingredients:

400 g dried fig
400 g dried natural product as an example b. plums, apricot, raisins
400 g nuts z. b. hazelnuts, almonds, pecans
5 eggs
125 g spread
200 g spelled flour type 1050
1 tbsp cinnamon
1 tsp clove stripped

Arrangement Steps

Roughly cleave the figs, dried organic products, and nuts. Separate the eggs and beat the egg whites until solid. Beat the spread until cushy, at that point include the egg yolks and flour and make a smooth batter. Ply in organic products, nuts, and flavors. Cautiously crease within the protein.

Fill the batter into a heating tin fixed with preparing the paper, smooth , and prepare within the broiler at 175 ° C (fan stove 150 ° C; gas: level 2) for around hour . Play out a stick test. Take the cake out of the stove and let it cool.

Chocolate Fruit Cake

Ingredients:

300 g prunes
300 g dried fig
200 g prepared organic product
200 g almond portions
150 g hazelnuts
5 eggs - 125 g spread
1 tbsp nectar
200 g spelled flour
1 squeeze ground carnation
½ tsp ground ginger
1 tbsp cinnamon
100 g dim chocolate
20 g coconut oil

Planning Steps

Roughly slash plums, figs, and heated organic products. Slash nuts with a blade or quickly put them during a Blitz hacker. Separate eggs beat egg whites with a hand blender to a firm day off. Whisk the margarine and nectar until cushioned, at that point include the ingredient and flour and blend to a smooth mixture. Ply the natural products, nuts, and flavors under the mixture and cautiously overlap within the egg whites. Line a heating tin with preparing paper and pour within the batter. Heat during a preheated broiler at 175 ° C (fan stove: 150 ° C; gas: speed 2) for around an hour.

Take the cake out of the broiler and let it cool. Within the interim, hack the chocolate and soften alongside coconut oil over a boiling water shower. Twist the cake with the chocolate.

Avocado mousse

Ingredients:

2 ready avocados
2 tbsp coconut milk
40 g chocolate

40 ml of nectar
½ tsp vanilla powder
½ tsp chia seeds (ground)
12 raspberries
1 tsp ground coconut

Planning Steps

Halve the avocados, stone them and spoon them into a blender.

Add coconut milk, chocolate, nectar, vanilla powder, and ground chia seeds.

Puree to a smooth mass.

Chill in any event half-hour or overnight before serving. Select

the raspberries, wash, and pat dry. Topping the avocado and mousse with raspberries and coconut chips.

Avocado Mint dessert with Chocolate

Ingredients:

400 ml coconut milk (can)
3 ready avocados
10 g mint (0.5 pack)
2 tbsp juice
50 g agave syrup
100 g chocolate drops produced using dim chocolate (cocoa content at any rate of 70%)

Arrangement Steps

Open the coconut milk and spoon out the strong part at the very best - don't shake the can previously - and place it during an enormous bowl. Whisk the firm coconut milk with a hand blender and afterward empty it into a cake or heating dish.

Halve the avocados, expel the stones, evacuate the mash, and put during a blender. Wash mint, shake dry, and pluck leaves. Puree the avocado mash with juice, agave syrup, and mint to a velvety and smooth mass.

Pour the avocado blend onto the foamy coconut milk, sprinkle with chocolate drops and blend the blend cautiously yet equitably. The surface of the mass got to be moderately smooth.

Place stick film on the yogurt mass and depress delicately so as that there is no air between the film and thus the dessert mass. Spot the ice within the cooler for at any rate 2 hours. 5. Let it defrost quickly and appreciate it.

Cottage cheese with Plums

Ingredients:

700 g potatoes
6 plums
45 g margarine (3 tbsp)
30 g nectar (2 tbsp)
2 squeezes cinnamon
250 g quark (20% fat in dry issue)
50 g coconut sugar
30 g raisins (2 tbsp)
150 g spelled flour type 1050
1 egg
1 squeeze cardamom powder
1 squeeze clove powder

Planning Steps

For the quark legs, strip, wash, hack the potatoes and cook delicately in bubbling water in around quarter-hour over medium warmth. At that point pour off and let cool for 10 minutes.

Within the interim, wash the plums, cut them down the middle, expel the stones, and cut the plums into cuts. Warmth 1 tablespoon of margarine during a touch pot. Include the plums and braise for 3 minutes over medium warmth. Include nectar and let it caramelize for five minutes. Season with a spot of cinnamon.

Press potatoes through a potato press into a bowl. Include the curd, sugar, raisins, flour, egg, and flavors to the potatoes and ply everything into a smooth mixture; on the off chance that it's excessively soggy, include some flour. Structure 18 little treats out of the batter.

Fry the quark balls in progression. Warmth 1 teaspoon margarine during a container. Include 4-5 batter heaps and prepare until brilliant on all sides in around 3-4 minutes over medium warmth; spend the rest of the mixture also. Organize the quark drumstick with the plums.

Coconut milk Cake with the Chocolate Base

Ingredients:

2 eggs
1 squeeze salt
80 g agave syrup
125 g margarine
220 g flour type 1050 or spelled flour 1050
½ parcel heating powder
30 g chocolate (vigorously oiled)
1 parcel custard powder
400 ml coconut milk (9% fat)
30 g coconut sugar
40 g coconut drops
4 sheets gelatin
150 ml topping
100 g dim chocolate
20 g coconut oil

Planning Steps

Separate eggs and beat egg whites with salt to egg whites. Mix agave syrup with spread and ingredient until foamy. Blend the flour, heating powder, and cocoa and sifter to the ingredient froth, at that point procedure to a smooth mixture and overlap within the egg whites cautiously.

Line or oil the spring form dish with heating material. Include the mixture, smooth and heat at 180 ° C (convection 160 ° C; gas: level 2) for around 25-30 minutes (make a stick test). At that point let the cake cool within the form.

Within the interim, mix the pudding powder with 5–6 tablespoons of coconut milk until smooth. Put the rest of the coconut milk, coconut bloom sugar, and 30 g coconut pieces during a pan and convey it to the bubble. Mix within the blended pudding powder and convey to the bubble while mixing and afterward let it cool.

Soak the gelatin in chilly water. Whip 100 ml of cream until solid. Warm the rest of the cream during a pot marginally and hack the all-around communicated gelatin in it. Mix in 4 tablespoons of the coconut milk and afterward increase the remainder of the coconut milk. Include the cream and smooth the cream on the chocolate base. Chill for at any rate hour.

Roughly cleave the dull chocolate and dissolve with the coconut oil over the water shower, let cool marginally. Meanwhile, cautiously expel the cake from the shape. Spread the cake with the chocolate icing. Sprinkle with outstanding coconut pieces and let it set. Serve dig pieces.

Zucchini Mint Popsicles

Ingredients:

2 zucchini
10 g ginger (1 piece)
30 g coconut bloom sugar (3 tbsp)
5 g mint (1 bunch)
50 ml of juice
2 tbsp nectar

Arrangement Steps

Clean, wash, and finely grind zucchini. Strip and finely grind the ginger.

Mix zucchini with coconut bloom sugar and ginger. Wash the mint leaves, shake dry, blend in with the zucchini blend, and spread quite 8 dessert molds.

Mix juice with 450 ml of water and nectar. Fill in ice forms and let freeze for around hour.

At that point embed wooden sticks and permit them to freeze for an extra 3 hours. Expel from the molds to serve.

Currant Skyr Popsicles

Ingredients:
250 g red currants
1 natural lemon (pizzazz)
3 tbsp syrup
200 g skyr
100 g Greek yogurt
100 g topping
Directions:
Pluck currants from the panicles, wash and finely puree alongside the lemon get-up-and-go, and a few of tbsp syrup. Spread the blend through a fine strainer into a bowl.
Mix the Skyr with yogurt in another bowl. Add 1/3 of it to this puree and blend.
Stir the remainder of the syrup into the remainder of the Skyr yogurt blend. Whip the cream until hardened and spread half over
all of the two masses and crease incautiously. Fill the blend on the other hand in 6 yogurt forms and blend delicately with a spoon. Freeze for around hour. At that point embed wooden sticks and permit them to freeze for an extra 3 hours.
To serve, expel ice from the molds and fill in as wanted on a soothing record plate.

Pineapple Popsicles

Ingredients:
600 g new pineapple mash
100 g raspberries
200 g coconut milk (without sugar)
50 g rice syrup
1 lime (juice)
Arrangement Steps
Cut the pineapple mash into pieces, set 100 g aside. Wash the raspberries cautiously and pat them dry.
Mix coconut milk with rice syrup. Acknowledged the pineapple with the coconut milk and thus the lime squeeze during a blender and crush finely.
Fill the blend into 8 yogurt molds, include 4-5 raspberries each, and let freeze for around hour. At that point embed wooden sticks and let it freeze for an extra 3 hours. To serve, expel ice from the molds and organize with the pineapple pieces put during a secure spot.

Coconut and Chocolate dessert with Chia Seeds

Ingredients:
400 ml of coconut milk
4 tbsp syrup
15 g chocolate (2 tbsp; vigorously oiled)
2 packs chai tea
12 g white chia seeds (2 tbsp)
250 g soy yogurt
30 g dim chocolate (in any event 70% cocoa)
Planning Steps
Put coconut milk during a pan. Include syrup and chocolate and warmth, however, don't bring back the bubble. Hang the tea sack in, spread, expel from the warmth, and let steep for half-hour. At that point remove the tea sack, pressing out the fluid. Blend in 1 1/2 tbsp chia seeds and yogurt. Fill the mass in 8 ice shapes and let freeze for around hour. At that point embed wooden sticks and permit them to freeze for an extra 3 hours. Chop the chocolate and dissolve over a warm water shower. Expel the dessert from the molds and brighten with the chocolate and thus the remaining chia seeds.

Sesame Vanilla dessert

Ingredients:
130 g dark sesame
1 favorer
300 ml milk (3.5% fat)

200 g topping
4 eggs
40 g coconut sugar

Directions:

Roast 120 g sesame seeds during a hot container without fat for five minutes over medium warmth. Expel from the container and let cool for five minutes. At that point pound finely with a processor or mortar.

Within the interim, split the vanilla case lengthways and cut out the mash with a blade. Carry rock bottom sesame to the overflow with vanilla mash, milk, and cream. Expel from the warmth and let cool for five minutes.

Within the interim, separate the eggs (utilize the proteins somewhere else). Beat egg yolks with coconut bloom sugar until feathery. Mix within the recent cream blend and warmth during a metal bowl over a high temp water shower with mixing to around 75 ° C until the blend thickens, this may take around 10 minutes. At that point let cool for around 20 minutes, blending every so often.

Then let the mass freeze smooth during a yogurt producer for around 40 minutes. Or on the other hand, fill a holder and freeze within the cooler for 3-4 hours. Mix at regular intervals. For serving, cut balls out of the ice and sprinkle with the rest of the sesame seeds.

Exotic Vegan Pancakes with Mango

Ingredients:

120 g spelled flour (type 630)
50 g coconut flour
2 tsp tartar preparing powder
1 squeeze salt
2 tbsp coconut sugar
450 ml rice drink (rice milk) with coconut
4 tsp rapeseed oil
½ mango
200 g coconut yogurt
2 tsp chia seeds

Arrangement Steps

Place every single dry element for the batter during a bowl and blend. Include the rice-coconut drink and blend it into a homogeneous mixture. On the off chance that the batter is excessively firm, include a scramble of rice and coconut drink.

Heat 2 teaspoons of oil during a covered container, add 1 tablespoon of spread to the skillet and prepare 4 to 6 hotcakes in around 3-4 minutes over medium warmth on the two sides until brilliant earthy colored.

Peel the mango, disengage from the center, and dig 3D squares. Spread the hotcakes on three plates, spread the yogurt elective produced using coconut on top, and present with the mango and chia seeds.

Halloween Desserts

Ingredients:

210 g whole meal spelled flour
7 tbsp entire natural sweetener
40 g spread
280 g dull chocolate (in any event 70% cocoa)
1 l milk (3.5% fat)
1 favorer
1 map. Orange strip
6 egg yolks
2 tbsp food starch
5 tsp chocolate

Directions:

For the bread rolls, rapidly manipulate 50 g of flour, 1 tbsp of entire unadulterated sweetener, and 25 g of margarine into a smooth short crust baked good. Chill enveloped by stick film for around half-hour. Roughly slash chocolate. Expel 10 tablespoons from the milk and put it during a secure spot. Cut the vanilla case lengthways and cut out the mash.

Put the rest of the milk during a pan with 240 g chocolate, vanilla mash, case, and orange pizzazz and warmth while blending. In a bowl, mix the egg yolks with 4 tablespoons of entire unadulterated sweetener until foamy, mix within the cornstarch and thus the milk put during a secure spot.
Stir within the recent cocoa drain and take back to the bubble within the pot and let it thicken. Expel the blend from the oven, keep beating quickly, evacuate the vanilla case, and let the pudding cool in glasses.
Sprinkle scone mixture with 1 tsp chocolate and add as a marbling. Reveal the batter and cut out headstones with an oval shaper. Spot treats on a heating sheet secured with preparing paper and prepares for 10–15 minutes during a preheated stove at 180 ° C (constrained air 160 ° C; gas: setting 2-3). Remove and let cool.
To reinforce, blend the rest of the Ingredients: (cocoa powder, flour, margarine, entire natural sweetener) and disintegrate. Dissolve the keep going 40 g of lifeless chocolate, fill it into slightly funneling sack and name it with the treats.
Sprinkle the pudding with the chocolate morsels, embed the named treats as a 'tombstone' and enhance them with blossoms as you would like

Cottage cheese with Raspberry Sauce

Ingredients:
400 g flour-bubbling potatoes (2-3 potatoes)
300 g raspberries
2 tbsp nectar
½ favorer
250 g low-fat quark
50 g coconut sugar
150 g spelled flour type 1050
1 egg cinnamon
15 g margarine (3 tsp)
30 g planed almond bits (2 tbsp)

Planning Steps

for the quark legs, strip, wash, slash the potatoes and cook delicately in bubbling water in around quarter-hour over medium warmth. At that point pour off and let cool for 10 minutes.
Within the interim, wash the raspberries cautiously and puree them with a hand blender. Push the mash through a sifter, blend in with nectar, and keep cool.
Within the interim, divide the vanilla case lengthways and cut out the vanilla mash with a blade.
Press potatoes through a potato press into a bowl. Include the curd, sugar, flour, egg, vanilla mash, and 1 spot of cinnamon to the potatoes and work everything into a smooth batter; within the event that it's excessively damp, include some flour. Structure 12 little treats out of the batter. Fry the quark balls in progression. Warmth 1 teaspoon margarine during a dish. Include 4 balls and prepare brilliant earthy colored on all sides in around 3-4 minutes; Bake remaining cups similarly.
Toast the almonds during a hot container without fat overmedium warmth for 3 minutes. Orchestrate the quark drumstick with the raspberry sauce and almonds.

Spelled Semolina Porridge with Elderberry Sauce and Roasted Hazelnuts

Ingredients:
300 ml elderberry juice
1 tbsp food starch
800 ml oat drink (oat milk)
1 squeeze salt
120 whole meal spelled semolina
100 g hazelnut bits
2 tbsp beet syrup

Directions:
Bring elderberry juice to a bubble with the exception of two tablespoons. Mix the rest of the juice with cornstarch until smooth, increase the pot, and mix. Stew for five minutes on a coffee to medium warmth and put during a secure spot.
Within the interim, put the oat drink with 1 touch of salt during a special pot and warmth. Mix within the spelled semolina with a whisk and convey it to the bubble. Lessen warmth and stew on low warmth with blending for around 5 minutes until it thickens.
Roast the hazelnut pieces during a container without oil over medium warmth for 3-4 minutes. Take out, let cool, and cleave generally.
Stir the syrup under the semolina porridge and separate it into four dishes. Shower elderberry sauce over it and serve sprinkled with hazelnuts.

Blackberry Quark Tartlets

Ingredients:
250 g whole meal spelled flour + 1 stacked tablespoon for handling
35 g chocolate (5 tbsp; intensely oiled)
1 squeeze salt
50 g crude natural sweetener
125 g cold, diced spread
2 eggs
250 g blackberry
1 natural lime
1 favorer
100 g crème fraiche cheddar
250 g low-fat quark - 1 tbsp syrup
15 g dull chocolate freely (at any rate 70% cocoa)
Directions:
Mix the flour with the chocolate, salt, and sugar. Include spread and 1 egg and utilize your hands to make a smooth batter. Spread and chill for half-hour.
Within the interim, cautiously wash the blackberries, channel, and cut them down the middle or quarter, contingent upon the size. Flush lime hot, rub dry, rub the strip; divide the lime, and press out the juice. Split the vanilla case lengthways and cut out the mash. Blend the crème fraiche with the quark, half the lime strip, 1–2 sprinkles of juice, syrup, vanilla mash, and thus the rest of the egg.
Divide the mixture into 4 equivalent pieces, turn them out on a floured surface (approx. 14 cm each) and put them in 4 tartlet molds. Spread the curd blend on the molds and pour the blackberries over it. Prepare the tartlets during a preheated broiler at 180 ° C (fan stove 160 ° C; gas: levels 2–3) for 30–35 minutes.
Remove the tartlets from the stove, allow them to chill for 10 minutes and expel them from the molds. Topping the blackberry quark tartlets with the rest of the lime strip and ground chocolate as wanted.

Strawberry Buckwheat salad

Ingredients::
1⁄3 cup (50g) buckwheat
One tablespoon ground turmeric
1⁄2 cup (80g) avocado
3⁄8 cup (65g) tomato
1⁄8 cup (20g) red onion
1⁄8 cup (25g) Medjool dates, pitted
One tablespoon capers
3⁄4 cup (30g) parsley
2⁄3 cup (100g) strawberries, hulled
one tablespoon extra virgin olive oil
Juice of 1⁄2 lemon
One ounce (30g) arugula

Directions:
Cook the buckwheat Cajanus cajan the turmeric according to the bundle instructions. Drain and set aside to sit back.
Finely chop the avocado, tomato, red onion, dates, capers, and parsley and mix with the cool buckwheat.
Slice the strawberries and twenty mix into the plate of mixed greens with the oil and lemon juice. Serve on a bed two arugula.

Dark Chocolate Protein Truffles

Total Time: twenty five thirty Serves: eight
Whey protein is one of the nourishments for building muscle, losing abundance weight and supporting good health. Instead of always golf shot golf shot in a golf shot, get your supermolecule with this Dark Chocolate Protein Truffles recipe! It's the proper treat to envision to envision to envision to envision what is more, get associate degree few sirtuin-activating foods as well.
Ingredients::
¼ cup medjool dates, chopped
¼ cup vanilla whey supermolecule supermolecule
¼ cup almond milk
⅛ Cup steel cut oats
Two tablespoon honey
One tablespoon coconut flour
Two dark chocolate bars, minimum eighty fifth eighty fifth
¼ cup coconut oil
Bearings:
Combine along the combine, supermolecule supermolecule, almond milk, nectar, oats, and coconut flour and kind into eight balls.
Melt chocolate and cubic centimeter oil over medium-low heat in a saucepan.
Once melted, stop working stop working stop working the chocolate cool for 5-10 thirty and allow provides to thicken. Dip each ball into the melted chocolate until completely secured.
Place them in the cooler Cajanus cajan solidify.

Matcha with Vanilla

Prep: five five, Easy Serves: one
Trade your commonplace tea or coffee for this coffee coffee green matcha and coffee coffee. It's perhaps to Cajanus cajan at home and takes just 5 5
Ingredients:
½ tsp matcha powder
Seeds from associate degree large portion of a coffee pod
Guidance:
Boil the kettle then pour 100ml of the water into associate degree estimating instrumentation. Pour half the hot water into a small bowl, to warm it, at that point embody the matcha powder and vanilla seeds to the rest of the water at intervals the instrumentation.
Whisk embody mixture with a bamboo match whisk or scaled down electric whisk till it's smooth, lump-free and slightly bubbly. Eliminate the water in the warmed coffee bowl, then pour in the prepared matcha tea.

Turmeric Tea

Ingredients:
Three heaped tsp ground turmeric
one tbsp go ground ginger
One small orange, energy pared
Agave and 0.5 slices, to serve
Instructions:
Boil 500ml water in embody kettle. Place embody turmeric, ginger and orange zest in to a tea kettle or instrumentation. Pour associate degree the effervescent cubic centimeter and effervescent to effervescent for effervescent five minutes.

Strain through a filter or tea strainer into 2 cups, add a slice two lemon and sweeten with agave, at intervals the event that you simply like.

Date and Walnut Cinnamon Bites

Ingredients::

Three walnut halves

Three pitted Medjool combine

Ground cinnamon, to taste

Instruction:

Carefully cut every VI 0.5 into 3 cuts, then do the same with the dates. Place a slice of vi on top of every date, dust with cinnamon and serve.

The Sirt Food Diet's Date and Walnut Porridge

Ingredients:

Two hundred cubic centimeter Milk or sans farm farm

One Medjool date, chopped

Thirty five g thirty five items

1 tsp. Pecan butter or four chopped walnut halves

fifty g Strawberries, hulled

Guidelines:

Place the milk and date throughout a pan, heat gently, embodyn add embody buckwheat flakes a large minutes the dish is your amount dish.

Stir in embody pecan butter or walnuts, prime with you'd and serve.

Add the kale and embody for a further five 5. At intervals the event that you just that you just that you just that you just that you just, essentially add associate degree embody water. Once your forty five options associate degree once made made, stir at intervals the parsley.

Make two very little wells in embody sauce and crack each egg into them. Decrease embody heat to its lowest setting and cover embody cooking pan with associate degree lid or foil. Leave the eggs to embody for 10–12 5, at which point the whites ought to be firm while the yolks are still liquid. Cook for an additional 3–4 minutes if you prefer the yolks Cajanus cajan be firm. Serve immediately – ideally straight from the instrumentation.

Chocolate Cupcakes With Matcha Icing

Preparation Time: 15 minutes

Cooking Time: 20 minutes

Servings: 12

Ingredients:

5 oz. self-rising flour 5 oz. caster sugar

2 oz. 60g cocoa

1/2 tsp salt

1/2 tsp. good espresso coffee

½ cup milk

½ tsp. vanilla extract, unsweetened

¼ cup vegetable oil 1 egg

3/8 cup boiling water

For the icing:

2 oz. butter at room temperature 2 oz. icing sugar

1 tbsp. matcha green tea powder

1/2 tsp. vanilla bean paste 50g soft cream cheese

Directions:

Preheat the oven to 350°F. Line a cupcake tin with silicone or paper muffin cups. Put the flour, cocoa, sugar, salt and espresso powder in a big bowl and mix.

Add the vanilla, vanilla extract, vegetable oil and egg into the dry ingredients beat with an electric mixer until well blended. Gently pour into the boiling water gradually until completely blended.

Keep mixing to add air bubbles to the batter. The batter will result much more liquid than a standard cake mixture.

Spoon the batter evenly in the cupcake tin, remember than each place must not be fuller than 3/4. Bake in the oven for about 15-18 minutes, until the mix bounces back when exploited.

Remove from the oven and let it cool completely before icing.

To make the icing, cream the butter and icing sugar together until smooth and soft. Add matcha powder vanilla and stir. Ice the cupcakes.

Nutrition Facts:

Calories: 220kcal Fat: 8g Carbohydrate: 33g Protein: 4g

Fruit Skewers & Strawberry Dip

Preparation Time: 15 minutes

Cooking Time: 0 minutes

Servings: 6

Ingredients:

5oz red grapes

2lb pineapple, peeled and diced 14oz strawberries

Directions:

Place 3½ oz. of the strawberries into a food processor and blend until smooth. Pour the dip into a serving bowl. Skewer the grapes, pineapple chunks and remaining strawberries onto skewers. Serve alongside the strawberry dip.

Nutrition Facts:

Calories: 131kcal Fat: 1g Carbohydrate: 30g Protein: 2g

Choc Nut Truffles

Preparation Time: 15 minute + 3 hours

Cooking Time: 0 minutes

Servings: 8

Ingredients:

5oz desiccated (shredded) coconut 2oz walnuts, chopped

1oz hazelnuts, chopped

4 medjool dates

2 tbsp. 100% cocoa powder or cacao nibs 1 tbsp. coconut oil

Directions:

Place all of the ingredients into a blender and process until smooth and creamy. Using a teaspoon, scoop the mixture into bite-size pieces then roll it into balls. Place them into small paper cups, cover them and chill for 3 hours before serving.

Nutrition Facts:

Calories: 41kcal Fat: 3g Carbohydrate: 4g Protein: 1g

No-Bake Strawberry Flapjacks

Preparation Time: 15 minutes + 4 hours

Cooking Time: 0 minutes

Servings: 8

Ingredients:

3 oz. porridge oats 4 oz. dates

2 oz. strawberries

2 oz. peanuts, unsalted 2 oz. walnuts

1 tbsp. coconut oil

2 tbsp. 100% cocoa powder

Directions:

Place all of the ingredients into a blender and process until they become a soft consistency. Spread the mixture onto a baking sheet or small flat tin. Press the mixture down and smooth it out. Put in the fridge 4 hours, then cut it into 8 pieces and serve.

Nutrition Facts:

Calories: 191kcal Fat: 11g Carbohydrate: 21g Protein: 2g

Chocolate Balls

Preparation Time: 15 minutes

Cooking Time: 0 minutes

Servings: 6

Ingredients:

2oz peanut butter (or almond butter) 1oz cocoa powder

1oz desiccated (shredded) coconut
1 tbsp. honey
1 tbsp. cocoa powder for coating

Directions:

Place the ingredients into a bowl and mix. Using a tsp scoop out a little of the mixture and shape it into a ball. Roll the ball in a little cocoa powder and set aside. Repeat for the remaining mixture. Can be eaten straight away or stored in the fridge.

Nutrition Facts:

Calories: 240 Carbs: 21g Fat: 15g Protein: 4g

Warm Berries & Cream

Preparation Time: 10 minutes
Cooking Time: 5 minutes
Servings: 4

Ingredients:

9oz blueberries 9oz strawberries 3½ oz. redcurrants 3½ oz. blackberries
4 tbsp. fresh whipped cream 1 tbsp. honey
Zest and juice of 1 orange

Directions:

Place all of the berries into a pan along with the honey and orange juice. Gently heat the berries for around 5 minutes until warmed through. Serve the berries into bowls and add a dollop of whipped cream on top.

Nutrition Facts:

Calories: 217kcal Fat: 2g Carbohydrates: 30g Protein: 2g

Chocolate Fondue

Preparation Time: 5 minutes
Cooking Time: 5 minutes
Servings: 4

Ingredients:

4oz dark chocolate 11oz strawberries 7oz cherries
2 apples, peeled, cored and sliced 3½ Fl. oz. double cream

Directions:

Place the chocolate and cream into a saucepan and warm it until smooth and creamy. Serve in the fondue pot or transfer it to a serving bowl. Scatter the fruit on a serving plate ready to be dipped into the chocolate.

Nutrition Facts:

Calories: 350kcal Fat: 10g Carbohydrates: 23g Protein: 2g

Walnut & Date Loaf

Preparation Time: 30 minutes
Cooking Time: 45 minutes
Servings: 12

Ingredients:

9oz self-rising flour
4oz medjool dates, chopped 2oz walnuts, chopped
8fl oz. milk 3 eggs
1 medium banana, mashed
1 tsp baking soda

Directions:

Sieve baking soda and flour into a bowl. Add in banana, eggs, milk and dates and mix well. Transfer the mixture to a lined loaf tin and smooth it out. Scatter the walnuts on top. Bake the loaf in the oven at 180C/360F for 45 minutes.

Transfer it to a wire rack to cool before serving.

Nutrition Facts:

Calories: 186kcal Fat: 5g Carbs: 33g Protein: 2g

Strawberry Frozen Yogurt

Preparation Time: 60 – 120 minutes
Cooking Time: 0 minutes
Servings: 4

Ingredients:

1lb plain yogurt 6oz strawberries Juice of 1 orange
1 tbsp. honey (optional)

Directions:
Place strawberries and orange juice into a food processor and blitz until smooth.
Filter the mixture through a sieve into a bowl to remove seeds. Stir in the honey and yogurt. Transfer the mixture to an ice-cream maker and follow the manufacturer's instructions. Alternatively pour the mixture into a container and place in the freezer for 1 hour. Use a fork to whisk it and break up ice crystals and freeze for other 2 hours.
Nutrition Facts:
Calories: 100kcal Fat: 0.6g Carbohydrate: 21g Protein: 4g

Chocolate Brownies

Preparation Time: 15 minutes
Cooking Time: 30 minutes
Servings: 14
Ingredients
7oz dark chocolate (min 85% cocoa) 70z medjool dates, pitted
3½oz walnuts, chopped
3 eggs
1fl oz. melted coconut oil 2 teaspoons vanilla essence
½ tsp baking soda
Directions:
Place the dates, chocolate, eggs, coconut oil, baking soda and vanilla essence into a food processor and mix until smooth.
Stir the walnuts into the mixture. Pour the mixture into a lined baking tray and bake at 350F for 25-30 minutes.
Allow it to cool. Cut into pieces and serve.
Nutrition Facts:
Calories: 188kcal Fat: 12g Carbohydrate: 19g Protein: 3g

Crème Brûlée

Preparation Time: 10 minutes
Cooking Time: 3 minutes
Servings: 4
Ingredients:
14oz strawberries
11oz plain low-fat yogurt 4oz Greek yogurt
3½oz brown sugar 1 tsp vanilla extract
Directions:
Divide the strawberries between 4 ramekin dishes.
In a bowl combine the plain yogurt with the vanilla extract. Spoon the mixture onto the strawberries.
Scoop the Greek yogurt on top. Sprinkle the sugar over each dish, completely covering the top.
Place the dishes under a hot grill (broiler) for around 3 minutes or until the sugar has caramelized.
Nutrition Facts:
Calories: 311kcal Fat: 25g Carbohydrate: 16g Protein: 5g

Pistachio Fudge

Preparation Time: 10 minutes
Cooking Time: 0 minutes
Servings: 6
Ingredients:
8oz medjool dates, pitted
3½ oz. pistachio nuts, shelled
2 oz. desiccated shredded coconut 1 oz. oats
2 tbsp. water
Directions:
Place the dates, nuts, coconut, oats and water into a food processor and process until the ingredients are well mixed.
Roll the mixture in a 1-inch thick roll a cut it into 6 pieces. Refrigerate 2 hours and serve.
Nutrition Facts:
Calories: 280kcal Fat: 12g Carbohydrate: 18g Protein: 4g.

Spiced Poached Apples

Preparation Time: 30 minutes
Cooking Time: 20 minutes
Servings: 4
Ingredients:
4 apples
2 tbsp. honey 4-star anise
2 cinnamon sticks 1 cup green tea
¼ cup Greek yogurt
Direction:
Place the honey and green tea into a saucepan and bring to the boil. Add apples, star anise and cinnamon. Reduce the heat and simmer gently for 15 minutes. Serve the apples with a dollop of Greek yogurt.
Nutrition Facts:
Calories: 180 Fat: 0.5g Carbohydrate: 25g Protein: 5g

Banana Pecan Muffins

Preparation Time: 30 minutes
Cooking Time: 40 minutes
Servings: 8
Ingredients:
3 Tbsp. butter softened 4 ripe bananas
1 Tbsp. honey
⅛ cup orange juice, unsweetened 1 tsp cinnamon
2 cups flour
1 tbsp. instant yeast 2 pecans, sliced
1 tbsp. vanilla
2 eggs
Directions:
Preheat the oven to 350°F. Lightly oil sides and bottom of a muffin tin and dust with flour. Tap to remove any excess flour.
Peel the bananas and mash them with a in a bowl. Add flour and mix.
Add orange juice, butter, eggs, vanilla, yeast and cinnamon and stir to combine.
Roughly chop the pecans onto a chopping board, add to the mix.
Fill each muffin tin until 3/4 and bake in the oven for approximately 40
minutes, or until golden.
Nutrition Facts:
Calories: 223kcal Fat: 9g Carbohydrates: 31g Protein: 7g

Banana And Blueberry Muffins

Preparation Time: 20 minutes
Cooking Time: 30 minutes
Servings: 12
Ingredients:
4 large ripe bananas, mashed 3/4 cup of sugar
1 egg, lightly beaten
1/2 cup of peanut butter, 2 cups of blueberries
1 tsp baking powder
1 tsp baking soda 1/2 tsp salt
1 cup of coconut, shredded 1/2 cup of flour
1/2 cup applesauce Dab of cinnamon
Direction:
Add mashed banana to a large mixing bowl. Insert sugar and egg and mix well. Add peanut butter and blueberries.
Add the dry ingredients into the wet mix and mix together lightly. Set into 12 greased muffin cups and bake for 20-25min at 350 F.
Nutrition Facts:
Calories: 250 Carbs: 39g Fat: 9g Protein: 4g

Golden Milk Ice Cream

Preparation Time: 8 hours
Cooking Time: 5 min
Servings: 5
Ingredients:
28 oz. Full-fat coconut milk 2 tbsp. Extra virgin olive oil 1/4 cup Maple syrup
2- inchFresh ginger, finely sliced A pinch of sea salt
½ tsp Ground cinnamon

1 tsp Ground turmeric 1/8 tsp Black pepper 1/8 tsp Cardamom

1 tsp pure vanilla extract, unsweetened

Directions:

Place your ice cream churn and bowl in the freezer a night before, to properly chill.

Add the maple syrup, turmeric, coconut milk, cardamom, fresh ginger, pepper, sea salt, and cinnamon into a large pot and heat over medium heat.

Allow to simmer, whisking continuously to mix the ingredients.

Then put off heat and add the vanilla extract. Stir once more to combine. Adjust flavor if needed, adding more maple syrup for sweetness, turmeric

for intense flavor, salt to balance the flavors, or cinnamon for warmth.

Transfer the mixture plus the ginger slices into a mixing bowl and allow to cool to room temperature.

Cover the bowl and place in the refrigerator to chill overnight or for a minimum of 4 to 6 hours.

The next day, use a strainer or a spoon to remove the ginger slices.

Then add the olive oil for more creaminess. Whisk to combine thoroughly.

Add the mixture to your ice cream maker and churn according to the instructions by the manufacturers – this should take about 30 minutes. In case you don't have an ice cream maker, skip this phase and go to the next one.

Move the ice cream to a freezer-safe container and smoothen the top with your spoon.

Cover with a lid and place in the freezer for about four to six hours, until firm. Bring out of the freezer ten minutes before serving to soften.

Nutrition Facts:

Calories: 140kcal Fat: 7g Carbohydrate: 17g Protein: 2g

Chocolate Cashew Truffles

Preparation Time: 10 minutes
Cooking Time: 35 minutes
Servings: 4
Ingredients:

1 cup ground cashews

1 tsp of ground vanilla bean

½ cup of coconut oil

¼ cup raw honey 2 flax meal

2 hemp hearts - 2 cacao powder

Directions:

Mix all ingredients and make truffles by rolling small amounts of mixture and balls. Sprinkle coconut flakes on top.

Nutrition Facts:

Calories: 187kcal Fat: 16.5g Carbohydrate: 6g Protein: 2.3g

Double Almond Raw Chocolate Tart

Preparation Time: 10 minutes
Cooking Time: 35 minutes
Servings: 4
Ingredients:

1½ cups of raw almonds

¼ cup of coconut oil, melted 1 raw honey

8 oz. dark chocolate, chopped 1 cup of coconut milk

½ cup unsweetened shredded coconut

Directions:

Crust:

Ground almonds and add melted coconut oil, raw honey and combine. Using a spatula spread this mixture into a pie pan.

Filling: Put the chopped chocolate in a bowl, heat coconut milk and pour over chocolate and whisk together. Pour filling into tart shell. Refrigerate. Toast almond slivers chips and sprinkle over tart.

Nutrition Facts:

Calories: 291 Fat: 9.4g Carbohydrate: 23.4g Protein: 12.4g

Bounty Bars

Preparation Time: 10 minutes
Cooking Time: 35 minutes
Servings: 4
Ingredients:
2 cups desiccated coconut 3 coconut oil - melted
1 cup of coconut cream - full fat
4 of raw honey
1 tsp ground vanilla bean
Coating:
Pinch of sea salt
½ cup cacao powder 2 raw honey
1/3 cup of coconut oil (melted)
Directions:
Mix coconut oil, coconut cream, and honey, vanilla and salt. Pour over desiccated coconut and mix well.
Mold coconut mixture into balls and freeze. Or pour the whole mixture into a tray, freeze and cut into small bars when frozen.
Prepare the coating by mixing salt, cocoa powder, honey and coconut oil. Dip frozen coconut balls/bars into the chocolate coating, put on a tray and freeze again.
Nutrition Facts:
Calories: 120 Fat: 4.3g Carbohydrates: 16.7g Protein: 1g

Chocolate Cream

Preparation Time: 10 minutes
Cooking Time: 35 minutes
Servings: 4
Ingredie ts:
1 avocado
2 coconut oil
2 raw honey
2 cacao powder
1 tsp ground vanilla bean Pinch of salt
¼ cup almond milk
¼ cup goji berries
Directions:
Blend all the ingredients in the food processor until smooth and thick.
Distribute in four cups, decorate with goji berries and put the fridge overnight.
Nutrition Facts:
Calories: 200kcal Fat: 4.3g Carbohydrate: 25.2g Protein: 12.8g

Peanut Butter Truffles

Preparation Time: 10 minutes
Cooking Time: 30 minutes
Servings: 4
Ingredients:
5 tbsp peanut butter 1 tbsp coconut oil
1 tbsp raw honey
1 tsp ground vanilla bean
¾ cup almond flour
Coating:
Pinch of salt 1 cocoa butter
½ cup 70% chocolate
Directions:
Mix peanut butter, c all ingredients in a dough. Roll the dough into 1-inch balls, place them on parchment paper and refrigerate for half an hour (yield about 12 truffles). Melted chocolate and cocoa butter, add a pinch of salt. Dip each truffle in the melted chocolate, one at the time. Place them back on the pan with parchment paper and put in the fridge.
Nutrition Facts:
Calories: 194 Fat: 8g Carbohydrate: 13.1g Protein: 4g

Chocolate Pie

Preparation Time: 10 minutes
Cooking Time: 30 minutes
Servings: 4
Ingredients:
2 cups flour
1 cup dates, soaked and drained 1 cup dried apricots, chopped 1½ tsp ground vanilla bean

2 eggs
1 banana, mashed
5 cocoa powder
3 raw honey
1 ripe avocado, mashed
2 tbsp. organic coconut oil
½ cup almond milk
Directions:
In a bowl, add flour, apricots and dates finely chopped and mix. Add the banana and the eggs lightly beaten and mix.
Add vanilla, cocoa, honey, avocado and coconut oil and mix.
Add almond milk bit by bit. You could need less than ½ cup to get the right "cake consistency".
Put in a greased baking tin and cook for 30-35 minutes at 350° F. Always
check the cake and allow a few more minutes if it's not done. Allow to cool before serving.
Nutrition Facts:
Calories: 380kcal Fat: 18.4g Carbohydrate: 50.2g Protein: 7.2g

Chocolate Walnut Truffles

Preparation Time: 10 minutes
Cooking Time: 35 minutes
Servings: 4
Ingredients:
1 cup ground walnuts 1 tsp cinnamon
½ cup of coconut oil
¼ cup raw honey 2 chia seeds
2 cacao powder
Directions:
Mix all ingredients and make truffles. Coat with cinnamon, coconut flakes or chopped almonds.
Nutrition Facts:
Calories: 120kcal Fat: 4.4g Carbohydrate: 10.2g Protein: 5.2g

Frozen Raw Blackberry Cake

Preparation Time: 10 minutes
Cooking Time: 45 minutes
Servings: 4
Ingredients:
Crust:
3/4 cup shredded coconut
15 dried dates soaked and drained 1/3 cup pumpkin seeds
1/4 cup of coconut oil Coconut whipped cream **Top filling:**
1 pound of frozen blackberries
¾ cup raw honey
1/4 cup of coconut cream 2 egg whites
Directions:
Grease the cake tin with coconut oil and mix all base ingredients in the blender until you get a sticky ball. Press the base mixture in a cake tin. Freeze. Make Coconut Whipped Cream. Freeze.
Blitz berries and then add honey, coconut cream and egg whites.
Pour middle filling - Coconut Whipped Cream in and spread evenly. Freeze. Pour top filling berries mixture-in the tin, spread, decorate with blueberries and almonds and return to freezer.
Nutrition Facts:
Calories: 472 Fat: 18g Carbohydrate: 15.8g Protein: 33.3g

Chocolate Hazelnuts Truffles

Preparation Time: 10 minutes
Cooking Time: 30 minutes
Servings: 12
Ingredients:
1 cup ground almonds
1 tsp ground vanilla bean
½ cup of coconut oil
½ cup mashed pitted dates 12 whole hazelnuts
2 cacao powder

Directions:
Mix all ingredients and make truffles with one whole hazelnut in the middle.
Nutrition Facts:
Calories: 70 Fat: 2.8g Net carbs: 16.9g Protein: 2.2g

Chocolate Pudding with Fruit

Preparation Time: 10 minutes
Cooking Time: 45 minutes
Servings: 2
Ingredients:
Chocolate cream:
1 avocado
2 tsp. raw honey
2 tbsp. coconut oil 3 tsp. cacao powder
1 tsp ground vanilla bean
Pinch of sea salt
¼ cup of coconut milk
Fruits:
1 chopped banana
1 cup pitted cherries 1 tbsp. coconut flakes
Directions:
Blend all chocolate cream ingredients and divide it in two cups. Put fruit chunks on top and sprinkle shredded coconut on top.
Put at least 2 hours in the fridge before serving.
Nutrition Facts:
Calories: 106kcal Fat: 5g Carbohydrate: 20.4g Protein: 14g

Chocolate Maple Walnuts

Preparation Time: 15 minutes
Cooking Time: 30 minutes
Servings: 15
Ingredients:
½ cup pure maple syrup, 2 cups raw, whole walnuts
½ cup dark chocolate, at least 85%
1 ½ tbsp. coconut oil, melted 1 tbsp. water
1 tsp. of vanilla extract

Directions:
Line a large baking sheet with parchment paper. In a medium to a large skillet, combine the walnuts and ¼ cup of maple syrup and cook over medium heat, stirring continuously, until walnuts are entirely covered with syrup and golden in color, about 3 – 5 minutes.
Pour the walnuts onto the parchment paper and separate it into individual pieces with a fork. Allow cooling completely; at least 15 minutes.
In the meantime, melt the chocolate with the coconut oil, add the remaining maple syrup and stir until combined. When walnuts are cooled, transfer them to a glass bowl and pour the melted chocolate syrup over the top.
Use a silicone spatula to mix until walnuts are entirely covered gently.
Transfer back to the parchment paper-lined baking sheet and, once again, separate each of the nuts with a fork.
Place the nuts in the fridge for 10 minutes or the freezer for 3 – 5 minutes, until chocolate has completely set. Store in an airtight bag in your fridge.
Nutrition Facts:
Calories 139 Fat 10 g Carbohydrate 19 g Protein 24 g

Matcha and Chocolate Dipped Strawberries

Preparation Time: 25 minutes
Cooking Time: 25 minutes
Servings: 5
Ingredients:
4 tbsp. cocoa butter
4 squares of dark chocolate,
¼ cup of coconut oil
1 tsp Matcha green tea powder
20 – 25 large strawberries, stems on

Directions:
Melt cocoa butter, dark chocolate, coconut oil and Matcha until smooth. Remove from heat and continue stirring until chocolate is completely melted.
Pour into a large glass bowl and continuously stir until the chocolate thickens and starts to lose its sheen, about 2 - 5 minutes.
One at a time, hold the strawberries by stems and dip into chocolatematcha mixture to coat. Let excess drip back into the bowl.
Place on a parchment-lined baking sheet and chill dipped berries in the fridge until the shell is set, 20–25 minutes.
Nutrition Facts:
Calories 188 Fat 5.3 g Carbohydrate 10.9 g Protein 0.2 g

Strawberry Rhubarb Crisp

Preparation Time: 10 minutes
Cooking Time: 45 minutes
Servings: 8
Ingredients:
1 cup white sugar
½ cup buckwheat flour + 3 tbsp. 3 cups strawberries, sliced
3 cups rhubarb, diced
½ lemon, juiced
1 cup packed brown sugar 1 cup coconut oil, melted
¾ cup rolled oats
¼ cup buckwheat groats
¼ cup walnuts, chopped
Directions:
Preheat oven to 375°F In a large bowl, mix white sugar, 3 tbsp. flour, strawberries, rhubarb, and lemon juice. Place the mixture in a 9x13 inch baking tray.
In a separate bowl, mix ½ cup flour, brown sugar, coconut oil, oats, buckwheat groats, and walnuts until crumbly.
Crumble on top of the rhubarb and strawberry mixture. Bake 45 minutes in the preheated oven, or until crisp and lightly browned.
Nutrition Facts:
Calories 167 Fat 3.1 g Carbohydrate 58.3 g Protein 3.5 g

Maple Walnut Cupcakes with Matcha Green Tea Icing

Preparation Time: 20 minutes
Cooking Time: 25 minutes
Servings: 24
Ingredients:
For the Cupcakes:
2 cups of All-Purpose flour
½ cup buckwheat flour
2 ½ teaspoons baking powder
½ tsp salt
1 cup of cocoa butter 1 cup white sugar
1 tbsp. pure maple syrup
3 eggs
2/3 cup milk
¼ cup walnuts, chopped
For the Icing:
3 tbsp. coconut oil, thick at room temperature
3 tbsp. icing sugar
1 tbsp. Matcha green tea powder
½ tsp vanilla bean paste
3 tbsp. cream cheese, softened
Directions:
Preheat oven to 350 degrees F. Place paper baking cups into muffin tins for 24 regular-sized muffins. In a medium bowl, mix flours, baking powder, and salt.
In a separate large bowl, mix sugar, butter, syrup, and eggs with a mixer. Add to the dry ingredients, mix and add milk. Pour batter into muffin cup until 2/3 full.
Bake for 20-25 minutes or until an inserted toothpick comes out clean. Cool completely before icing. To Make the Icing: Add the

coconut oil and icing sugar to a bowl and use a hand-mixer to cream until it's pale and smooth.

Fold in the matcha powder and vanilla. Finally, add the cream cheese and beat until smooth. Pipe or spread over the cupcakes once they're cool.

Nutrition Facts:

Calories 164 Fat 6 g Carbohydrate 21 g Protein 2 g

Dark Chocolate Mousse

Preparation Time: 10 minutes
Cooking Time: 2+ hours
Servings: 4
Ingredients:

1 (16 oz.) package silken tofu, drained
½ cup pure maple syrup 1 tsp pure vanilla extract
¼ cup of soy milk
½ cup unsweetened cocoa powder Mint leaves

Directions:

Place the tofu, maple syrup, and vanilla in a food processor or blender. Process until well blended.

Add remaining ingredients and process until the mixture is thoroughly blended.

Pour into small dessert cups or espresso cups. Chill for at least 2 hours. Garnish with fresh mint leaves just before serving.

Nutrition Facts:

Calories 175kcal Fat 24 g Carbohydrate 18 g Protein 5 g

Matcha Green Tea Mochi

Preparation Time: 10 min
Cooking Time: 20 min
Servings: 12 pieces
Ingredients:

2 tbsp. Matcha powder.
1 cup superfine white rice flour 1 tsp Baking powder
1 cup Coconut milk 1/2 cup Sugar
2 tbsp. Butter melted

Directions:

Heat your oven to 325 degrees F. Grease your baking tin with a non-stick spray. Mix all the dry ingredients plus the sugar.

Whisk to blend, then add the coconut milk and melted butter. Stir well.

Place the mixture into the baking tin and place in the oven to bake for approx. 2o minutes.

Nutrition Facts:

Calories: 100kcal Carbs: 13g Fat: 8g Protein: 2g

CPSIA information can be obtained
at www.ICGtesting.com
Printed in the USA
LVHW101933190121
676908LV00009B/289